Skull Base Surgery of the Posterior Fossa

William T. Couldwell

Editor

Skull Base Surgery of the Posterior Fossa

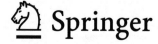 Springer

Editor
William T. Couldwell
Department of Neurosurgery
Clinical Neurosciences Center
University of Utah
Salt Lake City, UT, USA

ISBN 978-3-319-88368-7   ISBN 978-3-319-67038-6   (eBook)
https://doi.org/10.1007/978-3-319-67038-6

Printed on acid-free paper

This Springer imprint is published by Springer Nature
The registered company is Springer International Publishing AG
The registered company address is: Gewerbestrasse 11, 6330 Cham, Switzerland

Contents

Part I   Introduction

1   Surgical Anatomy of the Posterior Fossa   3
Jaafar Basma and Jeffrey Sorenson

Part II   Approaches

2   Retrosigmoid Craniotomy and Its Variants   27
Christian Bowers, Olaide O. Ajayi, Kevin A. Reinard,
Daniel R. Klinger, Johnny B. Delashaw, Shane Tubbs,
and Zachary Litvack

3   Middle Fossa and Translabyrinthine Approaches   37
Justin C. Sowder, Breanne L. Schiffer, Richard K. Gurgel,
and Clough Shelton

4   Posterior and Combined Petrosal Approaches   55
David Aum, Omar Arnaout, Marcio S. Rassi, Walid Ibn
Essayed, and Ossama Al-Mefty

5   Far Lateral Approach and Its Variants   65
Karolyn Au, Angela M. Richardson, and Jacques Morcos

**6   Endoscopic Endonasal Approach for Posterior
Fossa Tumors**   75
André Beer-Furlan, Alexandre B. Todeschini,
Ricardo L. Carrau, and Daniel M. Prevedello

Part III   Specific Diseases

7   Petroclival Meningiomas   89
Amol Raheja and William T. Couldwell

8   Meningiomas of the Cerebellopontine Angle   103
Stephen T. Magill, Philip V. Theodosopoulos,
Aaron D. Tward, Steven W. Cheung,
and Michael W. McDermott

9 Tentorial Meningiomas.............................. 115
Hiroki Morisako, Takeo Goto, and Kenji Ohata

10 Foramen Magnum Meningiomas 135
Angela M. Richardson, Karolyn Au, and Jacques Morcos

11 Vestibular Schwannomas 145
Gmaan Alzhrani, Clough Shelton, and William T. Couldwell

12 Epidermoid Cyst.................................... 165
Gmaan Alzhrani and William T. Couldwell

13 Metastasis to the Posterior Fossa...................... 177
Bradley D. Weaver and Randy L. Jensen

**14 Microsurgical Management of Posterior
Fossa Vascular Lesions** 195
M. Yashar S. Kalani and Robert F. Spetzler

Index.. 221

Contributors

Olaide O. Ajayi, MD Swedish Neuroscience Institute, Seattle, WA, USA

Ossama Al-Mefty, MD Department of Neurosurgery, Brigham and Women's Hospital, Boston, MA, USA

Gmaan Alzhrani, MD Department of Neurosurgery, Clinical Neurosciences Center, University of Utah, Salt Lake City, UT, USA

Omar Arnaout, MD Department of Neurosurgery, Brigham and Women's Hospital, Boston, MA, USA

Karolyn Au, MD, MSc Department of Neurological Surgery, University of Miami/Jackson Memorial Hospital, Miami, FL, USA

David Aum, MS University of South Florida Morsani College of Medicine, Tampa, FL, USA

Jaafar Basma, MD University of Tennessee, Memphis, TN, USA

André Beer-Furlan Neurological Surgery, Rush University Medical Center, Chicago, IL, USA

Christian Bowers, MD Swedish Neuroscience Institute, Seattle, WA, USA

Ricardo L. Carrau, MD Department of Otolaryngology, The Ohio State University Wexner Medical Center, Columbus, OH, USA

Steven W. Cheung, MD Department of Otolaryngology, University of California, San Francisco, San Francisco, CA, USA

William T. Couldwell, MD, PhD Department of Neurosurgery, Clinical Neurosciences Center, University of Utah, Salt Lake City, UT, USA

Johnny B. Delashaw, MD Swedish Neuroscience Institute, Seattle, WA, USA

Walid Ibn Essayed, MD Department of Neurosurgery, Brigham and Women's Hospital, Boston, MA, USA

Takeo Goto, MD, PhD Department of Neurosurgery, Osaka City University Graduate School of Medicine, Osaka, Japan

Richard K. Gurgel, MD Division of Otolaryngology – Head and Neck Surgery, University of Utah School of Medicine, Salt Lake City, UT, USA

Randy L. Jensen, MD, PhD Department of Oncological Sciences, Huntsman Cancer Institute, Salt Lake City, UT, USA

Department of Radiation Oncology, Huntsman Cancer Institute, Salt Lake City, UT, USA

Department of Neurosurgery, Clinical Neurosciences Center, University of Utah, Salt Lake City, UT, USA

M. Yashar S. Kalani, MD, PhD Department of Neurosurgery, Barrow Neurological Institute, St. Joseph's Hospital and Medical Center, Phoenix, AZ, USA

Daniel R. Klinger, MD Swedish Neuroscience Institute, Seattle, WA, USA

Zachary Litvack, MD Swedish Neuroscience Institute, Seattle, WA, USA

Stephen T. Magill, MD Department of Neurological Surgery, University of California, San Francisco, CA, USA

Michael W. McDermott, MD Department of Neurological Surgery, University of California, San Francisco, CA, USA

Jacques Morcos, MD, FRCS(Eng), FRCS(Ed), FAANS Department of Neurological Surgery, University of Miami/Jackson Memorial Hospital, Miami, FL, USA

Hiroki Morisako, MD, PhD Department of Neurosurgery, Osaka City University Graduate School of Medicine, Osaka, Japan

Kenji Ohata, MD, PhD Department of Neurosurgery, Osaka City University Graduate School of Medicine, Osaka, Japan

Daniel M. Prevedello Neurological Surgery, The Ohio State University, Columbus, OH, USA

Amol Raheja, MBBS, MCh Department of Neurosurgery, All India Institute of Medical Sciences, New Delhi, India

Marcio S. Rassi, MD Department of Neurosurgery, Brigham and Women's Hospital, Harvard Medical School, Boston, MA, USA

Kevin A. Reinard, MD Swedish Neuroscience Institute, Seattle, WA, USA

Angela M. Richardson, MD, PhD Department of Neurosurgery, University of Miami/Jackson Memorial Hospital, Miami, FL, USA

Breanne L. Schiffer, MD, MPH Division of Otolaryngology – Head and Neck Surgery, University of Utah School of Medicine, Salt Lake City, UT, USA

Clough Shelton, MD Division of Otolaryngology – Head and Neck Surgery, University of Utah School of Medicine, Salt Lake City, UT, USA

Jeffrey Sorenson, MD University of Tennessee, Memphis, TN, USA

Justin C. Sowder, MD Division of Otolaryngology – Head and Neck Surgery, University of Utah School of Medicine, Salt Lake City, UT, USA

Robert F. Spetzler, MD Department of Neurosurgery, Barrow Neurological Institute, St. Joseph's Hospital and Medical Center, Phoenix, AZ, USA

Philip V. Theodosopoulos, MD Department of Neurological Surgery, University of California, San Francisco, CA, USA

Alexandre B. Todeschini Neurological Surgery, Columbus, OH, USA

Shane Tubbs, PhD, PA-C Swedish Neuroscience Institute, Neurosurgery-Seattle Science Foundation, Seattle, WA, USA

Aaron D. Tward, MD, PhD Department of Otolaryngology, University of California, San Francisco, San Francisco, CA, USA

Bradley D. Weaver, BS University of Utah School of Medicine, Salt Lake City, UT, USA

Department of Oncological Sciences, Huntsman Cancer Institute, Salt Lake City, UT, USA

Part I

Introduction

Surgical Anatomy of the Posterior Fossa

1

Jaafar Basma and Jeffrey Sorenson

Abbreviations

AICA	Anterior inferior cerebellar artery
IAC	Internal auditory canal
ICA	Internal carotid artery
III	Oculomotor nerve
IV	Trochlear nerve
IX	Glossopharyngeal nerve
PCA	Posterior cerebral artery
PICA	Posterior inferior cerebellar artery
SCA	Superior cerebellar artery
SCC	Semicircular canal
V	Trigeminal nerve
VI	Abducens nerve
VII	Facial nerve
VIII	Vestibulocochlear nerve
X	Vagus nerve
XI	Spinal accessory nerve
XII	Hypoglossal nerve

in this region necessitates a wide variety of surgical approaches. Because small surgical errors here have the potential to cause significant morbidity, the posterior fossa surgeon must become an expert in this anatomy. The images used in this chapter were created in Dr. Al Rhoton Jr.'s laboratory with the express purpose of making surgery in the posterior fossa more "accurate, gentle, and safe." For more in-depth study, please refer to his textbook [1] or the online Rhoton Collection [2]. We will first examine the enclosure of the posterior fossa which is formed by the bowl-shaped skull base covered by the pitched tentorium. We will then review Dr. Rhoton's "rule of three," which divides the neurovascular contents of the posterior fossa into three groups of structures, each organized around a major posterior fossa artery. The cranial nerves, arachnoid cisterns, and special regions of the posterior fossa are then surveyed from the perspective of various surgical approaches.

Introduction

The posterior fossa is the most complex and surgically challenging region of human anatomy. The high density of eloquent neurovascular structures

J. Basma, MD • J. Sorenson, MD (✉)
University of Tennessee, 847 Monroe Avenue, Suite 427, Memphis, TN 38163, USA
e-mail: jbasma@uthsc.edu;
jsorenson@semmes-murphey.com

Enclosure of the Posterior Fossa

Skull Base

The posterior fossa is bounded primarily by three bones that form a bowl-shaped cavity (Fig. 1.1a). The occipital bone forms the rounded squamosal posterior wall of this cavity, as well as the floor, and most of the anterior wall (clivus). The sphenoid bone contributes the upper third of the clivus, which

© Springer International Publishing AG 2018
W.T. Couldwell (ed.), *Skull Base Surgery of the Posterior Fossa*,
https://doi.org/10.1007/978-3-319-67038-6_1

also forms the posterior wall of the sella turcica (dorsum sella). The lateral walls of the posterior fossa are formed by the mastoid and petrous portions of the temporal bone, which are angled inward to meet the relatively narrow clivus (Fig. 1.1a). The posterior fossa is thus larger posteriorly, where the cerebellum occupies the entire volume, but then tapers anteriorly as the anatomical landscape transitions to the brainstem and cranial nerves. Viewed from above, its outline resembles a semicircle topped by a rounded triangle. The relatively flat floor of the posterior fossa exists along the posterolateral portion of the foramen magnum, whereas the anterior part of the foramen magnum is the lower edge of the upward sloping clivus.

Neural Foramina

The bones of the posterior fossa are lined with dura mater, which often contains venous lakes between its layers. Anteriorly and laterally, there are five pairs of neural foramina into which a sleeve of posterior fossa dura follows, forming small or large CSF-filled dural caves (Fig. 1.1c). The trigeminal nerve exits the posterior fossa through an ostium formed by a depression of the petrous temporal bone below and the superior petrosal sinus above (Fig. 1.1b, d). The dura of this foramen continues into the middle fossa to form Meckel's cave – a CSF-filled space that also contains the trigeminal ganglion. More medially, the abducens nerve enters a narrow dural sleeve with CSF evagination (Dorello canal) that courses between the petrous apex and clivus before entering the cavernous sinus. The facial, cochlear, and vestibular nerves traverse the internal auditory canal, which is tapered toward its lateral fundus (Figs. 1.1b–d and 1.7e). Although the jugular foramen, which is formed by an opening between the petrous and occipital bones, is a large neural foramen, it harbors relatively little CSF (Figs. 1.1b–d and 1.2a, b). The hypoglossal canal passes through the superior aspect of the occipital condyle and travels anterolaterally (Figs. 1.1a–c and 1.2a, d). Often there are duplicated inlets that converge to a single outlet which then emerges near the medial aspect of the jugular foramen.

Tentorium

The "lid" covering the posterior fossa "bowl" is formed by the tentorium – an extension of dura that separates the cerebrum from the cerebellum with a central anterior opening (incisura) (Fig. 1.1f). The tentorium is anchored to the petrous ridge, where its layers separate to form the superior petrosal sinus, and to the occipital bone where it forms the transverse sinuses and torcula (Fig. 1.1e). It slopes downward from the incisura toward these lateral and posterior attachments. Additional venous channels often course between the layers of the tentorium. The falx cerebri joins the tentorium in the midline at the straight sinus, which communicates the vein of Galen at the incisura with the torcula (Figs. 1.1f and 1.5a). The tentorium extends anteriorly on either side of the incisura as the anterior and posterior petroclinoidal folds that attach to the anterior and posterior clinoidal processes, respectively. These two folds outline the posterior roof of the cavernous sinus, where the oculomotor nerve enters (Fig. 1.1f). The trochlear nerve is intimately related to the tentorial edge as it enters the posterior cavernous sinus, just medial to the anterior petroclinoidal fold (Fig. 1.4a).

Venous Sinuses

A rich anastomosing system of venous sinuses is organized around the inner walls of the posterior fossa [3]. Superiorly, the superior petrosal and transverse sinuses course along the edges of the tentorium. The two transverse sinuses meet at the torcula, along with the straight sinus and the superior sagittal sinus which flank the falx cerebri. A variable occipital sinus projects inferiorly from the torcula along the falx cerebelli. The sigmoid sinus begins at the junction of the transverse and petrosal sinuses and then courses in a sulcus of the mastoid bone (Fig. 1.1b), before emptying into the jugular bulb inferior to the petrous bone (Figs. 1.1d and 1.2a). The sigmoid sinus is more often larger on the right side. The inferior petrosal sinus courses along the petroclival fissure (Fig. 1.1b, d), transmitting flow to the jugular bulb posteriorly

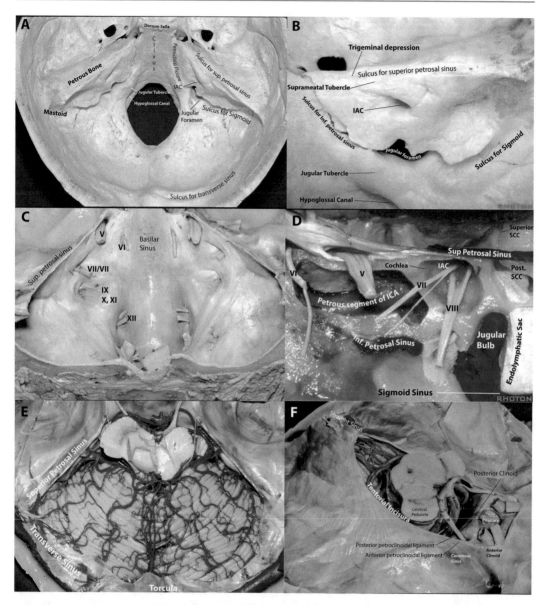

Fig. 1.1 Posterior fossa osseous and dural enclosure. (**a**) Superior view of the skull base. The posterior fossa is enclosed by the sphenoid, temporal, and occipital bones. The bony imprints of the major venous structures can be seen. (**b**) Medial view of the lateral bony wall of the posterior fossa. Sulci for venous sinuses encircling the medial face of the temporal bone are seen. The hypoglossal canal is bordered superiorly by the jugular tubercle, and the suprameatal tubercle is anterior and superior to the internal auditory canal (IAC). (**c**) Superior view of the posterior fossa dura. The dural lining of the posterior fossa invaginates into the neural foramina and forms venous channels between its layers. (**d**) Medial view of petrous temporal bone with internal structures exposed. The cochlea is located above the genu of the petrous carotid artery, and the semicircular canals are superior to the jugular bulb. The trigeminal nerve courses above the trigeminal depression of the petrous bone to enter Meckel's cave. (**e**) Superior view of the tentorium attachments. The tentorium is anchored to the petrous ridge at the superior petrosal sinus and to the occipital bone at the transverse sinus and torcula. (**f**) Right superior oblique view of the tentorium. The midbrain is continuous with the thalamus through the tentorial incisura. Anteriorly, the tentorium extends as the anterior and posterior petroclinoid folds which insert on the anterior and posterior clinoid processes. The oculomotor nerve enters the roof of the cavernous sinus between these folds

from the junction of the superior petrosal, basilar, and cavernous sinuses anteriorly (Fig. 1.2a). Thus, the superior and inferior petrosal sinuses, along with the sigmoid sinus and jugular bulb, form a venous ring around the medial face of the petrous bone (Fig. 1.2a). The petrosal and sigmoid portions of the jugular foramen empty into the jugular bulb, which occupies the lateral pars vascularis of the jugular foramen (Fig. 1.2c). The basilar sinus extends across the clivus, completing the anterior venous anastomosis of the posterior fossa. The posterior cavernous sinus of the middle fossa communicates with the posterior fossa venous circulation through the superior and inferior petrosal sinuses as well as the basilar sinus. This confluence of sinuses is often referred to as the petroclival venous confluence, through which the abducens nerve travels as it passes below the petrosphenoidal ligament (Fig. 1.2a).

Obstacles to Surgery

Several structures within the posterior fossa enclosure can result in significant morbidity if injured; therefore, these obstacles must be considered when designing surgical approaches. Smaller venous sinuses, such as the superior petrosal sinus, are sacrificed with rare consequences, but larger sinuses such as the transverse or sigmoid pose greater risk. Therefore, as an obstacle, the sigmoid sinus is a significant boundary between approaches even though it can be mobilized and retracted to increase exposure (Fig. 1.6b). Division of the tentorium rarely causes morbidity if care is taken to preserve the trochlear nerve and adequate venous outflow. Traversal of neural foramina should be avoided if preservation of nerve function is desired. In addition, the course of the facial nerve in the temporal bone must be appreciated as it passes through the tympanic cavity and then inferiorly into the anterior aspect of the mastoid (Fig. 1.8d). Manipulation of the greater superficial petrosal nerve or geniculate ganglion can also result in facial palsy when working through the middle fossa floor to access the posterior fossa (Fig. 1.11d). If hearing preservation is desired,

then the labyrinth, which lies posterior to the internal auditory canal, should be preserved (Fig. 1.8c–d). The cochlea is immediately anterior to the fundus of the internal auditory canal (Fig. 1.9c). The internal carotid artery enters the petrous bone anterior to the jugular foramen and runs vertically for a short distance before turning anteriorly below the cochlea into a horizontal orientation until it exits at the petrous apex (Figs 1.1d, 1.2d, and 1.9h). This presents a significant obstacle during anterior petrosectomy. Finally, the cavernous segment of the internal carotid artery can block lateral access from transnasal approaches (Fig. 1.12b, c).

Contents of the Posterior Fossa

The cerebellum and brainstem occupy most of the posterior fossa volume. The brainstem has three morphologically distinct regions in the posterior fossa: the midbrain, pons, and medulla oblongata. Each of these is bordered by arachnoid cisterns [4]. The mesencephalon (midbrain) is a transition from the functionally reflexive spinal cord and medulla to the correlative and associative diencephalon and forebrain. It extends from the thalamus to the pontomesencephalic sulcus. Anteriorly, the cerebral peduncles represent the array of corticospinal, corticobulbar, and corticopontine fibers descending from the internal capsule (Figs. 1.3a and 1.4a). These peduncles are separated by a gap, called the interpeduncular fossa, which contains a cistern of the same name that is bounded anteriorly by Liliequist's membrane. The lateral walls of this cistern give rise to the oculomotor nerves, and the posterior part contains the basilar apex and posterior cerebral artery perforators entering the posterior perforated substance (Fig. 1.3c). Relative to the dorsum sellae, the basilar apex can be high or low riding, which can influence the choice of surgical approach. The lateral midbrain is bordered by the crural cistern around the cerebral peduncle and the ambient cistern posterior to the peduncle (Fig. 1.4a). Posteriorly, the superior and inferior colliculi are bordered by the quadrigeminal cistern.

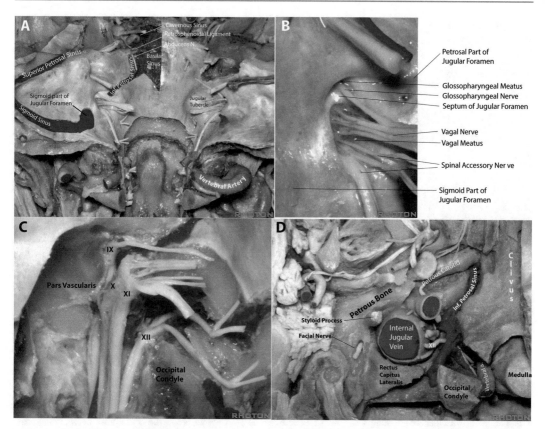

Fig. 1.2 Jugular foramen and skull base venous sinuses. (**a**) Posterior view. Venous drainage from the cavernous sinus and basilar sinus empties in the superior and inferior petrosal sinuses. The inferior petrosal sinus ends at the petrosal part of the jugular foramen. The sigmoid, superior, and inferior petrosal sinuses form a venous ring around the medial face of the petrous bones, bridged by the basilar sinus anteriorly. (**b**) Enlarged view of the intracranial jugular foramen. The septum of the jugular foramen separates the glossopharyngeal meatus from the vagal meatus. (**c**) Posterior view of the left jugular foramen which has been opened posteriorly. The cranial nerves occupy the medial aspect of the jugular foramen, while the jugular bulb is lateral. The hypoglossal nerve exits the cranial cavity inferior and medial to the jugular foramen before joining the other lower cranial nerves. (**d**) Inferior view of the right jugular foramen region. The jugular foramen is bordered by the petrous carotid anteriorly, the styloid process and facial nerve laterally, the occipital condyle medially, and the jugular process of the occipital bone and the rectus capitis lateralis posteriorly

The pons ("bridge") is developmentally a part of the medulla and is only distinguishable in mammals due to the pontine nuclei and the fibers of corticopontocerebellar and corticospinal tracts. It is a convex structure extending from the pontomesencephalic sulcus superiorly to the pontomedullary sulcus inferiorly. The descending corticospinal and corticobulbar fibers located in its anterior half are interrupted by transverse fibers coursing between the middle cerebellar peduncles. Intertwined between these are pontine nuclei involved in the corticopontocerebellar circuit. At the midlevel of the pons, the trigeminal nerve emerges anterior to the middle cerebellar peduncle (Figs. 1.3a and 1.4c). The posterior pons contains several cranial nerve nuclei, ascending tracts, and the floor of the fourth ventricle, where the abducens nucleus makes an impression called the facial colliculus (Fig. 1.5g). The pons is bordered anteriorly and laterally by the prepontine and cerebellopontine cisterns (Fig. 1.4b–d).

The medulla oblongata is the inferior segment of the brainstem. The pyramids represent its most anterior prominences and contain the corticospinal tract. At this level, 85% of the corticospinal fibers decussate. Lateral to the pyra-

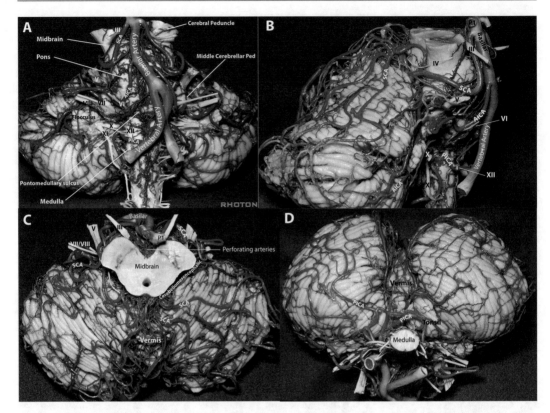

Fig. 1.3 Neurovascular relationships of the brainstem and cerebellum. (**a**) Anterior view of the brainstem and cerebellum. Following Rhoton's rule of three, the upper group of structures includes the mesencephalon, superior cerebellar artery (SCA), oculomotor nerve, and trigeminal nerve. The middle group includes the pons, anterior inferior cerebellar artery (AICA), cranial nerves VI–VIII, and the middle cerebellar peduncle. The inferior group holds the posterior inferior cerebellar artery, lower cranial nerves, and medulla. (**b**) Lateral view of the brainstem and cerebellum. Branches of the SCA are seen coursing around the midbrain and the superior cerebellar peduncle before supplying the superior surface of the cerebellum.

The SCA passes below the oculomotor nerve, which exits from the lateral aspect of the interpeduncular fossa. A caudal loop of the SCA may impinge upon the trigeminal nerve. The AICA supplies the middle cerebellar peduncle and the petrosal surface of the cerebellum. (**c**) Superior view of the midbrain and cerebellum. The SCA supplies the superior surface of the cerebellum, which conforms to the shape and slope of the posterior tentorium. The interpeduncular fossa is crowded by perforating branches of the basilar bifurcation. (**d**) Inferior view of the medulla and cerebellum. The suboccipital surface of the cerebellum and its tonsils are supplied by branches of PICA. The PICA forms a caudal loop near the cerebellar tonsil

mids, the inferior olive is bounded by the preolivary sulcus, where the hypoglossal rootlets emerge. Cranial nerves IX, X, and XI exit from the postolivary sulcus. The floor of the fourth ventricle at this level contains from medial to lateral: the hypoglossal nucleus, the dorsal nucleus of the vagus nerve, and the vestibular nuclei (Fig. 1.5g). The medulla is bounded anteriorly by the premedullary cistern and laterally by the cerebellomedullary cistern (Fig. 1.4e).

Arteries and Rule of Three

Dr. Albert Rhoton Jr. divided the neurovascular contents of the posterior fossa into three groups of structures, each organized around a major posterior fossa artery. These zones are stacked vertically, defining the main longitudinal axis of the posterior fossa. A separate important organizing scheme divides the CSF-filled spaces surrounding the brainstem into cisterns (Fig. 1.4). The brainstem and cerebellum are supplied by

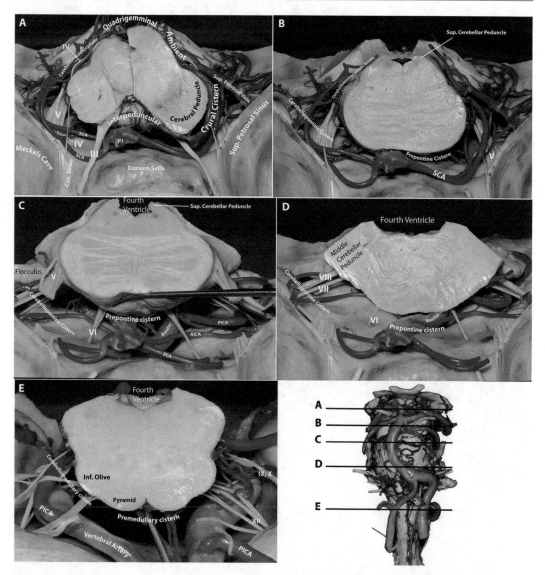

Fig. 1.4 Posterior fossa cisterns. Axial slices, though the brainstem and surrounding structures, superior view. (**a**) Section through the mesencephalon showing the surrounding interpeduncular, crural, ambient, and quadrigeminal cistern. (**b**) Upper pons surrounded by the prepontine and cerebellopontine cisterns. The superior cerebellar branches (SCA) course above the trigeminal nerves. (**c**) Midlevel pons. The prepontine cistern faces the clivus, and cerebellopontine cistern faces the petrous bone. The abducens nerve is seen piercing the clival dural to enter Dorello canal as the anterior inferior cerebellar artery (AICA) courses below it. (**d**) Lower pons. Cranial nerves VII, VIII, the flocculus, and the AICA are seen within the cerebellopontine cistern. (**e**) Section through the medulla showing the premedullary and cerebellomedullary cisterns. The hypoglossal nerve originates at the preolivary sulcus lateral to the pyramid, while cranial nerves IX–XI exit from the postolivary sulcus

branches of the vertebrobasilar system (Fig. 1.3). The vertebral arteries pierce the posterior fossa dura medial to the occipital condyles and pass inferior and then anterior to the lower cranial nerves before converging at the vertebrobasilar junction, near the pontomedullary sulcus (Figs. 1.2a and 1.3a). The basilar artery sends short and long circumflex arteries to the pons before it ultimately bifurcates into the posterior cerebral arteries at the level of the midbrain.

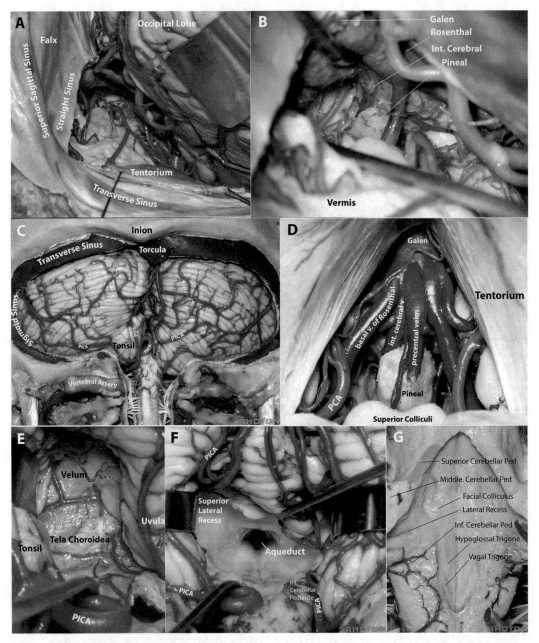

Fig. 1.5 Surgical views from posterior approaches. (**a**) The occipital transtentorial approaches exploit the corridor between the occipital lobe and falx-tentorium to access the posterior aspect of the tentorial incisura, dorsal mesencephalon, and pineal region. The vein of Galen complex is visualized deep in the surgical field. (**b**) Enlarged view of the occipital transtentorial approach. The pineal region and Galenian venous complex are exposed. (**c**) Posterior view of the suboccipital craniotomy. The suboccipital cerebellar surface is bordered by the transverse and sigmoid sinuses. (**d**) Posterior view of the supracerebellar infratentorial approach. The pineal gland and superior colliculi are exposed along with tributaries to the vein of Galen. The basal vein of Rosenthal, the internal cerebral veins, and the precentral veins are seen draining into the vein of Galen, which in turn empties

in the straight sinus at the midline of the tentorium. (**e**) Posterior inferior view of the telovelar approach. The cerebellar tonsil is retracted to expose the inferior roof of the fourth ventricle formed by the inferior medullary velum and tela choroidea, which anchors the fourth ventricle choroid plexus. (**f**) View of the fourth ventricle through the telovelar approach. Division of the tela choroidea and velum exposes the floor of the fourth ventricle, lateral recesses and the aqueduct of Sylvius. (**g**) Posterior view of the floor of the fourth ventricle. The protuberances identified in the floor of the fourth ventricle include the facial colliculus (abducens nucleus), the hypoglossal trigone, and the vagal trigone. The lateral recess communicates with the cerebellopontine angle through the foramen of Luschka. The superior and inferior cerebellar peduncles contribute to the lateral walls of the fourth ventricle

Three pairs of cerebellar arteries arise from the vertebrobasilar system. The course of the cerebellar arteries often includes loops and turns that are not confined to a single plane. Nonetheless, it can be useful to conceptualize three zones along the vertical axis of the posterior fossa defined by these three arteries (Fig. 1.3).

The upper zone follows the superior cerebellar artery (SCA) and includes the midbrain, upper pons, and superior cerebellum. After arising near the basilar apex, the SCA travels immediately inferior to the oculomotor nerve before curving around the brainstem close to the pontomesencephalic junction. It typically bifurcates into rostral and caudal branches. Laterally, these branches enter the cerebellomesencephalic fissure where they travel with the trochlear nerve. Before entering this fissure, one of its branches may loop inferiorly to contact the trigeminal nerve, possibly causing trigeminal neuralgia. After coursing posteriorly around the superior cerebellar peduncle (Fig. 1.4b), the branches emerge from the cerebellomesencephalic fissure to supply the vermis, superior cerebellar hemispheres, and dentate nucleus.

The middle zone follows the anterior inferior cerebellar artery (AICA) and includes the middle pons and cerebellopontine angle. The AICA usually originates from the lower half of the basilar artery (Figs. 1.3a–b). As it courses around the brainstem, it may pass near any of the cranial nerves emerging from the pontomedullary sulcus – the abducens, facial, cochlear, and vestibular nerves. Compression of the root entry zone of the facial nerve may cause hemifacial spasm. AICA enters the cerebellopontine angle to supply the middle cerebellar peduncle and the portion of the cerebellum facing the petrous temporal bone (Fig. 1.3a). Often, a loop of AICA can extend into the internal auditory canal (IAC) and impinge upon the nervus intermedius to cause geniculate neuralgia (Fig. 1.7e). AICA may also pass between the nerves of the 7/8 complex before they enter the IAC.

The lower zone follows the posterior inferior cerebellar artery (PICA) and includes the medulla and inferior cerebellum. PICA typically arises from the distal vertebral artery along the anterolateral medulla (Fig. 1.3a, b) but can arise from any part of the vertebral artery. Its origin can also be extradural. The PICA courses posteriorly from the anterior medulla above or below the hypoglossal nerve rootlets. As it reaches the lateral medulla, it turns inferiorly before encountering the cerebellar tonsil. It then passes anterior or posterior to the glossopharyngeal, vagus, and spinal accessory nerves in a variable manner (Fig. 1.3a). After forming its caudal loop, the PICA ascends along the inferior cerebellar peduncle, deep to the cerebellar tonsil, before bifurcating into branches supplying the inferior vermis and inferior hemisphere (Fig. 1.5c, e, f).

Veins

The veins of the posterior fossa are more variable than the arteries [3]. Deep veins include the vein of the cerebellomesencephalic fissure, the vein of the cerebellopontine angle, and the vein of the cerebellomedullary fissure. Also, one can commonly identify the veins of the superior, middle, and inferior cerebellar peduncles. The superficial cerebellar veins drain the tentorial, petrosal, suboccipital surfaces. The brainstem has a variable network of veins which are longitudinal or transverse. There are three major groups of bridging veins. The galenic group drains the internal cerebral vein and the basal vein of Rosenthal. The petrosal group includes the inferior petrosal sinus and jugular foramen, as well as the superior petrosal sinus that drains Dandy's vein. The tentorial group drains into the transverse sinus or directly into the tentorium.

Special Regions

Cavernous Sinus

The cavernous sinus borders the sella and sphenoid sinus laterally in the middle fossa. It provides a conduit for cranial nerves traveling from the posterior fossa into the orbit. These are situated laterally, and the carotid artery is located medially. The internal carotid artery enters the cavernous sinus after exiting the carotid canal of the temporal bone and turns vertically into the carotid sulcus of the sphenoid, which is flanked laterally by the lingual process of the sphenoid bone and the petrolingual ligament. This vertical paraclival portion then bends anteriorly below the posterior clinoid process before turning superiorly and posteriorly to exit the cavernous sinus below the anterior clinoid process. The cavernous sinus accepts venous drainage from the inferior and superior ophthalmic veins through the superior orbital fissure. It may drain sylvian and cortical veins directly or via the sphenoparietal sinus. It communicates with the contralateral cavernous sinus through the basilar plexus posteriorly and through the anterior and posterior intercavernous sinus superiorly. The cranial nerves enter the cavernous sinus at disparate angles and then converge at the superior orbital fissure. Lesions may involve both the cavernous sinus and posterior fossa through direct extension. The posterior portion of the cavernous sinus is often opened to expose the upper basilar artery region of the posterior fossa (Fig. 1.11f).

Clivus and Petroclival Region

The clivus (Latin, "slope") forms the anterior bony wall of the posterior fossa (Fig. 1.1a). The superior third is formed by the sphenoid bone (dorsum sellae). It is fused with the occipital part of the clivus through a synchondrosis at the level of the foramen lacerum. The occipital part of the clivus can be conceptually divided into middle and lower thirds which are at the level of the internal auditory canal and jugular foramen, respectively. These divisions correspond to Rhoton's rule of three.

The junction of the petrous bone and clivus at the petroclival fissure is marked by the inferior petrosal sinus. The petrous apex and foramen lacerum are at the superior end of this fissure, and the jugular tubercle and foramen are inferior to it (Fig. 1.1a, b). The inferior petrosal sinus communicates superiorly with the posterior aspect of the cavernous sinus (Fig. 1.2a). At this petroclival venous confluence, the abducens nerve travels

through Dorello canal, which is roofed by the petrosphenoidal ligament (Gruber's ligament), toward the inferior part of the cavernous sinus.

Given its anterior location, with anatomical barriers that may include temporal bone structures and several cranial nerves, the petroclival region is one of the most difficult areas to access. Approaches include retrosigmoid, posterior petrosal, anterior petrosal, orbitozygomatic, or pretemporal transcavernous. The posterior petrosal approaches offer a shorter working distance than the others, but the medial aspect of the petrous apex can sometimes become a blind spot due to the more lateral angle of attack. Anterior endoscopic approaches to this area have fewer neurovascular obstacles but are difficult exposures nonetheless.

Internal Auditory Meatus and Otological Structures

The internal auditory meatus is a CSF-filled space that invaginates into the petrous bone, gradually tapering from the wide medial porus to the narrow lateral fundus. It is divided horizontally at the fundus by the transverse crest, which separates the facial and superior vestibular nerve superiorly from the cochlear and inferior vestibular nerve below. The vertical crest (Bill's bar) separates the more anterior facial nerve from the posterior superior vestibular nerve (Fig. 1.7e). The labyrinthine artery is usually a branch of AICA, an injury of which can cause hearing loss. Superiorly, the suprameatal tubercle can be drilled to access Meckel's cave (Fig. 1.7b, c).

Drilling the posterior petrous temporal bone, whether from a posterior or middle fossa approach, may injure specialized structures for the transduction of sound and motion. The internal auditory meatus is flanked by the labyrinth posteriorly and the cochlea anteriorly (Figs. 1.1d, 1.8d, and 1.9c). The tympanic cavity lies between the internal and external auditory canals and contains the ossicles as well as a small segment of the facial nerve. The superior semicircular canal of the labyrinth protrudes toward the floor of the middle fossa as the arcuate eminence, but this is not always a reliable landmark. The posterior semicircular canal is directed toward the posterior fossa and can be violated when drilling the posterior wall of the internal auditory canal (Fig. 1.1d). The lateral semicircular canal is oriented toward the middle ear. Below its anterior portion, the facial nerve turns inferiorly from its tympanic segment to the mastoid segment (Fig. 1.8d). The mastoid air cells posterior to the labyrinth are drilled to reach the lateral semicircular canal (Fig. 1.8b–d). At this point in the exposure, car must be taken not to injure the facial nerve.

Jugular Foramen

The jugular foramen is formed by an opening between the petrous and occipital bones immediately inferior to the petroclival fissure (Fig. 1.1b). It begins less than a centimeter inferior to the internal auditory meatus and is superior to the hypoglossal canal. The petrous bone forms a dome over this foramen as it turns downward (Fig. 1.2c). As with the sigmoid sinus, the jugular foramen is often larger on the right side. It is bounded by the jugular process of the occipital bone and rectus capitis lateralis posteriorly, the occipital condyle medially, the petrous carotid canal anteriorly, and the styloid process and extracranial facial nerve laterally (Fig. 1.2d). The jugular bulb has a variable superior extent in the jugular fossa that may reach as high as the labyrinth. Hence, a high-riding jugular bulb may hinder infralabyrinthine and presigmoid approaches. At the posterior end of the petroclival fissure, the jugular bulb receives drainage from the inferior petrosal sinus, which becomes the petrosal part of the foramen. The posterior sigmoid part drains the sigmoid sinus. These two sinuses converge at the jugular bulb medial to the exiting lower cranial nerves, which then drain into the jugular vein (Fig. 1.2a–c). Cranial nerves IX, X, and XI travel through the medial portion of the jugular foramen. Branches of the ascending pharyngeal and occipital arteries may enter the jugular foramen and supply tumors in this location. The jugular tubercle is located medial and inferior to the jug-

ular foramen and is often removed to provide increased anterior exposure during far-lateral approaches (Figs. 1.1a and 1.2a).

Surgical Corridors and Related Anatomy

The significant number of anatomical barriers within the posterior fossa and its enclosure dictate a wide variety of approaches to avoid injuring important neurovascular structures. Approaches have been developed for nearly every angle into the posterior fossa, though some entail planned morbidity. We will review these approaches starting from the posterior perspective and moving stepwise anteriorly.

Posterior

Occipital Transtentorial
The occipital transtentorial approach is used to access pineal and third ventricle lesions, precentral cerebellar fissure, inferior colliculus, and anterior vermis. The trajectory is usually either through the occipital interhemispheric fissure lateral to the straight sinus or below the occipital lobe above the tentorium (Fig. 1.5a, b). The occipital lobe is retracted, and dissection proceeds to the tentorial incisura. The tentorium is then cut to gain access to the ambient and quadrigeminal cisterns and the precentral cerebellar fissure.

Supracerebellar Infratentorial
The natural corridor above the cerebellum and below the tentorium leads to the pineal region, tectal plate, and posterior third ventricle [5] (Fig. 1.5d). The inferior and medial temporal lobe may also be reached if the tentorium is cut to perform operations such as amygdalohippocampectomy. The patient is usually placed in the sitting position. The transverse sinus is retracted superiorly, and the cerebellum retracted inferiorly. Precentral cerebellar veins are often sacrificed, but other draining veins in this region should be preserved, particularly the internal cerebral veins and the veins of Rosenthal.

Suboccipital, Telovelar

The suboccipital craniotomy is one of the most common approaches in posterior fossa surgery (Fig. 1.5c). The occipital bone is removed to expose the suboccipital surface of the cerebellum as well as the transverse and sigmoid sinuses if wide exposure is needed. The cisterna magna is often opened to allow drainage of CSF before further dissection is done. The vermis presents an apparent surgical barrier to the fourth ventricle, and transvermian approaches were once common, but not without morbidity. Careful study of this anatomy led to the development of the telovelar approach, whereby the fourth ventricle is entered by cutting the tela choroidea and inferior medullary velum, which form the inferior roof of the fourth ventricle [6]. These thin membranes are exposed by separating the tonsil and uvula (Fig. 1.5e, f). This approach can expose the entire floor of the fourth ventricle, including the lateral recess and the cerebral aqueduct without morbidity.

Posterolateral: Retrosigmoid

A posterolateral perspective into the posterior fossa can be obtained through a presigmoid or retrosigmoid approach. The retrosigmoid approach is far more common, and it can provide exposure extending from the tentorium to the foramen magnum as well as cranial nerves IV through XII [7] (Fig. 1.7a, b). The asterion typically lies posterior to the sigmoid-transverse junction, which is often drilled early in the approach, though it has not been found to be a consistently reliable landmark (Fig. 1.6a). Another landmark for the transverse sinus is a line joining the occipital eminence, or the inion, with the upper margin of the zygomatic arch or the upper margin of the middle third of the ear. The transverse-sigmoid junction may also be predicted to be just posterior to the upper level of the mastoid notch, which can be easily palpated. Navigation technology has made localization of the sinuses a much easier task. Because this perspective is posterior to several cranial nerves and the lateral to medial trajectory is lim-

ited by the sigmoid sinus, access to the anterior brainstem is hindered (Fig. 1.7a, b). Additional bone removal over the sigmoid sinus allows more retraction of the sinus to increase anterior and medial visualization [8]. The superior petrosal vein may obscure the trigeminal nerve, so it is often divided, though a venous infarct may occasionally occur.

The retrosigmoid approach can be tailored for specific pathologies, such as vestibular schwannomas involving the internal auditory canal [9]

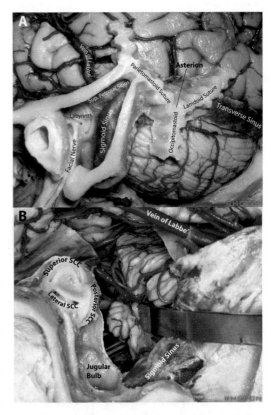

Fig. 1.6 Sigmoid sinus and related landmarks. (**a**) Lateral view of the left sigmoid sinus. The asterion represents the junction of the occipitomastoid, lambdoid, and parietomastoid sutures. It typically lies posterior to the sigmoid sinus and inferior to the transverse sinus, though it is not always a reliable localizing landmark. The retrosigmoid approaches are posterior to the sigmoid sinus and involve some retraction of the cerebellum. Note that the presigmoid space between the sigmoid sinus and the labyrinth can be very limited. (**b**) Division of the superior petrosal sinus allows the sigmoid sinus to be mobilized posteriorly, significantly enlarging the presigmoid corridor

(Fig. 1.8e). The superior lip of the IAC, known as the suprameatal tubercle, may also be drilled to enlarge the ostium of Meckel's cave, which is helpful for trigeminal tumors that extend from the posterior fossa into the middle fossa [10–12]. It also allows mobilization of the trigeminal nerve with further drilling of the petrous apex toward the petroclival fissure, similar to Kawase's approach. Extensive drilling risks injury to the posterior and superior semicircular canals, and their common crus, as well as the petrous carotid artery. Although this extension may open the space anteriorly to the ventral brainstem, the working area around the prepontine cistern remains limited.

Far-Lateral Approach

The retrosigmoid exposure may be extended more inferiorly by adding C1 and C2 hemilaminectomies so that the foramen magnum and spinal cord are visualized (Fig. 1.7f, g). Variants of the far-lateral approach provide exposure of the hypoglossal canal, vertebral artery, posterior inferior cerebellar artery (PICA), lower cranial nerves, lower clivus, and cervicomedullary junction [13, 14]. The suboccipital musculature is typically mobilized inferolaterally as a single flap. The exposure can be tailored by removing additional bone from the occipital and atlantal condyles to allow a more lateral to medial perspective. This often entails transposition of the vertebral artery out of the C1 transverse foramen (Fig. 1.7g). Removal of the posterior third of the condyle exposes the lateral aspect of the hypoglossal canal, but extensive condyle removal may destabilize the atlanto-occipital joint. Paracondylar bone can be drilled to access the posterior jugular foramen. Drilling of the jugular tubercle widens the surgical view of the lower clivus.

Posterolateral: Presigmoid

A trajectory through the mastoid bone anterior to the sigmoid sinus provides exposure of the brainstem with minimal or no retraction of the cerebel-

lum [15]. Because the petrous bone is directed anteriorly and medially toward the brainstem, the resulting angle of attack allows visualization of the anterior and medial aspects of the cranial nerves as they emerge from the brainstem better than a retrosigmoid approach. Additionally, the working distance to the brainstem is shorter. Once a mastoidectomy has been performed, removal of the labyrinth and cochlea further improves the view of the anterior brainstem and petroclival region but at the cost of hearing loss and facial nerve weakness. The retrolabyrinthine approach is often adequate, and it spares these structures.

The operative corridor is bounded inferiorly by the jugular bulb, which is sometimes located very close to the labyrinth, limiting the surgical corridor. The posterior boundary is the sigmoid sinus, but this can be retracted further posteriorly by additional bone removal. Further posterior mobilization of the sigmoid sinus is possible by dividing the superior petrosal sinus and tentorium (Fig. 1.6b). Division of the tentorium allows a combination of infratentorial and supratentorial access. Hence, optimal presigmoid approaches are often not purely infratentorial, because the corridor anterior to the sigmoid sinus is often very narrow unless it is retracted.

Mastoidectomy

The cortical bone in the area between the external auditory meatus, the supramastoid crest, and the mid-mastoid tip is progressively drilled [16] (Fig. 1.8). Alternatively, the superficial cortical layer may be disconnected and preserved for a more cosmetic closure. Drilling just below the supramastoid crest exposes the middle fossa dura, and the sigmoid sinus is skeletonized inferiorly to the level of the jugular bulb. The posterior fossa dura is found between the transverse-sigmoid junction (TSJ), the superior petrosal sinus, jugular bulb, and the labyrinth. Drilling deep in the suprameatal triangle opens the mastoid antrum, which is the biggest mastoid air cell. From there, the head of the incus can be identified in the epitympanic recess 1 cm deep to the spine of Henle, as well as the lateral semicircular canal (SCC).

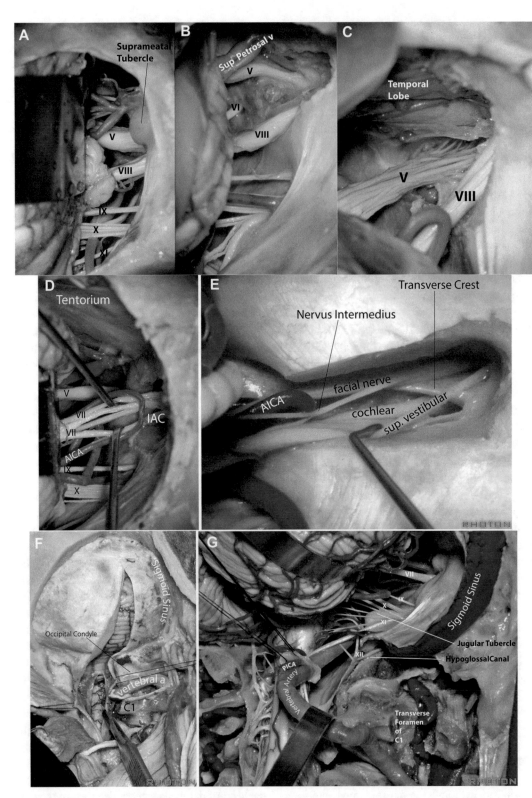

Fig. 1.7 Retrosigmoid and far-lateral approaches. (**a**) Posterior view of the right retrosigmoid approach. The retrosigmoid approach provides exposure extending from the tentorium to the foramen magnum, as well as the cerebellopontine angle. Structures identified include cranial nerves 4–12, flocculus, and internal auditory meatus. The superior petrosal bridging vein (Dandy's vein) is seen draining into the superior petrosal sinus. (**b**) The suprameatal tubercle, which lies superior and anterior to the internal auditory canal, can be drilled to access the proximal

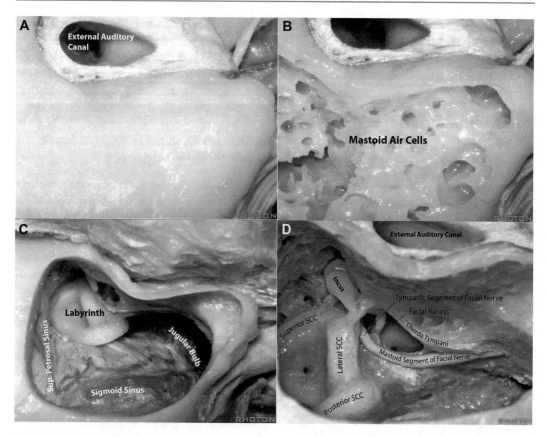

Fig. 1.8 Mastoidectomy. (**a**) Lateral view of the right mastoid process. The mastoid part of the temporal bone is posterior to the external auditory canal. The limits of the mastoidectomy are the asterion, the suprameatal crest, and the mastoid tip. (**b**) Mastoid air cells are drilled until the antrum is encountered, leading to the middle ear elements and the corticated labyrinthine structures. (**c**) The presigmoid posterior fossa dura is outlined by Trautman's triangle roughly between the superior petrosal sinus, the sigmoid sinus, and the jugular bulb. The posterior semicir-cular canal faces the posterior fossa dura and the superior semicircular canal faces the middle fossa dura. (**d**) Enlarged view of the labyrinth through a mastoidectomy exposure. The facial nerve bends inferiorly below the lateral semicircular canal to begin its mastoid segment in the anterior part of the mastoidectomy exposure. The short process of the incus points to this portion of the facial nerve. The chorda tympani courses further anterior than the facial nerve, and the space between them (facial recess) can be drilled to expose the tympanic cavity

Fig. 1.7 (continued) portion of Meckel's cave. (**c**) Extensive drilling of the suprameatal tubercle can be combined with division of the tentorium and superior petrosal sinus to increase exposure of Meckel's cave. (**d**) Posterior exposure of the internal auditory canal (IAC). The internal auditory meatus is opened, and the nerve rootlets have been identified. The anterior inferior cerebellar artery (AICA) often loops near these nerves. The labyrinthine artery also enters the IAC and its injury can lead to deafness. (**e**) Posterior view of the internal auditory canal and its nerves. The facial nerve is anterior and superior, and together with the superior vestibular nerve, is separated from the cochlear and inferior vestibular nerve by the transverse crest. The nervus intermedius carries sensory and parasympathetic fibers of the facial nerve. A loop of AICA often protrudes into the IAC and can cause geniculate neuralgia by impinging upon the nervus intermedius. (**f**) Posterior view of the far-lateral exposure. The far-lateral approach is an inferior continuation of the retrosigmoid approach, adding additional exposure through the foramen magnum, occipital condyle, and lamina of the atlas. (**g**) Far-lateral/transcondylar approach. The vertebral artery has been mobilized from the C1 transverse foramen, and the occipital and atlantal condyles have been drilled to expose the hypoglossal canal and to increase exposure of the lower clivus. An extradural PICA origin is seen. The jugular tubercle can be drilled to increase anterior exposure

Further drilling of mastoid air cells uncovers the compact bone of the digastric ridge inferiorly. The fallopian (or facial) canal can then be expected to course anteriorly to and in the same plane as a line joining the incus and the digastric ridge.

Transcrusal and Translabyrinthine Approaches

The translabyrinthine approach involves drilling the semicircular canals to expose the IAC, vestibule, and the different nerves directed to the ampullae (Fig. 1.9b). The IAC is accessed through the superior ampulla, and the superior vestibular nerve is encountered first posterior to Bill bar. This approach increases the surgical access to the anterolateral brainstem and clivus at the expense of hearing. The transcrusal, or partial translabyrinthine approach, has been devised to preserve most of the surgical advantages of the translabyrinthine approach without necessarily sacrificing hearing. Although it only entails drilling of the superior and posterior semicircular canals and their common crus, the risk of hearing loss is still significant.

Transcochlear and Transotic Approaches

In the transcochlear approach, the posterior petrous bone is completely drilled as well as parts of the tympanic bone [17] (Fig. 1.9c, d). To this end, the external auditory canal (EAC) is opened, the middle ear is accessed through the facial recess anterior to the facial nerve, and the latter is completely skeletonized. The GSPN and the chorda tympani are disconnected from the facial nerve to allow a posterior transposition of the nerve, which will result in permanent weakness. The cochlea is drilled above the petrous carotid artery. The transcochlear approach results in the widest access to the ventral brainstem with inferior extension to the jugular bulb. Because this approach carries the highest risk of facial nerve palsy, the transotic variant has been described to avoid manipulation of the nerve.

Combined Supra-/Infratentorial Petrosal Approaches

The petrosal exposures can be extended with a temporal craniotomy that crosses the transverse-sigmoid junction. The middle fossa dura is carefully incised while avoiding injury to the vein of Labbe before dividing the superior petrosal sinus and cutting the tentorium to communicate the posterior and middle fossae (Fig. 1.9e–h). The temporal lobe, tentorium, cerebellum, and sigmoid sinus can then all be retracted together to augment the combined presigmoid and subtemporal exposure [18].

Exposure of Jugular Foramen

The presigmoid mastoidectomy may be carried inferiorly and combined with a neck dissection to widely expose the jugular bulb and the infralabyrinthine area [19] (Fig. 1.10). The postauricular incision is extended inferiorly to expose the carotid artery, internal jugular vein, and the lower cranial nerves in the upper cervical region. The spinal accessory nerve may pass either anterior or posterior to the internal jugular vein near the C1 transverse process, and care must be taken not to

---

Fig. 1.9 (continued) of attack to the anterior brainstem and petroclival region. (**c**) Transposition of the facial nerve has been performed before drilling of the cochlea. (**d**) The transcochlear approach maximizes the presigmoid exposure of the deep anterior structures such as the trunk of basilar artery, the abducens nerve, and the clivus. (**e**) Left combined supra-/infratentorial petrosal approach. The mastoidectomy is combined with a temporal craniotomy. The superior petrosal sinus and the tentorium are cut to join the middle and posterior fossae, and the sigmoid sinus can be then be mobilized posteriorly to widen the presigmoid corridor. (**f**) View through a left retrolabyrinthine combined approach. (**g**) View through a left translabyrinthine combined approach. The vein of Labbe draining into the transverse-sigmoid junction must be identified and preserved. Its drainage into the superior petrosal sinus requires careful planning to preserve venous outflow. (**h**) View through a left transcochlear combined approach, which provides an extensive exposure ranging from the petrous carotid laterally, basilar trunk and pons anteriorly, oculomotor nerve superiorly, and jugular bulb inferiorly

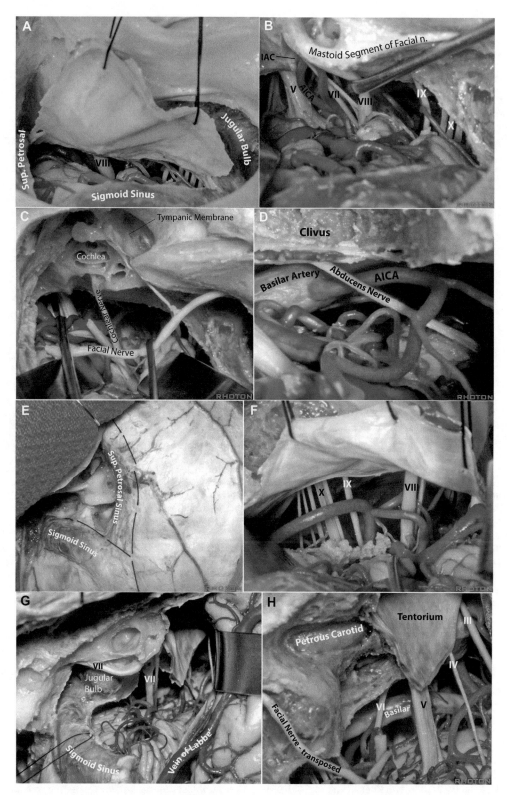

Fig. 1.9 Petrosal approaches. (**a**) Right retrolabyrinthine approach. The posterior fossa dura is opened posterior to the semicircular canals in the retrolabyrinthine approach. This exposes the cochlear, vestibular, facial, and lower cranial nerves, lateral pons and medulla above the jugular bulb, and elements of the posterior circulation. (**b**) Right translabyrinthine approach. Resecting the labyrinth exposes the internal auditory canal and widens the angle

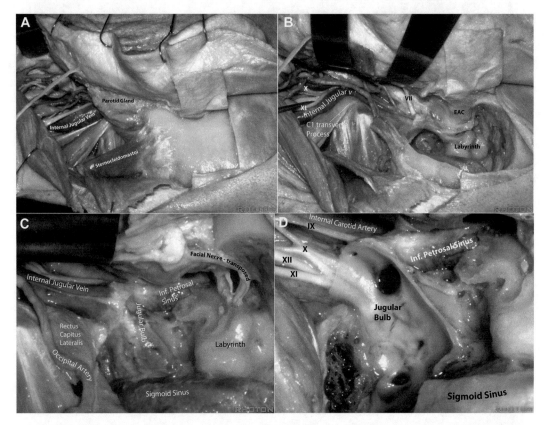

Fig. 1.10 Transtemporal postauricular approach to jugular foramen. (**a**) Left mastoid and cervical exposure. Lateral exposure of the jugular foramen involves a mastoidectomy approach combined with an upper neck dissection. It is important to recognize the different muscular layers and the diverging trajectories of the lower cranial nerves as they exit the cranium. (**b**) Mastoidectomy and internal jugular vein exposure. The transverse process of the atlas and its muscular relationships with the skull base is a crucial surgical landmark. The accessory nerve courses posteriorly toward the sternocleidomastoid muscle near the transverse process and may pass anterior or posterior to the jugular vein. The internal jugular vein passes immediately anterior to the transverse process. (**c**) Full exposure of left jugular bulb and infralabyrinthine area. Mobilization of the facial nerve anteriorly increases the exposure at a risk of irreversible weakness. Detachment of the rectus capitis lateralis muscle and removal of the jugular process of the occipital bone further exposes the posterior part of the jugular foramen. (**d**) The jugular vein is resected, and the medial wall of the jugular bulb is preserved to avoid damaging the medially located lower cranial nerves. The inferior petrosal sinus empties into the jugular foramen

injure it with posterior retraction of the sternocleidomastoid muscle. The facial nerve should be identified as it exits the stylomastoid foramen and passes lateral to the styloid process before entering the parotid gland anteriorly. The facial nerve may be transposed anteriorly to increase access to the petrosal portion of the jugular foramen, but this typically causes weakness. The styloid process can be removed if access to the high internal carotid and anterior aspect of the jugular foramen

is desired. Removal of the rectus capitis lateralis muscle opens the posterior edge of the jugular foramen (Fig. 1.2d).

Lateral

The simplest lateral trajectory to the posterior fossa is a subtemporal approach, which is limited inferiorly by the tentorium, but can expose the

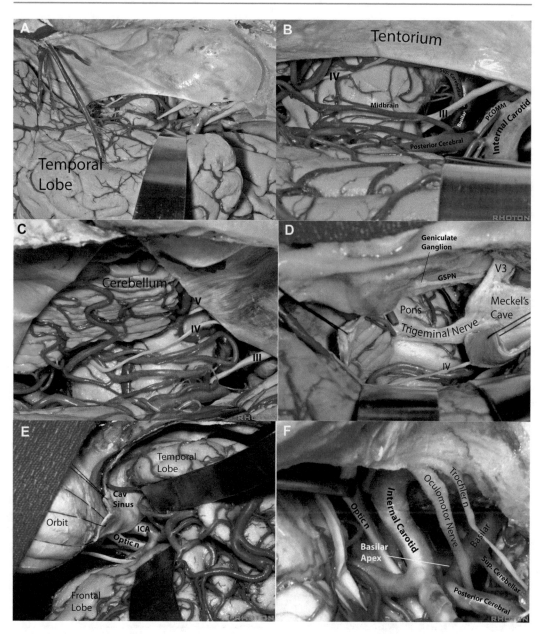

Fig. 1.11 Lateral and anterolateral approaches. (**a**) Left subtemporal approach. The subtemporal approach requires retraction of the temporal lobe to expose the lateral aspect of the tentorial incisura. Bridging temporal veins can be at risk of injury, which may cause a venous infarct of the temporal lobe. (**b**) View through a left subtemporal approach. The ambient, crural, and interpeduncular cisterns are exposed, and the basilar apex can be accessed. The oculomotor nerve is seen emerging between the superior cerebellar artery and the posterior cerebral artery. The trochlear nerve has a close relation with the superior cerebellar artery before it joins the tentorial edge near the cavernous sinus. (**c**) The tentorium is cut, taking care to preserve the trochlear nerve, to expose the tentorial surface of the cerebellum. Anterior brainstem exposure is blocked by the petrous temporal bone. (**d**) View through subtemporal transtentorial approach combined with an anterior petrosectomy. Kawase's rhombus is limited by the GSPN laterally, mandibular branch of the trigeminal nerve anteriorly, and the arcuate eminence posteriorly. (**e**) View through a right frontotemporal-orbitozygomatic approach. This allows for several operative corridors, including transsylvian, pretemporal, and subtemporal. (**f**) View through a right transcavernous exposure of the basilar apex region. The anterior clinoid has been removed, and the posterior cavernous sinus has been opened by skeletonizing the oculomotor and trochlear nerves. This facilitates mobilization of these nerves and drilling of the posterior clinoid and dorsum sella

basilar apex as well as the midbrain and its crural and ambient cisterns [20]. Care must be taken to preserve veins projecting to the transverse-sigmoid junction that may be avulsed with temporal lobe retraction (Fig. 1.11a, b). Division of the tentorium exposes the superior aspect of the cerebellum, but access to the pons is obstructed by the petrous temporal bone (Fig. 1.11c). The trochlear nerve may be injured when cutting the tentorium, especially anteriorly as it approaches the cavernous sinus. An anterior petrosectomy (Kawase's approach) extends the subtemporal exposure further into the posterior fossa, revealing the pons above and below the trigeminal nerve as well as the upper petroclival region [21] (Fig. 1.11d). Temporal bone drilling is typically limited by the greater superficial petrosal nerve and carotid artery laterally and the internal auditory canal and labyrinth posteriorly. The abducens nerve may be injured in Dorello canal if drilling is continued deep to the petrous apex.

Anterolateral

The interpeduncular fossa may be accessed through the pterional approach and its variants, such as the frontotemporal-orbitozygomatic or orbitozygomatic, which can be tailored for a subtemporal or pretemporal corridor to allow a transcavernous exposure. This results in an anterolateral perspective. The optic-carotid and the carotid-oculomotor windows can be opened through a classic pterional approach, and Liliequist's membrane is then dissected to reach the interpeduncular fossa and the basilar tip as taught by Yasargil. The view of midline anterior structures in the upper posterior fossa is limited by the posterior cavernous sinus, tentorium, dorsum sellae, clinoidal processes, carotid artery, optic nerve, oculomotor nerve, and the posterior communicating artery (Fig. 1.11e). The transcavernous approach involves opening the posterior cavernous sinus while preserving the oculomotor and trochlear

nerves. This facilitates drilling of the posterior clinoidal processes and dorsum sella to increase medial exposure [22–24] (Fig. 1.11f).

Anterior

Anterior approaches to the posterior fossa typically involve removal of midface sinuses to access the clivus. The most superior perspective can be provided by a transbasal approach [25] to remove the frontal, ethmoid, and sphenoid sinuses as well as the nasal cavity so that the clivus can be opened (Fig. 1.12a). The superior posterior fossa is obstructed by the pituitary gland. Olfaction is at risk but can be preserved with osteotomies of the cribriform plate.

The most common anterior approach to the posterior fossa today is the expanded endonasal approach (Fig. 1.12b). Removal of sinuses allows endoscopic exposure ranging from the frontal sinus to the odontoid process. The maxillary sinuses can be opened to expose more laterally, but lateral exposure is also limited by the Eustachian tubes. The petrous apex can be exposed by drilling through the pterygoid process. Transclival approaches can also be performed endoscopically through a transoral approach, though the view is foreshortened by the more extreme angle (Fig. 1.12c). Maxillotomy approaches can provide excellent transclival exposure of the posterior fossa as well as exposure of the middle and infratemporal fossa [26] (Fig. 1.12d). These are rarely performed in the era of skull base endoscopy.

Credits

All images are from the online Rhoton Collection. Dissections by Hiroshi Abe, Toshiro Katsuta, Antonio Mussi, Eduardo Seoane, Ryusui Tanaka, Helder Tedeschi, Tsutomu Hitotsumatsu, and Hung Wen.

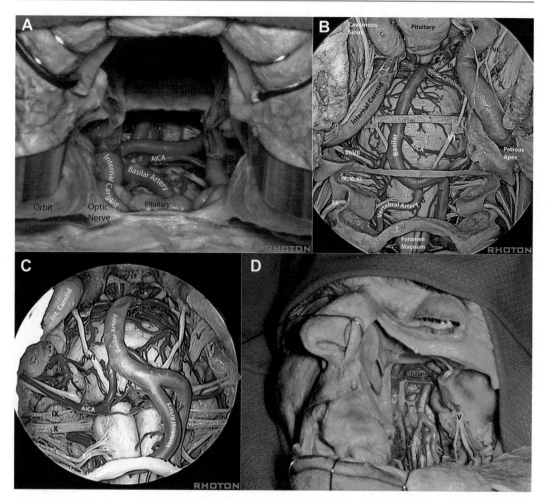

Fig. 1.12 Anterior approaches. (**a**) The transbasal approach through the anterior skull base, midface sinuses and nasal cavity can provide exposure of the clivus and pterygopalatine fossa. The clivus can then be opened ·to expose the posterior fossa. In this specimen, the prepontine cistern and the pontomedullary junction are visualized. The cavernous segment of the carotid is seen laterally. (**b**) The expanded endonasal approach through the clivus can expose the anterior aspect of the posterior fossa from the interpeduncular fossa to the foramen magnum. Exposure of lateral structures seen in this dissection is more challenging. (**c**) The endoscopic transoral approach provides a similar exposure to the endonasal approach, though with a more foreshortened perspective superiorly due to a more extreme angle. (**d**) The transmaxillary approach provides a slightly lateral perspective through the maxillary sinus to expose the anterior aspect of the posterior fossa, the pterygopalatine fossa, and the infratemporal fossa. A facial incision has been made in this specimen, but a degloving incision is also possible

References

1. Rhoton AL Jr. Rhoton's cranial anatomy and surgical approaches. 1st ed. Philadelphia: Lippincott Williams & Wilkins; 2007.
2. http://rhoton.ineurodb.org.
3. Rhoton AL Jr. The posterior fossa veins. Neurosurgery. 2000;47:69–92.
4. Yasargil MG, Kasdaglis K, Jain KK, Weber HP. Anatomical observations of the subarachnoid cisterns of the brain during surgery. J Neurosurg. 1976;44:298–302.
5. Stein BM. Supracerebellar-infratentorial approach to pineal tumors. Surg Neurol. 1979;11:331–7.
6. Mussi A, Rhoton AL Jr. Telovelar approach to the fourth ventricle: microsurgical anatomy. J Neurosurg. 2000;92:812–23.
7. Rhoton AL Jr. The cerebellopontine angle and posterior fossa cranial nerves by the retrosigmoid approach. Neurosurgery. 2000;47:93–129.
8. Quinones-Hinojosa A, Chang EF, Lawton MT. The extended retrosigmoid approach: an alternative to radical cranial base approaches for posterior fossa lesions. Neurosurgery. 2006;58:208–14.

9. Ojemann RG. Retrosigmoid approach to acoustic neuroma (vestibular schwannoma). Neurosurgery. 2001;48:553–8.
10. Seoane E, Rhoton AL Jr. Suprameatal extension of the retrosigmoid approach: microsurgical anatomy. Neurosurgery. 1999;44:553–60.
11. Samii M, Tatagiba M, Carvalho GA. Retrosigmoid intradural suprameatal approach to Meckel's cave and the middle fossa: surgical technique and outcome. J Neurosurg. 2000;92:235–41.
12. Cheung S, Jackal R, Pitts L, Gutti P. Interconnecting the posterior and middle cranial fossae for tumors that traverse Meckel's cave. Am J Otolaryngol. 1995;16:200–8.
13. Wen HT, Rhoton AL Jr, Katsuta T, de Oliveira E. Microsurgical anatomy of the transcondylar, supracondylar and paracondylar extensions of the far lateral approach. J Neurosurg. 1997;87:555–8.
14. Al-Mefty O, Borba LA, Aoki N, Angtuaco E, Pait TG. The transcondylar approach to extradural nonneoplastic lesions of the craniovertebral junction. J Neurosurg. 1996;84:1–6.
15. Al-Mefty O, Ayoubi S, Smith RR. The petrosal approach: indications, technique, and results. Acta Neurochir Suppl (Wien). 1991;53:166–70.
16. Nelson RA. Temporal bone surgical dissection manual. 2nd ed. Los Angeles: House Ear Institute; 1991.
17. House WF, Hitselberger WE. The transcochlear approach to the skull base. Arch Otolaryngol. 1976;102:334–42.
18. Cho CW, Al-Mefty O. Combined petrosal approach to petroclival meningiomas. Neurosurgery. 2002;51:708–18.
19. Gardner G, Cocke EW, Robertson JH, Plmer RE, Bellott AL, Hamm CW. Skull base surgery for glomus jugulare tumors. Am J Otolaryngol. 1985;November Suppl:126–34.
20. Drake CG. The surgical treatment of aneurysms of the basilar artery. Clin Neurosurg. 1968;29:436–46.
21. Kawase T, Shiobara R, Toya S. Anterior transpetrosal-transtentorial approach for sphenopetro-clival meningiomas: surgical method and results in 10 patients. Neurosurgery. 1991;28:869–76.
22. Dolenc VV, Skrap M, Sustersic J, Skrbec M, Morina A. A transcavernous- transsellar approach to the basilar tip aneurysms. Br J Neurosurg. 1987;1:251–9.
23. Seoane E, Tedeschi H, de Oliveira E, Wen HT, Rhoton AL Jr. The pretemporal transcavernous approach to the interpeduncular and prepontine cisterns: micro- surgical anatomy and technique application. Neurosurgery. 2000;46:891–9.
24. Krisht AF. Transcavernous approach to diseases of the anterior upper third of the posterior fossa. Neurosurg Focus. 2005;19:E2.
25. Derome PJ. Surgical management of tumors invading the skull base. Can J Neurol Sci. 1985;12:345–7.
26. James D, Crockard HA. Surgical access to the base of skull and upper cervical spine by extended maxillotomy. Neurosurgery. 1991;29:411.

Part II
Approaches

Retrosigmoid Craniotomy and Its Variants

2

Christian Bowers, Olaide O. Ajayi,
Kevin A. Reinard, Daniel R. Klinger,
Johnny B. Delashaw, Shane Tubbs,
and Zachary Litvack

Background

The retrosigmoid craniotomy is a modification of the traditional suboccipital craniotomy, which was first described in the literature by Frankel et al. in 1904 [1, 2]. The suboccipital craniotomy provides a wide view of the posterior cranial fossa from the tentorium cerebelli to the foramen magnum. Although new technologies and techniques have been introduced to make the approach safer, it is a testament to its versatility that this surgical approach continues to be used nearly unchanged from its original description over a century ago [1].

Indications

The retrosigmoid craniotomy provides for exposure and access to extra-axial lesions in the cerebellopontine (CP) angle; lesions arising from the underside of the tentorium, vascular, and cranial nerve pathology of cranial nerves (CNs) V–XI;

C. Bowers, MD (✉) • O.O. Ajayi, MD
K.A. Reinard, MD • D.R. Klinger, MD
J.B. Delashaw, MD • Z. Litvack, MD
Swedish Neuroscience Institute, Seattle, WA, USA
e-mail: christian.bowers@wmchealth.org;
jdelashawjr@gmail.com

S. Tubbs, PhD, PA-C
Swedish Neuroscience Institute, Neurosurgery-
Seattle Science Foundation, Seattle, WA, USA

and intrinsic pathology of lateral cerebellar hemisphere and brainstem from mesencephalon to pontomedullary junction [1, 3]. Pathologies routinely accessed through this approach include meningioma, vestibular schwannoma, and neurovascular compression syndromes [4–7].

Anatomy

Cranial and Extradural Anatomy

The retrosigmoid craniotomy is a versatile approach, and the position and extent of the craniotomy (or craniectomy) is defined by the exact position and type of pathology in the CP angle. The limits of exposure are defined superiorly by the transverse sinus, inferiorly by the foramen magnum, medially by the anatomic midline, and laterally by the sigmoid sinus. The surgical keyhole for this approach is defined relative to the asterion. Analogous to a pterional craniotomy, the retrosigmoid approach may also be thought of as an "asterional" craniotomy.

The asterion, a consistent bony landmark for finding the junction of the transverse and sigmoid sinuses, is defined as the junction of the lambdoid, occipitomastoid, and parietomastoid sutures. The lambdoid suture travels obliquely from its origin at the caudal terminus of the sagittal suture, separating the parietal and occipital bones. It continues past the asterion as

© Springer International Publishing AG 2018
W.T. Couldwell (ed.), *Skull Base Surgery of the Posterior Fossa*,
https://doi.org/10.1007/978-3-319-67038-6_2

the occipitomastoid suture, separating the petrous temporal bone from the occipital bone, terminating at the jugular foramen. The parietomastoid suture separates the mastoid portion of the temporal bone from the parietal bone (Fig. 2.1).

A burr hole placed just anterior to the asterion typically exposes the junction of the transverse and sigmoid sinuses, a key anatomic landmark that defines the superior and ventral extent of exposure, respectively. Tubbs et al. [8] further studied the relationship between the superficial bony landmarks and the location of the venous sinuses in 100 adult cadaver skulls and defined this keyhole relative to the intersection of the "zygomatic line" and a "mastoid line" (Fig. 2.2). The zygomatic line parallels the superior border of the zygomatic arch and extends posteriorly from the root of the zygoma to the inion. The mastoid line connects the mastoid notch to the squamosal suture. In 80/100 cases, irrespective of laterality, the transverse-sigmoid junction lies within 1 cm of a burr hole placed inferior to the zygomatic line and dorsal to the mastoid line [8].

Intradural Anatomy

The CP angle is bordered by the tentorium cerebelli; the superior and inferior limbs of the angular cerebellopontine fissure; the petrosal surface of the cerebellum, lateral pons, and middle cerebellar peduncle; the petrous temporal bone; and, at its deep extent, the prepontine cistern, the petrous apex, and Meckel's cave. CNs V–XI are found within the CP angle, as well as branches of the superior cerebellar artery, anterior inferior cerebellar artery, and posterior inferior cerebellar artery. Rhoton et al. divided the contents of the CP angle into three neurovascular complexes, which have a relatively fixed position at the brainstem and skull base, and thus can be reliably identified even in the presence of distorting pathology such as tumors or vascular malformations [9–12].

The upper neurovascular complex consists of CN V, superior cerebellar peduncle, origin of the SCA (often duplicated), and superior petrosal venous complex (i.e., Dandy's vein). CN V exits the lateral surface of the pons at its midportion and runs obliquely toward the petrous apex to enter Meckel's cave. Typically, the SCA travels around the pons rostral to CN V but may send a caudal loop that comes in close proximity or contacts the CN V. The superior petrosal vein is often

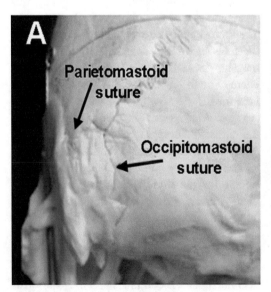

Fig. 2.1 Skull model with parietomastoid and occipitomastoid sutures identified and labeled

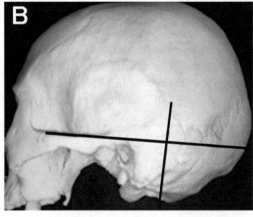

Fig. 2.2 Horizontal "zygomatic line" and vertical "mastoid line" demonstrate the intersection where a burr hole placed at the inferior aspect of the zygomatic line and the dorsal aspect of the mastoid line will be within 1 cm of the transverse-sigmoid junction 80% of the time

a complex of two to three veins that drain the lateral cerebellar surface before converging to insert into the petrosal sinus [7]. These veins may lie adjacent to CN V or may enter the tentorium separate from CN V, effectively tethering the lateral cerebellar hemisphere [7]. The middle neurovascular complex consists of the AICA, middle cerebellar peduncle, and cranial nerves VI–VIII. CN VII arises from the brainstem at the level of the pontomedullary junction 1–2 mm ventral to the vestibulocochlear entry point (Fig. 2.3). The facial and vestibulocochlear nerves course together as they travel laterally to the internal acoustic meatus. AICA typically forms a loop just below the CN VII–VIII complex with labyrinthine, recurrent perforating and subarcuate branches arising from this loop to course with CN VIII into the internal acoustic meatus [9–12]. The lateral recess of the fourth ventricle transitions into the foramen of Luschka, which is situated posteroinferior to the junction of CNs VII–VIII with the brainstem and is often not visualized, but may be identified by a tuft of choroid plexus protruding into the CP angle [11]. The flocculus, which projects from the lateral recess, forms a bulge of cerebellar tissue sitting superficial to CNs VII–VIII and adjacent to the choroid plexus [11].

The lower complex consists of CNs IX–XI, the inferior cerebellar peduncle, and the PICA [10]. CNs IX–XI arise as rootlets along the posterior edge of the medullary olive in the groove of the postolivary sulcus (Fig. 2.3). CN IX is typically one or two rootlets arising from the upper medulla just caudal to CN VII, whereas CN X comprises a line of tightly packed rootlets just inferior to this. The rootlets of CN XI are more widely separated, running from the lower two-thirds of the olive to the upper cervical cord, its cranial roots often being difficult to distinguish from vagal fibers. CNs IX–XI exit at the jugular foramen with the glossopharyngeal exiting more anteromedially at the pars nervosa and CNs X–XI exiting posterolaterally at the larger pars vascularis. CN XII exits the medulla along the anterior margin of the caudal olive, its roots running anterolaterally to reach the hypoglossal canal. Both branches of PICA and the vertebral artery may pass through or contact rootlets of the lower cranial nerves [10].

Surgical Technique

Positioning

The three-quarter prone position is our position of choice because it maximizes the working space between the patient's head and ipsilateral shoulder, thus providing adequate working space for the surgical corridor (Fig. 2.4a, b) [13]. Several other positions have been described for a retrosigmoid approach, each with its own relative advantages and disadvantages, including the sitting position [14], supine position with the head maximally rotated to the contralateral side [7], or the lateral position with the head turned 90° [15].

A series of stepwise maneuvers are undertaken to place the patient in this position. If utilized, a vacuum positioner [i.e., "beanbag"] is prepositioned on the bed. Alternatively, pillows and bolsters may be used to support the torso. A minimum of four surgical personnel are required to safely perform these maneuvers, with the neurosurgeon typically in control of the head, assistants at each side controlling shoulders and hips, and one assistant in control of the legs and feet. Our preference is to pin the head with the skull

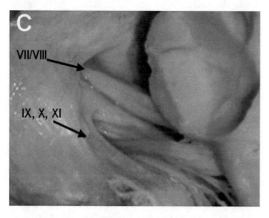

Fig. 2.3 Cadaveric specimen demonstrating the right CN VII–VIII complex and CNs IX, X, and XI as they exit the brainstem

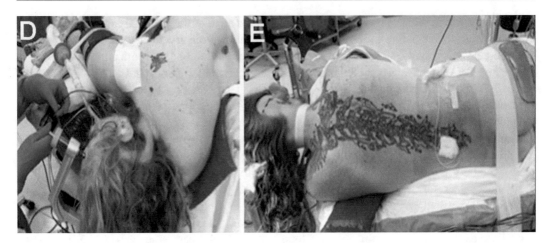

Fig. 2.4 (**a, b**) Photographs showing two patients in a three-quarter prone position, with the pressure points padded and the patients secured to the operating tables

clamp after the body is positioned and maintain direct manual control of the head.

Starting from a supine position, the patient is translated such that the shoulders are 2–4 cm above the end of the bed. The patient is then translated laterally such that the contralateral hip lies past the midline of the bed, often with the ipsilateral hip (temporarily) suspended by an assistant off the edge of the bed. Simultaneous with this translation, the torso is rotated to bring the ipsilateral shoulder up and over midline into the three-quarter prone position. Alternatively, if a lumbar drain is to be placed, the rotation may be paused at true lateral for insertion and then continued to three-quarter prone. An axillary roll is placed one handbreadth below the axilla, at the mid-nipple line. The dependent arm may be left extended and supported on a bed-rail arm board or may be slung in the armature of the head clamp, suspended hanging over the edge of the bed [16]. The independent arm is supported on pillows or an elevated arm board, with care to minimize pressure in the brachial fossa (Fig. 2.4a, b). The dependent leg is left extended, with care to pad the fibular head to prevent a peroneal nerve palsy. The independent leg is flexed at the hip and knee, allowing the iliac crest to roll over, and the pelvis is positioned with the same degree of rotation as the shoulders and torso.

The whole bed is then placed into a 10–15° reverse Trendelenburg position. This elevation increases venous outflow from the head. Combined with subarachnoid drainage, this should provide a significant working corridor without the need for hyperosmolar agents (e.g., saline or mannitol). If not already done, the head is placed into three-point skull clamp pin fixation, with one pin on the contralateral forehead (taking care not to pin the temporal branch of the facial nerve) and two pins at the contralateral asterion and inion. The head is then titled 5–10° toward the contralateral shoulder, opening the angle between the cardinal axis of the cranium and the torso. The head is rotated 10–15° to the contralateral shoulder, and the chin is flexed toward the sternum, taking care not to compromise the airway or contralateral jugular vein. Prior to locking the pin clamp to the bed, anesthesia should confirm the patency and position of the airway. Rotation and flexion of the head may dislodge a shallow intubation. If the head is over-rotated or over-flexed, the contralateral internal jugular vein may be compressed, leading to an increase in intracranial pressure and intraoperative cerebellar swelling.

The patient's body is securely restrained so that the operating table can be rotated liberally to maximize the angle of approach for the microscope. This usually involves a vacuum positioner and reinforcement with nonperforated cloth tape across the shoulder, torso, and hips. In larger patients, the ipsilateral shoulder is taped down across the long axis of the arm to open up the angle between head and shoulders, maximizing the surgeon's angles of attack and visualization of the operative space during the operation (Fig. 2.4a, b).

We utilize a C-shaped, retroauricular incision about two fingerbreadths medial to the mastoid process, which extends from the pinna to the tip of the mastoid (Fig. 2.5a, b). In most cases, we prefer to raise a single myocutaneous flap with a combination of electrocautery and sharp dissection. Although many authors prefer to raise a subgaleal flap and take the combined fascia/periosteum at the insertion of the sternocleidomastoid as a separate local periosteal flap, we harvest a separate free flap (temporoparietal fascia or fascia lata) as necessary. The subperiosteal dissection is carried down, and the asterion is identified (which may also be confirmed with intraoperative neuronavigation).

Craniotomy Technique

Prior to the marking of the skin incision, the positions of the transverse and sigmoid sinuses should be approximated with anatomic landmarks or confirmed with neuronavigation. A straight line drawn from the root of the zygoma to the poste-rior occipital protuberance (inion) defines the course of the transverse sinus (Fig. 2.5b) [8]. The asterion and digastric grooves are identified (Fig. 2.6a). The "zygomatic line" and a "mastoid line" as described by Tubbs et al. [8] and demonstrated in Fig. 2.6b are marked with a surgical marker at the time of surgery to approximate the transverse-sigmoid junction.

In our experience, there is a lower likelihood of tearing the dura or the lateral wall of a sinus with craniectomy as opposed to a craniotomy. A high-speed cutting burr such as a 6 mm fluted ball or acorn bit is used to fashion a craniectomy tailored to the size and scope of the lesion. Care is taken to expose the sigmoid-transverse junction at the superolateral margin of the craniectomy without violating the venous sinuses. Often, the mastoid emissary vein (Fig. 2.7a) or a complex of emissary veins (Fig. 2.7b) may be skeletonized and followed ventrally and superiorly to its insertion near the junction of the sinuses. Invariably, the mastoid air cells will be entered prior to thinning out the bone over the sigmoid sinus ("blue lining") and should be packed with wax during exposure (and again during reconstruction) to prevent a postoperative CSF leak ("wax in, wax out").

Kerrison rongeurs are used to remove 4–6 mm of bone overlying the sigmoid sinus (Fig. 2.8) to

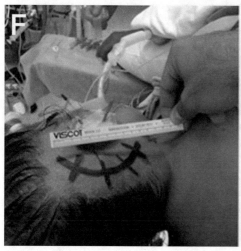
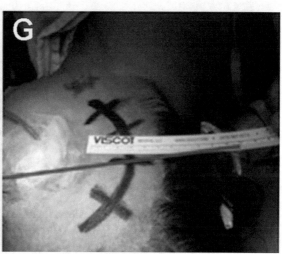

Fig. 2.5 (**a, b**) A C-shaped retroauricular incision two fingerbreadths medial to the mastoid process, extending from the pinna to the tip of the mastoid. Figure **b** has a *red* *line* drawn from the root of the zygoma to the inion, approximating the course of the transverse sinus

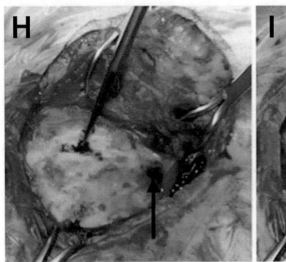
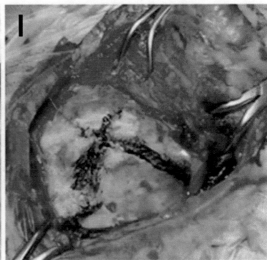

Fig. 2.6 (a) The asterion is identified on a right retrosigmoid approach. The last centimeter of the three sutures, whose intersection forms the asterion, has been marked in black surgical marker with a pointer identifying it (lambdoid suture, occipitomastoid suture, and parietomastoid suture). The beginning of the digastric groove has been marked with black surgical marker as well (*black arrow*). (**b**) The "zygomatic line" and a "mastoid line" marked out on a right retrosigmoid approach as described by Tubbs et al. [8]

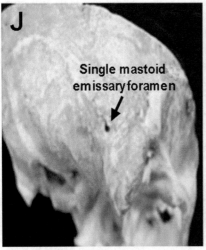
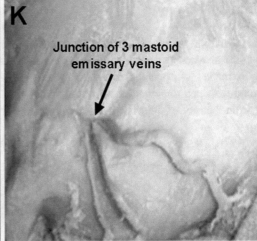

Fig. 2.7 (a) Cadaveric specimen demonstrating large single mastoid emissary foramen feeding the right sigmoid sinus deep to the foramen. (**b**) Cadaveric specimen showing the convergence of three mastoid emissary veins as they drain eventually into the sigmoid sinus

maximize visualization of the cerebellopontine angle and minimize retraction on the cerebellum. For pathology that involves the foramen magnum, caudal extension of the exposure and extensive bone removal as well as cerebrospinal fluid (CSF) drainage from the cisterna magna provides excellent exposure of the craniocervical junction.

There are multiple methods of opening the dura that are permissible as long as a watertight dural closure is obtained. Although a single curvilinear opening is probably the most popular

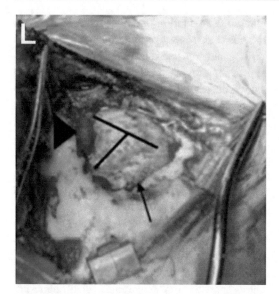

Fig. 2.8 A large right retrosigmoid craniectomy has been performed, so the transverse sinus is completely exposed (*black arrow*). The sigmoid sinus is exposed and covered with thrombin-soaked Gelfoam pieces (*black arrowhead*) for hemostatic purposes. The dural opening is outlined with *thick black lines*

method of dural opening because of the potential of closing the dura with a running suture, we also sometimes utilize a T-shaped dural opening to allow for maximal visualization with the bottom part of the T coming right up to the transverse-sigmoid junction (Fig. 2.8, black lines). Once the cerebellum is exposed, tenting sutures are placed along the superior and ventral margins to increase the angles and degree of exposure. Care should be taken though, as these may completely occlude the sinuses during the case, resulting in a transverse sinus thrombosis.

Handheld retractors can be used to help with the exposure of the petrous temporal bone and the tentorium cerebelli, permitting sharp dissection/division of arachnoid tethering the cerebellar hemisphere. If a lumbar drain was not prepositioned into the subarachnoid space preoperatively, the arachnoid around the foramen magnum may be sharply dissected, and additional brain relaxation can be obtained by further drainage of CSF from this cistern. Although retractionless surgery is preferred, placement of a self-retaining retractor over the surface of the cerebellum may be required early on for visualization of key

neurovascular structures in the cerebellopontine angle. The other key maneuver (aside from CSF relaxation) for safely increasing exposure is to control and divide the petrosal (veins) early in the case. For large lesions or lesions within the superior third of the CPA cistern, these veins may be sacrificed with relative impunity to further untether the hemisphere. The veins should be divided closer to the cerebellar surface, leaving a "tail" off their insertion into the sinus/tentorium; amputating the complex at its insertion results in a hole in the wall of the petrosal sinus, which may be difficult to control without packing it off with oxidized cellulose.

Reconstruction and Closure

Obtaining watertight dural closure is important to reduce the incidence of postoperative CSF leak. In cases where the dura is thin or compromised, the use of a dural patch with dural substitutes as well as abdominal fat graft may be of benefit. Regardless of type of dural opening, care should be taken to keep the dural folds moist during the case to help with future closure and utilize dural grafts as needed to obtain a watertight dural closure (Fig. 2.9).

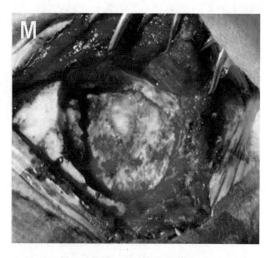

Fig. 2.9 Right-sided watertight dural closure with a suturable dural graft after a retrosigmoid craniectomy was performed for an acoustic neuroma resection

Alternatively, temporalis fascia may be harvested, or a free fascial graft may be harvested from the abdominal wall or tensor lata. Additionally, the use of dural sealants may be necessary to ensure a watertight seal and prevent postoperative CSF leak. All bony surfaces and mastoid air cells are carefully waxed to limit the risk of postoperative CSF rhinorrhea or otorrhea.

Several studies have shown a lower incidence of postoperative headaches and better cosmetic outcomes when the dura is separated from the overlying soft tissues, preventing tension on the dura as the suboccipital muscular contracts [17]. We use a combination of titanium mesh and hydroxyapatite cement impregnated with antibiotic powder to fashion a cranioplasty prior to skin closure. This also serves to tamponade and secures the dural reconstruction.

Complications

Aside from the typical complications associated with any craniotomy, such as infection, postoperative hematoma, and parenchymal and/or neurovascular injury, the retrosigmoid approach is significantly associated with higher rates of CSF leaks and postoperative headaches when compared with other cranial surgical approaches [18, 19]. One recent meta-analysis of the three approaches for acoustic neuroma surgery (translabyrinthine, middle fossa, and retrosigmoid) found that in >5000 patients in 35 studies, the only significant complication differences between the approaches were higher rates of CSF leak and postoperative headache with the retrosigmoid approach [18]. CSF leak is a known risk of posterior fossa cranial procedures because of the need for watertight dural closure. In addition to the main concern for leaking from the dura and through the incision or pseudomeningocele development, the air cells of the mastoid are frequent sources of CSF leak and must be waxed off so that CSF cannot enter through them.

Postoperative headaches are also common with the retrosigmoid approach; two of the more common explanations are bone dust entering into the posterior fossa from internal acoustic meatus drilling and muscle-dural attachment and adhesion after surgery [18]. Multiple studies have shown decreased rates of postoperative retrosigmoid headaches when a cranioplasty is performed at the time of closure so that the muscles cannot attach to the dura, but this benefit is only seen after 1 year of increased headaches after surgery [18–22]. Transverse and/or sigmoid sinus occlusion after a retrosigmoid approach is a potentially serious problem as it has been associated with headaches, increased intracranial pressure, seizures, and even intracranial hemorrhage [23]. There is a paucity of data involving rates of sinus occlusion after retrosigmoid craniectomy. One report in the otolaryngological literature suggests it is not even of clinical significance, and therefore they do not monitor for it or treat it when it occurs [24]; however, reports in the neurosurgical literature treat it as potentially lethal and thus recommend treating it with anticoagulation when it occurs. Pseudotumor cerebri can occur occasionally after transverse-sigmoid sinus occlusion, requiring subsequent treatment [24, 25]. Although more research needs to be done, standard practice is to avoid sinus occlusion at all costs, with some authors advocating initiating non-bolus systemic heparin 24 h after surgery once occlusion has been documented on postoperative imaging [23].

Conclusions

The retrosigmoid approach is a workhorse for CP angle pathology and lateral skull base surgery. We review the anatomy of the various regions accessed by this approach and demonstrate how we position, pin, and perform the key surgical steps while describing helpful surgical pearls. For example, although the extent and size of craniectomy varies depending on the pathology of each particular case, anatomical studies have shown that a burr hole placed inferior and dorsal to the junction of the "mastoid line" and "zygomatic line" will usually be within 1 cm of the transverse-sigmoid junction [8]. While recognizing that there are a multitude of acceptable methods for performing this surgery, we review some key techniques that can help to lower the complication rates of CSF leak, postoperative headaches, and transverse-sigmoid sinus occlusion, which are seen at increased rates with the retrosigmoid approach.

References

1. Cohen NL. Retrosigmoid approach for acoustic tumor removal. 1992. Neurosurg Clin N Am. 2008;19(2):239–50. vi
2. Fraenkel J, Hunt JR, Woolsey G, Elsberg CA. I. Contribution to the surgery of neurofibroma of the acoustic nerve: with remarks on the surgical procedure. Ann Surg. 1904;40(3):293–319.
3. Amenta PS, Morcos JJ. Left-sided retrosigmoid craniotomy for the resection of a vestibular schwannoma. Neurosurg Focus. 2014;36(1 Suppl):1.
4. Yamahata H, Tokimura H, Hirahara K, Ishii T, Mori M, Hanaya R, et al. Lateral suboccipital retrosigmoid approach with tentorial incision for petroclival meningiomas: technical note. J Neurol Surg B Skull Base. 2014;75(4):221–4.
5. Raza SM, Quinones-Hinojosa A. The extended retrosigmoid approach for neoplastic lesions in the posterior fossa: technique modification. Neurosurg Rev. 2011;34(1):123–9.
6. Nash B, Carlson ML, Van Gompel JJ. Microvascular decompression for tinnitus: systematic review. J Neurosurg. 2017 Apr;126(4):1148–1157.
7. Broggi G, Broggi M, Ferroli P, Franzini A. Surgical technique for trigeminal microvascular decompression. Acta Neurochir. 2012;154(6):1089–95.
8. Tubbs RS, Loukas M, Shoja MM, Bellew MP, Cohen-Gadol AA. Surface landmarks for the junction between the transverse and sigmoid sinuses: application of the "strategic" burr hole for suboccipital craniotomy. Neurosurgery. 2009;65(6 Suppl):37–41. discussion
9. Hardy DG, Peace DA, Rhoton AL Jr. Microsurgical anatomy of the superior cerebellar artery. Neurosurgery. 1980;6(1):10–28.
10. Lister JR, Rhoton AL Jr, Matsushima T, Peace DA. Microsurgical anatomy of the posterior inferior cerebellar artery. Neurosurgery. 1982;10(2):170–99.
11. Matsushima T, Rhoton AL Jr, Lenkey C. Microsurgery of the fourth ventricle: part 1 microsurgical anatomy. Neurosurgery. 1982;11(5):631–67.

12. Matsushima T, Rhoton AL Jr, de Oliveira E, Peace D. Microsurgical anatomy of the veins of the posterior fossa. J Neurosurg. 1983;59(1):63–105.
13. Ausman JI, Malik GM, Dujovny M, Mann R. Three-quarter prone approach to the pineal-tentorial region. Surg Neurol. 1988;29(4):298–306.
14. Duke DA, Lynch JJ, Harner SG, Faust RJ, Ebersold MJ. Venous air embolism in sitting and supine patients undergoing vestibular schwannoma resection. Neurosurgery. 1998;42(6):1282–6. discussion 6–7
15. Jung S, Kang SS, Kim TS, Kim HJ, Jeong SK, Kim SC, et al. Current surgical results of retrosigmoid approach in extralarge vestibular schwannomas. Surg Neurol. 2000;53(4):370–7. discussion 7–8
16. Rhoton AL Jr. The cerebellopontine angle and posterior fossa cranial nerves by the retrosigmoid approach. Neurosurgery. 2000;47(3 Suppl):S93–129.
17. Pabaney AH, Reinard KA, Asmaro K, Malik GM. Novel technique for cranial reconstruction following retrosigmoid craniectomy using demineralized bone matrix. Clin Neurol Neurosurg. 2015;136:66–70.
18. Ansari SF, Terry C, Cohen-Gadol AA. Surgery for vestibular schwannomas: a systematic review of complications by approach. Neurosurg Focus. 2012;33(3):E14.
19. Fetterman BL, Lanman TH, House JW. Relief of headache by cranioplasty after skull base surgery. Skull Base Surg. 1997;7(1):1–4.
20. Ruckenstein MJ, Harris JP, Cueva RA, Prioleau G, Alksne J. Pain subsequent to resection of acoustic neuromas via suboccipital and translabyrinthine approaches. Am J Otolaryngol. 1996;17(4):620–4.
21. Schaller B, Baumann A. Headache after removal of vestibular schwannoma via the retrosigmoid approach: a long-term follow-up-study. Otolaryngol Head Neck Surg. 2003;128(3):387–95.
22. Schessel DA, Nedzelski JM, Rowed D, Feghali JG. Pain after surgery for acoustic neuroma. Otolaryngol Head Neck Surg. 1992;107(3):424–9.
23. Moore J, Thomas P, Cousins V, Rosenfeld JV. Diagnosis and management of dural sinus thrombosis following resection of cerebellopontine angle tumors. J Neurol Surg B Skull Base. 2014;75(6):402–8.
24. Zanoletti E, Cazzador D, Faccioli C, Martini A, Mazzoni A. Closure of the sigmoid sinus in lateral skull base surgery. Acta Otorhinolaryngol Ital. 2014;34(3):184–8.
25. Keiper GL Jr, Sherman JD, Tomsick TA, Tew JM Jr. Dural sinus thrombosis and pseudotumor cerebri: unexpected complications of suboccipital craniotomy and translabyrinthine craniectomy. J Neurosurg. 1999;91(2):192–7.

Middle Fossa and Translabyrinthine Approaches

3

Justin C. Sowder, Breanne L. Schiffer,
Richard K. Gurgel, and Clough Shelton

Abbreviations

AAO-HNS	American Academy of Otolaryngology-Head and Neck Surgery
ABR	Auditory brainstem response
CPA	Cerebellopontine angle
dB	Decibel
DVT	Pulmonary embolism
EAC	External auditory canal
GSPN	Greater superficial petrosal nerve
GTR	Gross-total resection
HB	House-Brackmann
IAC	Internal auditory canal
ICH	Intracerebral hemorrhage
MRI	Magnetic resonance imaging
NTR	Near-total resection
PE	Pulmonary embolism
POD	Postoperative day
PTA	Pure-tone average
SDS	Speech discrimination score
SNHL	Sensorineural hearing loss
SRT	Speech reception threshold
STR	Subtotal resection

J.C. Sowder, MD • B.L. Schiffer, MD, MPH
R.K. Gurgel, MD • C. Shelton, MD (✉)
Division of Otolaryngology – Head and Neck
Surgery, University of Utah School of Medicine,
50 N. Medical Dr. SOM 3C120, Salt Lake City,
UT 84113, USA
e-mail: Justin.Sowder@hsc.utah.edu; Breanne.
Schiffer@hsc.utah.edu; Richard.Gurgel@hsc.utah.edu;
clough.shelton@hsc.utah.edu

Introduction

Surgical approaches to the internal auditory canal (IAC) and cerebellopontine angle (CPA) for the treatment of acoustic neuromas have improved dramatically since their inception. While early surgical techniques were used primarily for debulking of large tumors and relieving pressure on the brainstem, modern skull base surgery has evolved to focus more on functional preservation, particularly with regard to serviceable hearing and facial nerve function.

The middle fossa approach is an example of a surgical approach to the skull base that was developed to preserve function. The middle fossa approach was originally reported in 1904 to gain access for vestibular nerve sectioning. This was prior to the introduction of the operating microscope and modern microsurgical techniques, and the facial nerve was at high risk for injury during these procedures [1]. The approach was further developed when William F. House revised it in 1961. Through cadaver studies, it was realized that it would be a viable option for the removal of acoustic neuromas [2]. Through this approach, the entirety of the contents of the internal auditory canal (IAC) can be visualized, and the facial nerve can be positively identified in the fallopian canal without tumor involvement [3, 5]. While initially used to remove tumors of all sizes, through Dr. House's first ten clinical cases as well the observations of John B. Doyle, Jr., it was realized that in all but the smallest of tumors a labyrinthectomy was required to gain the appropriate access to the cerebellopontine angle (CPA) [6]. It was also noted to be a technically challenging operation as the exposure is limited, there is a lack of definitive landmarks, and the facial nerve is often submitted to more manipulation than in other approaches [7, 8]. Limitations in early detection of acoustic neuromas at the time led to relatively infrequent use of the middle fossa approach; however, House and Hitselberger did determine through their series of patients that hearing and facial nerve function could be preserved if tumors were small [9]. With the eventual development of gadolinium-enhanced magnetic resonance imaging (MRI), there was an increased identification of patients with small tumors and serviceable hearing [3]. Consequently, an approach that could preserve hearing became desirable, leading to more widespread adoption of the technique. The middle fossa approach has been utilized for repair of superior semicircular canal dehiscence, encephaloceles, access to the petrous apex, decompression of the facial nerve for Bell's palsy or trauma, and other IAC lesions [1–13]. Prior to the technological advances that made the middle fossa approach more feasible, House and Hitselberger also developed the translabyrinthine approach, which gave a direct route to the CPA through the temporal bone [14, 15]. While hearing is sacrificed because the vestibular portion of the inner ear is obliterated, this approach provides wide exposure with potential identification of the facial nerve from the brainstem to the stylomastoid foramen. The CPA and IAC are also widely exposed via translabyrinthine exposure. The approach is primarily extradural, and there is minimal to no brain retraction. Due to the wide exposure, the translabyrinthine approach is also used for facial nerve decompression when hearing does not need to be preserved, facial nerve repair and the removal of other CPA lesions, including meningiomas, intracranial epidermoids, and paragangliomas [16]. As compared to the classic suboccipital approach, the patient is in the supine position (versus sitting), which reduces the risk of air embolism as well as the rare but serious complication of spinal cord infarction and quadriplegia [17]. The translabyrinthine approach has also been found by some authors to have a lower incidence of postoperative CSF leak and headache as compared to the retrosigmoid approach, while others have found the rate of CSF leaks to be similar [18, 19].

Preoperative Evaluation

Patients with an acoustic neuroma most often present with complaints of unilateral hearing loss, followed by tinnitus, vertigo, and, rarely, facial hypesthesia in descending order [20]. Once a complete clinical history and physical exam have been performed, pure-tone and speech audiometry are important diagnostic tests to perform. The auditory brainstem response (ABR) was long considered the most sensitive diagnostic modality, with the interaural wave V latency being greater than 0.2 ms considered abnormal [21]. However, the use of enhanced MRI has found the false negative rate of ABR to be 18-30% for intracanalicular tumors [22]. We do not routinely perform ABR to screen for acoustic neuromas at our institution because of the limited clinical utility. If sufficient clinical suspicion exists based on symptoms and audiometry, the imaging modality of choice is a gadolinium-enhanced MRI. As an alternative to using contrast-enhanced MRI, a screening protocol with a fast spin-echo MRI sequence is highly sensitive and specific and provides ultrahigh-resolution images of the IAC, making it possible to determine the nerve of origin of very small tumors [23]. We found there was no difference in diagnostic accuracy compared to traditionally enhanced sequences and that the diagnostic accuracy is more sensitive and specific than brainstem audiometry (ABR) at a similar cost and is significantly cheaper than contrasted MRI [23, 24].

Indications for Surgery

Once an acoustic neuroma has been diagnosed and the patient has elected to undergo surgical resection, the most important factors when considering the surgical approach are preoperative hearing status and tumor size. We use the middle fossa approach for patients who have a small tumor, primarily located in the lateral portion of the internal auditory canal and good preoperative hearing. The retrosigmoid approach is used for patients with a small tumor, primarily located in the cerebellopontine angle that does not extend to the lateral portion of the internal auditory canal and good preoperative hearing. The translabyrinthine approach is used for patients with large tumors or patients with poor preoperative hearing.

Since 1995, the American Academy of Otolaryngology-Head and Neck Surgery (AAO-HNS) has broken down hearing status into four classifications (A–D), as shown in Table 3.1 [25]. Class A and B hearing (PTA >50 dB, SDS >50%) are considered "serviceable" hearing, and if preserved will facilitate, the use of amplification postoperatively [26]. More recent guidelines by the AAO-HNS have recommended a new minimal standard of reporting hearing results by plotting a scattergram relating average pure-tone thresholds to word recognition scores; however, few studies evaluating acoustic neuroma outcomes have been published to date using these guidelines [27]. The audiometric criteria to perform hearing conservation surgery vary from surgeon to surgeon, and the indications must be individualized to the needs of each patient [28]. Many use serviceable hearing, or the "50/50 rule," as the cutoff to attempt hearing preserva-

tion. Jackler and Pitts consider those with "good hearing" (>70% SDS, <30 dB speech reception threshold (SRT)), a CPA component <1 cm, and shallow IAC involvement as excellent candidates for hearing conservation surgery. Conversely, those with what they called "poor" hearing (<30% SDS, >70 dB SRT), a large (>3 cm) CPA component, and deep penetration of the IAC are considered poor candidates for hearing conservation and undergo a translabyrinthine approach [29]. In our practice, we use the arbitrary audiometric criteria of a SRT <50 dB and a SDS >70% as criteria to perform hearing conservation surgery. We do not routinely perform middle fossa surgery on patients older than 65 years, as they do not tolerate temporal lobe retraction as well as younger patients and have more fragile dura than younger patients.

As has been shown in multiple studies, the smaller the tumor, the easier it is to remove and the greater the likelihood that hearing will be preserved [30–32]. The middle fossa approach is ideal for resection of tumors isolated to the IAC (intracanalicular) with no or limited extension into the CPA when there is serviceable hearing. Extension of the tumor further than 1–1.5 cm into the CPA is a relative contraindication to this approach, with exceptions made for those with serviceable hearing in the operative ear and either poor contralateral hearing or bilateral tumors [16, 20]. In contrast, hearing preservation is very unlikely with tumors that have a CPA component measuring greater than 2 cm in its greatest dimension [33, 34]. In such tumors, the translabyrinthine approach is ideal because it is associated with the highest rate of preserving facial nerve function [20]. The retrosigmoid approach (discussed elsewhere) can be used in an attempt to preserve serviceable hearing in tumors smaller than 2 cm, so long as they do not extend to the fundus of the IAC [35].

Table 3.1 AAO-HNS hearing classification system

Class	PTA (dB)	SDS (%)
A	≤ 30 and	≥ 70
B	> 30, ≤50 and	≥ 50
C	> 50 and	≥ 50
D	Any level	< 50

PTA 4-frequency pure-tone average of 500, 1000, 2000, and 3000 dB, *dB* decibel, *SDS* speech-discrimination score

Patient Counseling

A thorough discussion includes reviewing the relative anatomy and the options of observation and stereotactic radiation, in addition to surgery.

We routinely use graphic diagrams of the anatomy and provide pamphlets to our patients to take home. Patients who are candidates for hearing preservation surgery are informed that there is an approximately 50% chance that their hearing will be "saved"; however it is unlikely that it will improve after tumor removal [36]. It is reiterated in those undergoing the translabyrinthine approach that the operation will result in complete loss of hearing in the operative ear. The patient is counseled that with the middle fossa approach, there is approximately a 90% chance that the facial nerve function will be normal or near normal (House-Brackmann grade I or II) in the long term. They are informed that there is, however, a 20–30% chance of having temporary facial paresis in the immediate to early postoperative period. Those undergoing a translabyrinthine approach are told that the facial nerve integrity is preserved in 90% of patients, and our best and most consistent results are seen with smaller tumors removed via the translabyrinthine approach. As the tumor size increases, the rate of postoperative facial nerve dysfunction increases as well. Those with preoperative tinnitus are told that while their symptoms may get better, it is unlikely to disappear. It is divulged to those with no preoperative tinnitus that there is a 25% chance of developing it postoperatively [37]. The rare but serious complications of CSF leak, meningitis, brain injury, stroke, and death are discussed, and the patient's wishes regarding possible blood transfusion are documented. The expected recovery, including 4–6 weeks of downtime from work, is outlined. We stress that dizziness is expected postoperatively, and that the rapidity and degree of central compensation is influenced greatly by early patient ambulation.

Surgery

General Preoperative Preparation

Long acting muscle relaxants are avoided at induction and throughout the procedure to prevent interference with facial nerve monitoring. A Foley catheter is placed to monitor urine output, and central arterial and venous lines are inserted, if indicated. A preoperative antibiotic with adequate CSF penetration is given prior to skin incision, and a single dose of intravenous dexamethasone is given at the beginning of the procedure. The patient's head is supported by a "donut" or a Mayfield head holder and is rotated toward the contralateral shoulder. For middle fossa craniotomies, the head can be secured with pins or simply turned to the side contralateral to the tumor. The electrodes for the facial nerve monitor and intraoperative ABR, when hearing is monitored in middle fossa approaches, are positioned and confirmed to be functioning. The preplanned surgical incisions are injected with 1% lidocaine with epinephrine 1:100,000. If abdominal fat is to be harvested, the lower abdomen is shaved if necessary, the skin is cleaned with Betadine, and the area is draped with sterile towels and Ioban.

Surgical Technique: Middle Fossa Approach

For the middle fossa craniotomy, the surgeon sits at the head of the table, and the microscope is off to the side. The ipsilateral scalp is shaved to accommodate the incision, which begins at the pretragal area and extends superiorly 7–8 cm with a gentle curve anteriorly (Fig. 3.1). The incision should begin at the inferior border of the tragus and be immediately anterior to the tragus, placed in a pretragal skin crease. The pretragal skin crease placement minimizes the cosmetic impact of this facial incision. By extending the incision to the inferior border of the tragus, one can expose the floor of the middle fossa more easily. Plastic adhesive drapes are applied; the skin and plastic drapes are scrubbed with Betadine and blotted dry. Towels are placed encompassing the temporoparietal scalp, including the auricle and zygomatic arch. An adhesive craniotomy drape is placed and cut away to expose the skin prior to making the skin incision. Intraoperative mannitol is given to decrease intracranial CSF pressure and to facilitate temporal lobe retraction. The skin incision is made with a No. 15 blade, and the temporalis muscle and fascia are divided with electrocautery and retracted

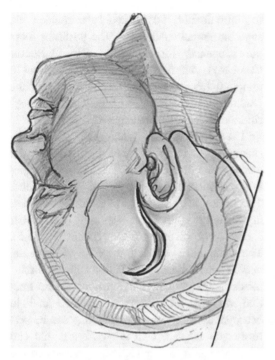

Fig. 3.1 A preauricular curvilinear incision is made that extends into the temporal scalp. Extension of this incision to the inferior border of the tragus allows exposure of the floor of the middle fossa

with an Adson Cerebellar Retractor to expose the calvarium. The craniotomy opening is made in the squamous portion of the temporal bone, measuring approximately 5 × 5 cm and located approximately two thirds anterior and one third posterior to the external auditory canal (EAC) or centered at the root of the zygoma. Anterior and inferior placement of the craniotomy is critical to ensure adequate exposure, particularly when operating on the left ear. The bone flap is based at the root of the zygoma as close to the floor of the middle fossa as possible and can be fashioned with a high-speed drill using a footplate attachment to protect the underlying dura. The dura is initially exposed in two corners of the bone flap diagonal to one another, which allows separation of the dura from the flap and introduction of the footplate drill. Care must be taken when creating the bone flap to avoid lacerating the dura, and the extradural position of the footplate should be confirmed periodically while drilling. It is sometimes necessary to remove additional bone along

the middle fossa floor with a cutting burr or rongeur once the craniotomy window is removed. An alternative technique is to outline the entire craniotomy flap with a high-speed drill using standard cutting followed by diamond burrs. The bone flap is set aside for replacement later.

The dura is elevated from the floor of the middle fossa with a suction irrigator and a blunt dural elevator, with the initial landmark being the middle meningeal artery. This marks the anterior extent of the dissection. If venous bleeding is encountered in the area, it can be controlled with either a slurry of powdered absorbable gelatin sponge (Gelfoam) and thrombin or absorbable knitted fabric (Surgicel). Dissection of the dura proceeds in a posterior-to-anterior direction to protect against injury to a potentially dehiscent geniculate ganglion, which is seen in 5% of cases. The petrous ridge is then identified posteriorly, and the superior petrosal sinus is elevated from its groove at the time the true ridge is identified. The arcuate eminence and greater superficial petrosal nerve (GSPN) are identified, which are the major landmarks in the intratemporal portion of the dissection.

Once the dura is elevated, the Layla retractor is placed over the medial ridge of the superior petrosal sinus and locked in place to support the temporal lobe. An alternative is the House-Urban retractor, however the Layla retractor has a lower profile and dual retractor blades to support the widely elevated temporal lobe (Fig. 3.2) [38]. The GSPN is located medial to the middle meningeal artery (Fig. 3.3). A large diamond drill with continuous suction irrigation is used to identify the superior semicircular canal. Once this is skeletonized and followed anteriorly, the geniculate ganglion is identified. As described by Garcia-Ibanez, the IAC is located at the bisection of the angle formed by the GSPN and the superior semicircular canal [39]. Bone is removed at the medial aspect of the petrous ridge at this bisection, identifying the IAC. This is taken laterally in the same axis of the external auditory canal, exposing the dura of the posterior fossa widely (2 cm), and the porus acusticus is exposed for 270° circumferentially. As the lateral IAC is approached, the surgical field tightens with the labyrinthine portion of the facial nerve lying immediately posterior to the basal turn of the cochlea. The dissection must consequently narrow

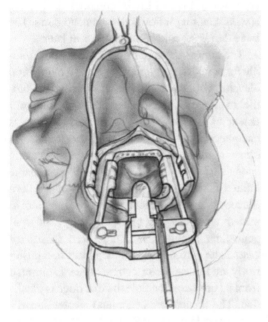

Fig. 3.2 The craniotomy window is placed two thirds anterior to the external auditory canal. A variety of retractors can be used to support the temporal lobe

to approximately 90° to avoid the cochlea and superior semicircular canal. The posterior fossa dura is opened with a microblade (No. 59; Beaver Company), and the CSF is released, resulting in temporal lobe relaxation. At the fundus of the IAC, the vertical crest (Bill's bar) and the labyrinthine facial nerve are exposed.

The dura of the IAC is incised along the posterior aspect, and the facial nerve is identified in the anterior portion of the IAC (Fig. 3.4). The superior vestibular nerve is divided at its lateral end. The tumor is separated from the facial nerve under high magnification, beginning at Bill's bar and dissecting from medial to lateral (Fig. 3.5). The arachnoid is divided, the edge of the facial nerve identified, and the facial-vestibular anastomosis is sharply cut. This prevents excess traction on the facial nerve that can lead to neuropraxia. Intracapsular debulking can be performed, if needed, with microscissors and cup forceps. Again, tumor removal proceeds in the medial to lateral direction, here to prevent traction on the cochlear nerve and its blood supply as it enters the modiolus. The inferior vestibular nerve can be left in place if uninvolved in an

Fig. 3.3 The greater superficial petrosal nerve is visible on the floor the middle fossa. It is immediately medial to the middle meningeal artery. The superior semicircular canal is medial to the arcuate eminence. The internal auditory canal can be located by bisecting the angle formed by the greater superficial petrosal nerve and the superior semicircular canal

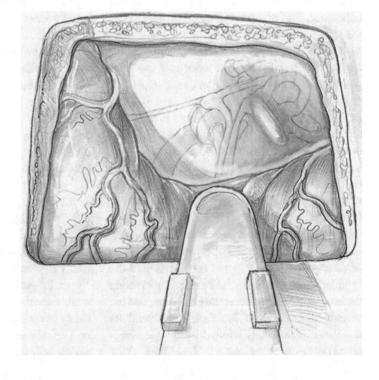

Fig. 3.4 The internal auditory canal is exposed and the facial nerve is identified adjacent to Bill's bar. The dura of the internal auditory canal is opened on its posterior surface with a micro knife

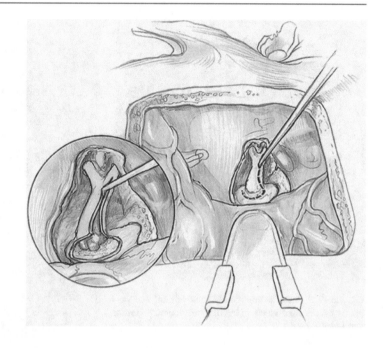

Fig. 3.5 The arachnoid surrounding the facial nerve is divided with a right-angle hook. The facial nerve is separated from the tumor from medial to lateral. It is important to identify the vestibular-facial nerve anastomoses and divide them sharply, to avoid traction injury to the facial nerve

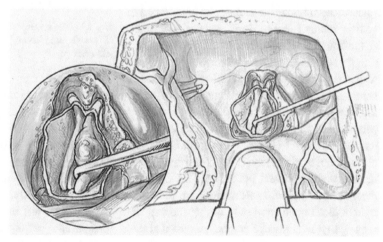

attempt to preserve the labyrinthine artery; however partial vestibulopathy from a retained inferior vestibular nerve can result in persistent unsteadiness in some patients. For this reason, we recommend cutting the inferior vestibular nerve medial to the Scarpa's ganglion, but not dissecting it at the fundus of the IAC (Fig. 3.6).

Once the tumor is removed, the tumor bed is irrigated and hemostasis is obtained. Papaverine-soaked Gelfoam is placed along the cochlear nerve to prevent vasospasm. Abdominal fat is used to close the defect in the IAC. The retractor

is removed, and the temporal lobe is allowed to re-expand. The craniotomy flap is replaced with titanium mini-plates, the wound is closed with absorbable sutures in layers, and a mastoid-type pressure dressing is placed.

Surgical Technique: Translabyrinthine Approach

For the translabyrinthine approach, the operating room setup is identical to that for a standard mastoidectomy. The ipsilateral scalp is shaved four fingerbreadths above and behind the postauricular

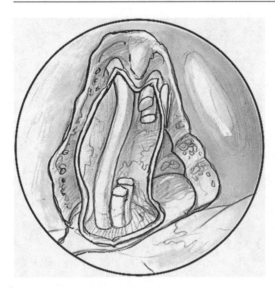

Fig. 3.6 The tumor is completely removed and the vestibular nerves are divided, to avoid a postoperative partial vestibulopathy

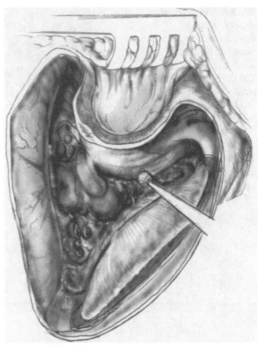

Fig. 3.7 The mastoidectomy is carried out with exposure of the sigmoid sinus, vertical facial nerve course, and labyrinth

sulcus. The surgical site is prepped and draped in similar manner as the middle fossa approach. A hockey stick-shaped retroauricular skin incision that extends behind the mastoid tip is made with a No. 15 blade down to the temporalis fascia, hemostasis is obtained, and an anterior-based skin flap is elevated. A standard anterior-based periosteal flap is elevated with a Lempert elevator, and the mastoid cortex is exposed. Care must be taken not to violate the EAC skin when elevating the flap to prevent postoperative CSF otorrhea. Adson Cerebellar Retractors are placed at right angles to one another to retract the soft tissues. Temporalis muscle can be harvested at this time and placed on the back table to use for eustachian tube packing, if planned. A cortical mastoidectomy is performed with a high-speed drill, large cutting burrs, and suction irrigation. The dura should be exposed along the sigmoid sinus and tegmen at the sinodural angle, which is the deepest point of the dissection. The bone is removed 2 cm posterior to the sigmoid sinus to adequately expose the posterior fossa dura. A thin shell of bone is left over the sigmoid sinus (Bill's island) to protect it from the shaft of the burr during the labyrinthectomy (Fig. 3.7). Some surgeons decompress the sigmoid sinus completely to facilitate retraction to improve

exposure. The sinodural angle should be opened as far posteriorly as possible to facilitate a tangential view of the vestibule, which lies medial to the facial nerve [40]. We routinely open the facial recess, remove the incus, and pack the eustachian tube to prevent a route of egress of CSF. Alternatively, the facial recess bone and incus can be left intact. After tumor dissection, muscle can be packed around the incus in an effort to seal off the middle ear from the temporal bone defect and posterior fossa CSF flow [41]. The mastoid facial nerve is identified and followed down to the stylomastoid foramen.

A labyrinthectomy is performed with small (3–4 mm) cutting burrs (Fig. 3.8). The semicircular canals initially are skeletonized. The canals are then serially fenestrated and opened completely on a broad front, beginning with the horizontal semicircular canal. It is important to open on a broad front to provide continuous landmarks. The horizontal canal is opened down to its intersection with the posterior canal. The posterior canal is opened in a similar fashion up to its

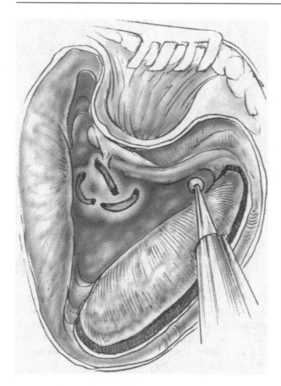

Fig. 3.8 The labyrinthectomy is carried out, the facial nerve is skeletonized, and the bone is removed between the jugular bulb and the internal auditory canal

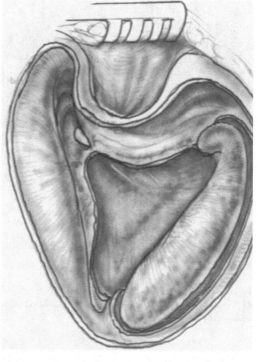

Fig. 3.9 The posterior fossa and middle fossa dura are exposed. Exposure of the middle fossa dura is important to allow for extradural retraction of the cerebellum

intersection with the superior canal (crus commons) superiorly and its ampullated end anterior-inferiorly, which marks the inferior border of the IAC. Caution must be taken to prevent damage to the mastoid segment of the facial nerve here. Bony removal proceeds inferiorly until the jugular bulb is identified at the same level as the IAC. The superior canal is opened along its entire path toward its ampulla, taking care not to violate the temporal lobe dura superiorly. The subarcuate artery is often encountered in the center of the arch of the superior canal, marking the superior border of the IAC [16]. All of the remaining bone between the vestibule and the jugular bulb is removed (Fig. 3.9).

Prior to opening the IAC, which begins deep to the vestibule and runs anteriorly away from the surgeon, its dura must be exposed in 270°. The cochlear aqueduct enters the posterior fossa in between the IAC and the jugular bulb and marks the inferior limit of bone removal. The bone is removed anterior to the cochlear aqueduct

between the inferior IAC and jugular bulb to facilitate exposure to the inferior aspect of the tumor. Care is taken not to remove bone deep to the cochlear aqueduct to prevent injury to contents of the jugular foramen [42]. Bone superior to the IAC is removed last due to its location near the facial nerve in order to expose the superior aspect of the tumor (Fig. 3.10).

Prior to opening the dura, we vigorously irrigate the cavity with bacitracin solution to remove the bone dust. The posterior fossa dura is incised sharply over the midportion of the IAC with a microblade (No. 59; Beaver Company) and scissors. This incision is extended along the IAC and arches superiorly and inferiorly around the porus acusticus in a Y shape. For large tumors, the incision may need to be extended toward the sigmoid sinus [16]. Hemostasis is obtained with bipolar electrocautery. The arachnoid is opened with a sharp hook, allowing the egress of some CSF. At this point, only fenestrated suction tips should be used.

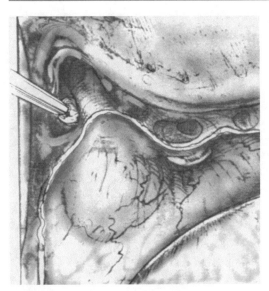

Fig. 3.10 The internal auditory canal is exposed in 270° of it is circumference. The facial nerve is identified adjacent to Bill's bar

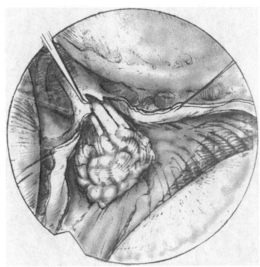

Fig. 3.11 The dura of the internal auditory canal is opened. The facial nerve is identified in the anterior lateral portion of the internal auditory canal. The superior vestibular nerve is immediately posterior to the facial nerve. The facial nerve is separated from the tumor, the dissection proceeds from medial to lateral

The facial nerve is again identified using stimulation and followed using a sharp right-angle hook, and Bill's bar is palpated. The superior vestibular nerve and vestibulofacial fibers can be transected with this instrument. The inferior vestibular nerve is identified and cut. Once an adequate plane between the tumor and the facial nerve is developed, a blunt hook is used to continue the dissection. The motion of the dissection is from medial to lateral, to avoid traction on the facial nerve at its exit through the distal internal auditory canal (Fig. 3.11). The arachnoid enveloping the facial nerve is divided with a sharp right-angle hook. This is sometimes adequate to facilitate complete removal of small tumors (Fig. 3.12) [43]. If the tumor is large, the capsule can be incised, and the tumor can be debulked with either microsurgical instruments or an ultrasonic dissector. The tumor is followed to the brainstem, developing a plane with both blunt and sharp instrumentation. Cottonoids should be placed along the cerebellum and brainstem as they are exposed to protect the underlying structures. Intratumoral bleeding is controlled with bipolar cautery or topical hemostatics (as above), and only vessels that enter the tumor capsule are ligated.

Once the tumor is removed and hemostasis is complete, abdominal fat is harvested and cut into various-sized strips. The abdominal wound is closed with absorbable sutures and Steri-Strips, and a Penrose drain is left in place. The fat is soaked in bacitracin solution and packed tightly into the CPA, IAC, and mastoid cavity. Some surgeons advocate placing a titanium mesh or absorbable cranioplasty plate over the fat. The periosteal flap is reapproximated with 3–0 Vicryl sutures in a horizontal mattress fashion, ensuring a watertight closure. The subcutaneous tissues are reapproximated with buried interrupted 3-0 Vicryl sutures, and the skin is closed with either subcuticular absorbable sutures or a running locking 4-0 nylon suture. A standard mastoid-type pressure dressing is applied.

Postoperative Care

The patient is typically extubated in the operating room and observed in the intensive care unit overnight. The Foley catheter, arterial and central venous lines, and Penrose drains are typically removed on the morning of postoperative day (POD) #1. The mastoid dressing is removed on

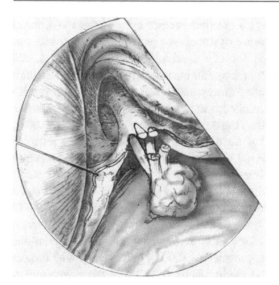

Fig. 3.12 Small tumor separated from the facial nerve. We usually section both branches of the vestibular nerve and the cochlear nerve (Permission to use figures from chapters 49–50, Brackmann et al. [75]; granted by Elsevier)

POD #1. If stable, the patient is transferred to the surgical floor on POD #1. Early ambulation is encouraged at this point to facilitate vestibular compensation. It is important at this point to have all but one peripheral IV removed and to only spot-check pulse oximetry to prevent excess lines that impede mobilization. Incentive spirometry is begun on POD #1 and continued until discharge. The typical hospital course is 3–5 days.

Postoperative pain is generally mild and controlled with routine analgesics. The middle fossa approach is often associated with more severe pain due to muscle spasms from division of the temporalis muscle and can be associated with mild, temporary trismus. Severe vertigo with nausea is common in the postoperative period due to sectioning of the vestibular nerves. Patients with smaller tumors, such as those removed by the middle fossa approach, often have more severe symptoms as they had more retained vestibular function going in to surgery. Control of these symptoms is important for patient comfort, and we have found good success with Phenergan (promethazine), Compazine (prochlorperazine), and Haldol (haloperidol). It is important to note that we have seen poor symptomatic control with

Zofran (ondansetron) in this setting, unless the nausea is related to anesthesia in the first 24 h postoperatively only. We have found that most patients have severe dizziness for the first 24–48 h postoperatively. By the end of the first postoperative week, they are often left with residual unsteadiness, but most are able to ambulate without assistance. Patients are to abstain from driving until no longer dizzy. We do prescribe vestibular physical therapy for a small subset of patients, most of who are elderly or had preoperative vestibular symptoms. Patients are advised to avoid getting their incisions wet until 7 days after surgery and to avoid vigorous activity or heavy lifting for 6 weeks.

Outcomes

Hearing Preservation

The rate of hearing preservation has improved over time in patients who undergo tumor resection via the middle fossa approach. In a study of 106 patients followed over 25 years published in 1989, hearing was preserved in 59% of patients and was maintained at preoperative levels in 35% of patients [32]. Brackmann and coworkers published their results of 333 patients followed for 7 years in 2000 and found a hearing preservation rate of 80%, with hearing preserved near the preoperative level (within 15 dB PTA and 15% SDS) in 50% [26]. We recently evaluated 78 consecutive patients with intracanalicular acoustic neuromas removed via middle fossa approach. Of those with functional preoperative hearing (AAO-HNS class A/B), 75% had functional hearing postoperatively with an average follow-up of 15 months [44]. In comparing outcomes between hearing conservation approaches, a recent systematic review found the middle fossa approach to be superior to the retrosigmoid approach for hearing preservation in patients with tumors <1.5 cm (hearing loss in 43.6% vs 64.3%, $P < 0.001$). However, no difference in rate of hearing loss was found between these two approaches for intracanalicular tumors (40.6% vs 44.3%, $P = 0.492$) [19].

The increased rate of hearing preservation over time is likely due to a combination of technical improvements as well as increased experience, thanks to the growing number of smaller tumors found on imaging [45]. Several authors have found that preserved hearing in patients who underwent middle fossa tumor resection deteriorates over time. One study published in 1990 found that 56% of patients followed for at least 3 years had a significant loss of hearing (mean loss of 2% SDS and 12 dB SRT) [46]. In a recently published series of 57 patients followed for 5 years, 55% of patients had serviceable hearing in the immediate postoperative period and 75% of those maintained it at their 5-year follow-up. We hypothesize that this improvement is due to a change from packing the IAC defect with temporalis muscle to abdominal fat, which likely results in less fibrosis and preserved cochlear blood supply [47].

Facial Nerve Function

Many consider the preservation of facial nerve function during acoustic neuroma resection as second in importance only to tumor removal, particularly when the patient does not have serviceable hearing preoperatively. In our recent series of 78 patients with acoustic neuroma removed via middle fossa approach, 90% had facial nerve function of House-Brackmann (HB) grade I or II [44]. This is consistent with the long-term outcomes published in previous studies [47–49]. Slattery et al. [50] reported 95% of 151 patients were HB grade I or II at year 1, and Woodson et al. found that 96% of their 49 patients were HB grade I and 4% were HB grade II at 2 years from surgery [51]. In a systematic review including 35 studies of over 5,000 patients who underwent surgical removal of acoustic neuromas in which facial nerve dysfunction was defined as HB grade III or higher at last follow-up, facial nerve dysfunction was seen in 16.7% in those treated with a middle cranial fossa approach and 4% of those treated with a retrosigmoid approach ($P < 0.001$) with intracanalicular tumors. When tumors were ≤1.5 cm (but extended out of the IAC), facial nerve dysfunction was seen in 3.3%, 7.2%, and 11.5% of the middle fossa, retrosigmoid, and translabyrinthine groups, respectively. The middle fossa approach was associated with significantly lower rates of facial nerve dysfunction than the translabyrinthine approach ($P < 0.001$), but no difference was seen between retrosigmoid approach and the other two approaches. When tumors were 1.5–3.0 cm, facial nerve dysfunction was seen in 17.3% of those treated with a middle cranial fossa approach, 6.1% of those treated with a retrosigmoid approach, and 15.8% of those treated with a translabyrinthine approach ($P < 0.001$). In the group with tumors >3 cm in diameter, 30.2% of those who underwent a retrosigmoid approach and 42.5% of those who underwent translabyrinthine approach had facial nerve dysfunction ($P < 0.001$) [19]. As one would expect, as tumor size increases, so does the risk to the facial nerve during surgical resection. In cases of large tumors (defined as ≥2.5 cm maximal or extrameatal cerebellopontine angle diameter), subtotal resection can be considered in order to increase the chance of facial nerve preservation [52, 53]. However, such an approach must be weighed against the risk of tumor recurrence [52]. In another systematic review evaluating facial nerve outcomes following the resection of tumors ≥2.5 cm, good facial nerve outcomes (HB grade I or II) were seen in 62.5% of the 555 translabyrinthine approaches and in 65.2% of the 601 retrosigmoid approaches ($P > 0.05$). When broken down by degree of resection, good facial nerve outcomes were seen in 92.5% who underwent subtotal resection (STR; $n = 80$), compared with 74.6% ($n = 55$) and 47.3% ($n = 336$) of those who underwent near-total (NTR) and gross-total resections (GTR), respectively ($P < 0.001$) [54]. In a recently published study prospectively evaluating 73 patients with large acoustic neuromas with at least 1 year of follow-up, 14 (19%) cases showed regrowth on MRI, 1 who underwent GTR (8.3%), 2 who underwent NTR (9.1%), and 11 who underwent STR (28.2%). This difference was statistically significant ($P = 0.01$) [53].

Complications

Complications are relatively rare for any approach, however the rate increases with tumor size, as one would expect.

Cerebrospinal Fluid Leak and Meningitis

Historical series report postoperative CSF leak in 2–7 % of patients who underwent middle fossa approach for tumor resection [32, 50]. In our most recent series of patients who underwent middle fossa tumor removal, none had a postoperative CSF leak. This is likely due to continuous flushing while drilling and copious irrigation to prevent bone dust from plugging arachnoid granulations, as well as meticulous dural plugging with abdominal fat, attention to plugging any air cells around the IAC, and cautious wound closure techniques [44]. In a review of all of their translabyrinthine approaches since 1974, the House group found an initial rate of CSF leak of 20% when using temporalis muscle to close the dura [15]. This improved to 7% with the use of abdominal fat and to 4% once they began using titanium mesh cranioplasty plates in 2003 [16, 55]. In a prospective study of 71 patients compared to historic controls, we found that there was no difference in incidence of CSF leak between fat graft and resorbable mesh cranioplasty (13.4% vs 12.7%, $P = 0.88$) [56]. A large systematic review published in 2012 found a rate of CSF leaks of 5.3% for the middle fossa approach and 7.1% for the translabyrinthine approach, consistent with previously published incidences [19].

Meningitis is becoming increasingly rare, due to the consistent use of perioperative antibiotics and reduced operative times. Smaller series published in the 1990s found rates of 2–5% in patients who underwent the middle fossa approach, however not all of those cases were culture proven [32, 50]. A review of 512 patients who underwent translabyrinthine approach from 2000 to 2004 found a rate of postoperative meningitis of only 0.6% [16]. It is important to note that patients can experience meningismus secondary to chemical meningitis in the postoperative setting. It is crucial to obtain a lumbar puncture in this setting to rule out a bacterial etiology.

Hemorrhage

A rare, but serious and potentially fatal complication is a hematoma in the CPA. This presents in the early postoperative period with signs of increased intracranial pressure. Such a scenario is managed by immediate exploration with removal of the fat packing, evacuation of the hematoma, and control of the source. This can be accommodated rapidly if the patient underwent the translabyrinthine approach. Incidences are isolated to individual case reports with the middle fossa approach, often in the forms of epidural or subdural hematomas [3, 45]. In their series of 512 patients, the House group found incidences of 0.8% and 0.6% for subdural and CPA hematomas, respectively, with the translabyrinthine approach [16].

Sigmoid Sinus Thrombosis

Sigmoid sinus thrombosis is an uncommon but well-recognized and potentially devastating complication of surgical approaches to the CPA. Risk factors for developing dural sinus thrombosis in the postoperative setting include mechanical injury during surgery, excessive manipulation and prolonged retraction of the sinus, dehydration, pregnancy, oral contraceptive use, infection, and hematologic disease [57, 58]. Though not always symptomatic, manifestations in those who develop this complication include headaches, altered mental status, seizures, focal neurologic deficits, papilledema, intracranial hemorrhage (ICH), and infarction [39, 57, 60]. While there is an abundance of literature discussing the treatment options and outcomes of sigmoid sinus thrombosis that is spontaneous or secondary to infection or trauma, there are only small, isolated case series discussing it in the postoperative period. In one of the largest series of 107 patients who underwent suboccipital or translabyrinthine resection of a CPA tumor, 5 (4.6%) developed transverse sinus thrombosis and symptomatic papilledema [61]. Three patients were treated with shunting and two were treated with acetazolamide and dexamethasone, and all patients' symptoms resolved. No patients were treated with anticoagulation. The number of patients who had asymptomatic thrombosis was not divulged. In a more recent series by Moore et al. [62], 5 out of 43 patients (11.6%) who underwent resection of acoustic neuroma developed transverse or sigmoid sinus thrombosis. All who developed thrombosis underwent tumor removal via translabyrinthine approach. Four were asymptomatic and diagnosed on routine postoperative imaging, and the fifth was diagnosed 5 weeks postoperative after developing ataxia and a cerebellar infarction. Those who developed thrombosis had larger tumors (3.24 cm vs 1.8 cm, $P < 0.001$) and underwent a longer operation (10 h vs 8 h, $P = 0.07$), though surgical duration fell just short of reaching significance. All were treated with systemic anticoagulation for 6 months, and none developed intracranial hemorrhage. A Cochrane review of two small prospective studies found that systemic anticoagulation for venous sinus thrombosis had a nonsignificant absolute reduction in the risk of death and dependency of 13%, suggesting anticoagulation in these patients is safe [63]. However, some reserve systemic anticoagulation for patients with clot propagation or symptom progression [58, 59, 61]. In those patients who are clinically deteriorating despite systemic anticoagulation, chemical or mechanical thrombectomy are options, particularly when a preexisting ICH is present [59].

Venous Thromboembolism

Patients undergoing craniotomy are known to be at moderate to high risk for developing postoperative deep vein thrombosis (DVT) and pulmonary embolism (PE). A meta-analysis by Kimmell and Jahromi [64] of 4,844 patients who underwent craniotomy found an incidence of venous thromboembolism (VTE) of 3.5%, including 2.6% with DVT and 1.4% with PE. Significant predictors of VTE on multivariate analysis in this study included craniotomy for tumor, transfer from acute care hospital, age ≥ 60 years, dependent functional status, tumor involving the CNS, sepsis, emergency surgery, surgical duration ≥ 4 h, postoperative urinary tract infection, postoperative pneumonia, ≥ 48 h of postoperative mechanical ventilation, and return to the operating room. Patients were assigned one point for each of these factors for a cumulative VTE score ranging from 0 to 12, with a higher score associated with a higher risk of VTE and mortality, as well as a longer hospital stay. Specifically, those with a score of ≥ 5 were 20 times more likely to develop a VTE compared with patients with a VTE score of 0. While chemical VTE prophylaxis is commonplace following most general surgical and orthopedic procedures, its use still remains infrequent by neurosurgeons and otolaryngologists who perform craniotomies. Numerous prospective trials and meta-analyses have failed to definitively demonstrate the safety of heparin products following craniotomy [65–72]. One such meta-analysis by Hamilton et al. [73] found an absolute risk reduction of symptomatic and asymptomatic VTE of 9.1% with heparin prophylaxis, compared to an absolute risk increase of 0.7% for ICH and 2.8% for minor bleeding. This translates to a likelihood of preventing 13 symptomatic and asymptomatic VTE for every ICH caused when using prophylactic heparin. However, when broken down by symptomatic or proximal VTE and PE, which are more clinically relevant, this ratio changes to 5 to 1 for proximal VTE and PE and 2 to 1 for symptomatic VTE. Currently, the American College of Chest Physicians only recommends the use of heparin in craniotomy patients who are "very high risk," with a risk of VTE ≥ 10, specifically in patients with a malignancy [74].

Major Neurological Complications

Ansari et al. defined major neurological complications in their systematic review as arterial or venous infarcts, seizures, or persistent cerebellar dysfunction. When grouped together, they found these occurred at a rate of 2.4% in the middle fossa approach and 2.6% in the translabyrinthine approach ($P = 0.512$) [19]. Seizures are more commonly seen following the middle fossa approach and are thought to be related to temporal lobe retraction. Limiting the time of temporal lobe retraction to 60–90 min can help to avoid this complication [3].

Summary

With the development of the operating microscope and microsurgical techniques, the approach to removing acoustic neuromas has evolved and improved over the years. Continued technical refinements have led to a low rate of complications and rare mortality. The incorporation of routine gadolinium-enhanced MRI has facilitated early diagnosis of small lesions and made hearing conservation surgery a possibility in these cases.

The primary considerations when deciding on the surgical approach are preoperative hearing status and tumor size. In patients with small lesions and serviceable hearing, use of the middle fossa approach can lead to preservation of preoperative hearing in up to 80% of patients with as many as 95% of patients being left with a normal or near-normal facial nerve function. In patients with poor preoperative hearing and/or large acoustic neuromas, the translabyrinthine approach has excellent exposure and has shown to be safe. As tumors increase in size, the rate of postoperative complications and facial nerve dysfunction increases. In acoustic neuromas larger than 2.5 cm, consideration can be given to subtotal tumor resection and facial nerve preservation, knowing that this may result in tumor regrowth over time.

References

1. Parry RH. A case of tinnitus and vertigo treated by division of the auditory nerve. 1904. J Laryngol Otol. 1991;105(12):1099–100.
2. House WF. Surgical exposure of the internal auditory canal and its contents through the middle, cranial fossa. Laryngoscope. 1961;71:1363–85.
3. Brackmann DE, Shelton C, House WF. Middle fossa approach. In: Shelton C, Brackmann D, Arriaga MA, editors. Otologic surgery. 4th ed. Philadelphia: Elsevier; 2016. p. 512–9.
4. Shelton C, Hitselberger WE. The treatment of small acoustic tumors: now or later? Laryngoscope. 1991;101(9):925–8.
5. Wade PJ, House W. Hearing preservation in patients with acoustic neuromas via the middle fossa approach. Otolaryngol Head Neck Surg. 1984;92(2):184–93.
6. Kurze T, Doyle JB Jr. Extradural intracranial (middle fossa) approach to the internal auditory canal. J Neurosurg. 1962;19:1033–7.
7. Brackmann D. Middle cranial fossa approach. In: House W, Luetje C, editors. Acoustic tumors management, vol. 2. Baltimore: University Park Press; 1979.
8. Glasscock ME, Poe DS, Johnson GD. Hearing preservation in surgery of cerebellopontine angle tumors. In: Fisch U, Valavanis A, Yasargil MG, editors. Neurological surgery of the ear and skullbase. Amsterdam: Kugler & Ghedini; 1989.
9. House F, Hitselberger WE. The middle fossa approach for removal of small acoustic tumors. Acta Otolaryngol. 1969;67(4):413–27.
10. Minor LB, Solomon D, Zinreich JS, Zee DS. Sound-and/or pressure-induced vertigo due to bone dehiscence of the superior semicircular canal. Arch Otolaryngol Head Neck Surg. 1998;124(3):249–58.
11. Baugh RF, Basura GJ, Ishii LE, Schwartz SR, Drumheller CM, Burkholder R, et al. Clinical practice guideline: bell's palsy. Otolaryngol Head Neck Surg. 2013;149(3 Suppl):S1–27.
12. Cannon RB, Gurgel RK, Warren FM, Shelton C. Facial nerve outcomes after middle fossa decompression for Bell's palsy. Otol Neurotol. 2015;36(3):513–8.
13. Cannon RB, Thomson RS, Shelton C, Gurgel RK. Long-term outcomes after middle fossa approach for traumatic facial nerve paralysis. Otol Neurotol. 2016;37:799–804.
14. House WF. Transtemporal bone microsurgical removal of acoustic neuromas. Evolution of trans-temporal bone removal of acoustic tumors. Arch Otolaryngol. 1964;80:731–42.
15. House WF. Translabyrinthine approach. In: House WF, Luetje C, editors. Acoustic tumors management, vol. 2. Baltimore: University Park Press; 1979. p. 43–87.
16. Goddard JC, McRackan TR, House JW. Translabyrinthine approach. In: Brackmann DE, Shelton C, Arriaga MA, editors. Otolgoic surgery. 4th ed. Philadelphia: Elsevier; 2016. p. 520–30.
17. Hitselberger WE, House WF. A warning regarding the sitting position for acoustic tumor surgery. Arch Otolaryngol. 1980;106(2):69.
18. Jackler R, Sim D. Retrosigmoid approach to tumours of the cerebellopontine angle. In: Brackmann DE,

Shelton C, Arriaga MA, editors. Otologic surgery. 3rd ed. Philadelphia: Elsevier; 2010. p. 603–20.

19. Ansari SF, Terry C, Cohen-Gadol AA. Surgery for vestibular schwannomas: a systematic review of complications by approach. Neurosurg Focus. 2012;33(3):E14.

20. Arriaga MA, Brackmann DE. Neoplasms of the posterior fossa. In: Flint PW, Haughey BH, Lund VJ, Niparko JK, Robbins KT, Thomas JR, et al., editors. Cummings otolaryngology – head and neck surgery, vol. 3. Philadelphia: Saunders; 2015. p. 2748–77.

21. Selters WA, Brackmann DE. Acoustic tumor detection with brain stem electric response audiometry. Arch Otolaryngol. 1977;103(4):181–7.

22. Wilson DF, Hodgson RS, Gustafson MF, Hogue S, Mills L. The sensitivity of auditory brainstem response testing in small acoustic neuromas. Laryngoscope. 1992;102(9):961–4.

23. Abele TA, Besachio DA, Quigley EP, Gurgel RK, Shelton C, Harnsberger HR, et al. Diagnostic accuracy of screening MR imaging using unenhanced axial CISS and coronal T2WI for detection of small internal auditory canal lesions. AJNR Am J Neuroradiol. 2014;35(12):2366–70.

24. Shelton C, Harnsberger HR, Allen R, King B. Fast spin echo magnetic resonance imaging: clinical application in screening for acoustic neuroma. Otolaryngol Head Neck Surg. 1996;114(1):71–6.

25. Committee on Hearing and Equilibrium guidelines for the evaluation of hearing preservation in acoustic neuroma (vestibular schwannoma). American Academy of Otolaryngology-Head and Neck Surgery Foundation, INC. Otolaryngol Head Neck Surg. 1995;113(3):179–80.

26. Brackmann DE, Owens RM, Friedman RA, Hitselberger WE, De la Cruz A, House JW, et al. Prognostic factors for hearing preservation in vestibular schwannoma surgery. Am J Otolaryngol. 2000;21(3):417–24.

27. Gurgel RK, Jackler RK, Dobie RA, Popelka GR. A new standardized format for reporting hearing outcome in clinical trials. Otolaryngol Head Neck Surg. 2012;147(5):803–7.

28. Shelton C, Brackmann DE, House WF, Hitselberger WE. Acoustic tumor surgery. Prognostic factors in hearing conversation. Arch Otolaryngol Head Neck Surg. 1989;115(10):1213–6.

29. Jackler RK, Pitts LH. Selection of surgical approach to acoustic neuroma. Otolaryngol Clin N Am. 1992;25(2):361–87.

30. Frerebeau P, Benezech J, Uziel A, Coubes P, Segnarbieux F, Malonga M. Hearing preservation after acoustic neurinoma operation. Neurosurgery. 1987;21(2):197–200.

31. Glasscock ME, McKennan KX, Levine SC. Acoustic neuroma surgery: the results of hearing conservation surgery. Laryngoscope. 1987;97(7 Pt 1):785–9.

32. Shelton C, Brackmann DE, House WF, Hitselberger WE. Middle fossa acoustic tumor surgery: results in 106 cases. Laryngoscope. 1989;99(4):405–8.

33. Shelton C. Hearing preservation in acoustic tumor surgery. Otolaryngol Clin N Am. 1992;25(3):609–21.

34. Yates PD, Jackler RK, Satar B, Pitts LH, Oghalai JS. Is it worthwhile to attempt hearing preservation in larger acoustic neuromas? Otol Neurotol. 2003;24(3):460–4.

35. Blevins NH, Jackler RK. Exposure of the lateral extremity of the internal auditory canal through the retrosigmoid approach: a radioanatomic study. Otolaryngol Head Neck Surg. 1994;111(1):81–90.

36. Shelton C, House WF. Hearing improvement after acoustic tumor removal. Otolaryngol Head Neck Surg. 1990;103(6):963–5.

37. Berliner KI, Shelton C, Hitselberger WE, Luxford WM. Acoustic tumors: effect of surgical removal on tinnitus. Am J Otolaryngol. 1992;13(1):13–7.

38. Chen DA, Arriaga MA, Fukushima T. Technical refinements in retraction for middle fossa surgery. Am J Otolaryngol. 1998;19(2):208–11.

39. Garcia-Ibanez E, Garcia-Ibanez JL. Middle fossa vestibular neurectomy: a report of 373 cases. Otolaryngol Head Neck Surg. 1980;88(4):486–90.

40. Buchman CA, Adunka OF. Translabyrinthine vestibular neurectomy. In: Brackmann DE, Shelton C, Arriaga MA, editors. Otologic surgery. 4th ed. Philadelphia: Elsevier; 2016. p. 397–407.

41. Goddard JC, Oliver ER, Lambert PR. Prevention of cerebrospinal fluid leak after translabyrinthine resection of vestibular schwannoma. Otol Neurotol. 2010;31(3):473–7.

42. Brackmann DE, Green JD. Translabyrinthine approach for acoustic tumor removal. Otolaryngol Clin N Am. 1992;25(2):311–29.

43. Wilkinson EP, Fayad JN, Lupo JE. Otologic instrumentation. In: Brackmann DE, Shelton C, Arriaga MA, editors. Otolgoic surgery. 4th ed. Philadelphia: Elsevier; 2016. p. 10–2.

44. Raheja A, Bowers CA, MacDonald JD, Shelton C, Gurgel RK, Brimley C, et al. Middle fossa approach for vestibular schwannoma: good hearing and facial nerve outcomes with low morbidity. World Neurosurg. 2016;92:37–46.

45. Brackmann DE, House JR 3rd, Hitselberger WE. Technical modifications to the middle fossa craniotomy approach in removal of acoustic neuromas. Am J Otolaryngol. 1994;15(5):614–9.

46. Shelton C, Hitselberger WE, House WF, Brackmann DE. Hearing preservation after acoustic tumor removal: long-term results. Laryngoscope. 1990;100(2 Pt 1):115–9.

47. Quist TS, Givens DJ, Gurgel RK, Chamoun R, Shelton C. Hearing preservation after middle fossa vestibular schwannoma removal: are the results durable? Otolaryngol Head Neck Surg. 2015;152(4):706–11.

48. Holsinger FC, Coker NJ, Jenkins HA. Hearing preservation in conservation surgery for vestibular schwannoma. Am J Otolaryngol. 2000;21(5):695–700.

49. Kutz JW Jr, Scoresby T, Isaacson B, Mickey BE, Madden CJ, Barnett SL, et al. Hearing preservation using the middle fossa approach for the treat-

ment of vestibular schwannoma. Neurosurgery. 2012;70(2):334–40. discussion 40–1

50. Slattery WH 3rd, Brackmann DE, Hitselberger W. Middle fossa approach for hearing preservation with acoustic neuromas. Am J Otolaryngol. 1997;18(5):596–601.

51. Woodson EA, Dempewolf RD, Gubbels SP, Porter AT, Oleson JJ, Hansen MR, et al. Long-term hearing preservation after microsurgical excision of vestibular schwannoma. Otol Neurotol. 2010;31(7):1144–52.

52. Gurgel RK, Theodosopoulos PV, Jackler RK. Subtotal/near-total treatment of vestibular schwannomas. Curr Opin Otolaryngol Head Neck Surg. 2012;20(5):380–4.

53. Monfared A, Corrales E, Theodosopoulos P, Blevins NH, Oghalai JS, Selesnick SH, et al. Facial nerve outcome and tumor control rate as a function of degree of resection in treatment of large acoustic neuromas: preliminary report of the acoustic neuroma subtotal resection study. Neurosurgery. 2015;79(2):194–203.

54. Gurgel RK, Dogru S, Amdur RL, Monfared A. Facial nerve outcomes after surgery for large vestibular schwannomas: do surgical approach and extent of resection matter? Neurosurg Focus. 2012;33(3):E16.

55. Rodgers GK, Luxford WM. Factors affecting the development of cerebrospinal fluid leak and meningitis after translabyrinthine acoustic tumor surgery. Laryngoscope. 1993;103(9):959–62.

56. Hillman TA, Shelton C. Resorbable plate cranioplasty after the translabyrinthine approach. Otol Neurotol. 2011;32(7):1171–4.

57. Nimjee SM, Powers CJ, Kolls BJ, Smith T, Britz GW, Zomorodi AR. Endovascular treatment of venous sinus thrombosis: a case report and review of the literature. J Neurointerv Surg. 2011;3(1):30–3.

58. Ohata K, Haque M, Morino M, Nagai K, Nishio A, Nishijima Y, et al. Occlusion of the sigmoid sinus after surgery via the presigmoidal-transpetrosal approach. J Neurosurg. 1998;89(4):575–84.

59. Medel R, Monteith SJ, Crowley RW, Dumont AS. A review of therapeutic strategies for the management of cerebral venous sinus thrombosis. Neurosurg Focus. 2009;27(5):E6.

60. Wasay M, Kojan S, Dai AI, Bobustuc G, Sheikh Z. Headache in cerebral venous thrombosis: incidence, pattern and location in 200 consecutive patients. J Headache Pain. 2010;11(2):137–9.

61. Keiper GL Jr, Sherman JD, Tomsick TA, Tew JM Jr. Dural sinus thrombosis and pseudotumor cerebri: unexpected complications of suboccipital craniotomy and translabyrinthine craniectomy. J Neurosurg. 1999;91(2):192–7.

62. Moore J, Thomas P, Cousins V, Rosenfeld JV. Diagnosis and management of dural sinus thrombosis following resection of cerebellopontine angle tumors. J Neurol Surg B Skull Base. 2014; 75(6):402–8.

63. Coutinho JM, de Bruijn SF, de Veber G, Stam J. Anticoagulation for cerebral venous sinus thrombosis. Stroke. 2012;43(4):e41–e2.

64. Kimmell KT, Jahromi BS. Clinical factors associated with venous thromboembolism risk in patients undergoing craniotomy. J Neurosurg. 2015;122(5):1004–11.

65. Agnelli G, Piovella F, Buoncristiani P, Severi P, Pini M, D'Angelo A, et al. Enoxaparin plus compression stockings compared with compression stockings alone in the prevention of venous thromboembolism after elective neurosurgery. N Engl J Med. 1998;339(2):80–5.

66. Bostrom S, Holmgren E, Jonsson O, Lindberg S, Lindstrom B, Winso I, et al. Post-operative thromboembolism in neurosurgery. A study on the prophylactic effect of calf muscle stimulation plus dextran compared to low-dose heparin. Acta Neurochir. 1986;80(3–4):83–9.

67. Cerrato D, Ariano C, Fiacchino F. Deep vein thrombosis and low-dose heparin prophylaxis in neurosurgical patients. J Neurosurg. 1978;49(3):378–81.

68. Collen JF, Jackson JL, Shorr AF, Moores LK. Prevention of venous thromboembolism in neurosurgery: a metaanalysis. Chest. 2008;134(2):237–49.

69. Dickinson LD, Miller LD, Patel CP, Gupta SK. Enoxaparin increases the incidence of postoperative intracranial hemorrhage when initiated preoperatively for deep venous thrombosis prophylaxis in patients with brain tumors. Neurosurgery. 1998;43(5):1074–81.

70. Goldhaber SZ, Dunn K, Gerhard-Herman M, Park JK, Black PM. Low rate of venous thromboembolism after craniotomy for brain tumor using multimodality prophylaxis. Chest. 2002;122(6):1933–7.

71. Macdonald RL, Amidei C, Baron J, Weir B, Brown F, Erickson RK, et al. Randomized, pilot study of intermittent pneumatic compression devices plus dalteparin versus intermittent pneumatic compression devices plus heparin for prevention of venous thromboembolism in patients undergoing craniotomy. Surg Neurol. 2003;59(5):363–72. discussion 72–4

72. Nurmohamed MT, van Riel AM, Henkens CM, Koopman MM, Que GT, d'Azemar P, et al. Low molecular weight heparin and compression stockings in the prevention of venous thromboembolism in neurosurgery. Thromb Haemost. 1996;75(2):233–8.

73. Hamilton MG, Yee WH, Hull RD, Ghali WA. Venous thromboembolism prophylaxis in patients undergoing cranial neurosurgery: a systematic review and meta-analysis. Neurosurgery. 2011;68(3):571–81.

74. Gould MK, Garcia DA, Wren SM, Karanicolas PJ, Arcelus JI, Heit JA, et al. Prevention of VTE in nonorthopedic surgical patients: antithrombotic therapy and prevention of thrombosis, 9th ed: American College of chest physicians evidence-based clinical practice guidelines. Chest. 2012;141(2 Suppl):e227S–77S.

75. Brackmann DE, Shelton C, Arriaga MA, Pazos A, Illustrator. In: Otologic surgery, 2nd ed. Philadelphia: W.B. Saunders Company; 2001.

Posterior and Combined Petrosal Approaches

David Aum, Omar Arnaout, Marcio S. Rassi,
Walid Ibn Essayed, and Ossama Al-Mefty

Introduction

The petrosal approach, as an initial concept, was described by Habuka et al. [1] in 1977 who performed the approach on a case of clival meningioma in a combined supra- and infratentorial craniotomy with a partial labyrinthectomy [2]. The modern petrosal approach, also referred to as the "posterior petrosal," was described by Al-Mefty et al. [3] and is centered on the petrous bone and offers simultaneous access to the petroclival junction, middle clivus, the apical petrous bone, Meckel's cave, and the cavernous sinus. The petrosal approach offers a wide exposure while eliminating the need for temporal or cerebellar retraction and is made possible by retro-displacement of the sigmoid sinus following sectioning the tentorium. The approach also shortens the operative distance to the clivus while potentially preserving the inner ear structures and allowing for resection of affected skull base bone. Other advantages include that the vascular supply to the tumor is made accessible early in the dissection and the approach affords multiple angles of attack to the lesion [4]. Finally, the approach is easily combined with other skull base approaches including the orbito-zygomatic, the total petrosectomy, and the transcondylar as the individual situation dictates.

The petrosal and combined petrosal approach may be used to expose a variety of skull base lesions including:

- Petroclival meningiomas, which arise in the upper two thirds of the clivus at the petroclival junction medial to the trigeminal nerve. Smaller tumors that remain medial to as low as the internal auditory meatus and cross midline could be approached via a zygomatic approach and an anterior petrosectomy [5, 6].
- Sphenopetroclival meningiomas, which extend into the middle cranial fossa by way of Meckel's cave or the cavernous sinus. These lesions frequently require a combined petrosal approach in order to achieve total excision. Alternatively, in patients who have already

D. Aum, MS (✉)
University of South Florida Morsani College of Medicine, Tampa, FL, USA
e-mail: aum@health.usf.edu

O. Arnaout, MD • W. Ibn Essayed, MD
O. Al-Mefty, MD
Department of Neurosurgery, Brigham and Women's Hospital, Boston, MA, USA
e-mail: oarnaout@bwh.harvard.edu;
wibnessayed@bwh.harvard.edu;
oalmefty@partners.org;
almeftyossama@bwh.harvard.edu

M.S. Rassi, MD
Department of Neurosurgery, Brigham and Women's Hospital, Harvard Medical School,
Boston, MA, USA
e-mail: rassima@hotmail.com

© Springer International Publishing AG 2018
W.T. Couldwell (ed.), *Skull Base Surgery of the Posterior Fossa*,
https://doi.org/10.1007/978-3-319-67038-6_4

lost functional hearing, a total petrosectomy (with drilling of the labyrinth and sometimes cochlea) can be considered.

- Posterior petrosal meningiomas, which can arise anterior or posterior to the internal auditory canal (IAC) but are lateral to the trigeminal nerve. Those arising anteriorly can be addressed either via a zygomatic approach or a petrosal approach depending on size, whereas those confined to the posterior petrosal surface can be addressed via a transmastoid approach to the cerebellopontine angle (CPA) [7].
- Medial tentorial meningiomas, which can originate anywhere along the tentorium. Those with significant infra- and supratentorial components can be approached via the petrosal approach which also allows for excision of the affected dura.

In addition to extra-axial pathology, other lesions are amenable to resection via a petrosal approach including suprasellar lesions such as retro-chiasmatic craniopharyngiomas [8], trigeminal schwannomas, posterior circulation aneurysms [9], brainstem vascular malformations [10], and large epidermoids spanning the posterior and middle cranial fossae.

Preoperative Planning

The main consideration in selection of surgical approach is based on careful study of the lesion as well as the surrounding normal anatomy. In particular, the structure and pattern of venous drainage should be considered especially when the approach involves planned transection of the tentorium and ligation of the superior petrosal sinus (SPS) [11]. Areas deserving of special attention include the point of insertion of the vein of Labbe, the dominance of the SPS, and the presence of other venous structures such as tentorial veins that would prohibit the approach.

Hearing evaluation should be performed preoperatively in order to establish a baseline and evaluate candidacy for total petrosectomy.

Furthermore, attention should be paid to tumor involvement of the temporal bone and in particular the petrous apex; the approach selected must allow for removal of involved bone.

Role of Intraoperative Monitoring

The incidence of cranial nerve injury can be mitigated by using intraoperative neuromonitoring [12]. Intraoperative neuromonitoring is employed for all skull base cases in our institution and includes, at minimum, somatosensory evoked potentials (SSEP), brainstem auditory evoked potentials (BAER), and motor evoked potentials (MEP). Additional cranial nerves are monitored depending on the anticipated extent of involvement with the lesion. For extensive sphenopetroclival lesions, we routinely monitor the trigeminal (V), oculomotor (III), abducens (VI), and facial nerves (VII). The lower cranial (IX, X, XI) nerves are also monitoring should the lesion extend near, or extend past, the jugular fossa.

Petrosal Approach (or Posterior Petrosal Approach)

Patient Positioning

The patient is placed supine with the operating table slightly flexed to elevate the head slightly above the level of the heart. The head is fixed in a three-pin head holder and turned to the side contralateral to the tumor with the vertex tilted toward the floor and the head tilted slightly toward the contralateral shoulder. A shoulder roll is required to achieve the optimal position. Intraoperative navigation is routinely used, with preoperative magnetic resonance (MR) and computed tomography (CT) imaging co-registered, for confirmation of anatomical landmarks. Intraoperative neuromonitoring is also routinely used as described in the preceding section. An area of the abdomen wall is marked and prepped for anticipated fat graft harvest.

Skin Incision and Craniotomy

The skin incision is made starting from the zygomatic arch approximately 1 cm anterior to the tragus and extending superiorly just behind the hairline to the level of the superior temporal line. The incision curves posteriorly about two finger breadths above the pinna and two finger breadths behind the mastoid before curving caudally and stopping approximately 4 cm below the level of the mastoid tip (Fig. 4.1). The skin flap is elevated in a plane superficial to the temporalis fascia and retracted inferiorly and anteriorly; the superficial temporal artery is preserved. Next, the temporalis fascia is dissected off the muscle and kept in continuity with the sternocleidomastoid (SCM) muscle forming a pedicled flap to be used for the closure. The SCM muscle is released from its attachment to the occipital bone and the mastoid and reflected down along with the pedicled temporalis fascia. The temporalis muscle is then elevated via subperiosteal dissection that preserves its deep vascular supply [13] and is retracted anteriorly and inferiorly. At this point, the temporal fossa, the lateral aspect of the posterior fossa and the mastoid along with the root of the zygoma, is well exposed.

Burr holes are placed rostral and caudal to the transverse sinus, one set laterally just behind the level of the sigmoid sinus and one set medially as allowed by the exposure for a total of four burr holes. A drill with a footplate attachment is used to liberate the temporal and occipital portions of the craniotomy, while a drilling burr is used to connect the cuts overlying the sinus. Once the craniotomy is completed and the bone flap is elevated, a mastoidectomy is pursued in order to fully skeletonize the sigmoid sinus to the level of

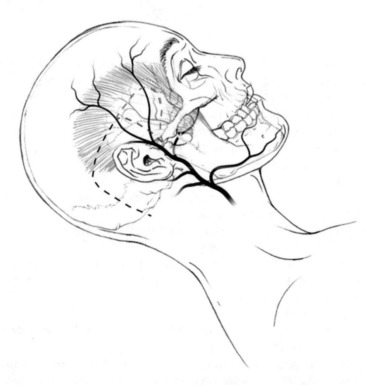

Fig. 4.1 The skin incision is made starting from the zygomatic arch approximately 1 cm anterior to the tragus and extending superiorly just behind the hairline. The incision curves posteriorly about two finger breadths above the pinna and two finger breadths behind the mastoid before curving caudally. For the combined petrosal approach, the incision is carried anteriorly to provide additional access to the middle cranial fossa (*blue dotted line*); for the posterior petrosal approach, the incision does not need this additional curve and is carried up from the zygoma (*red dotted line*). Both incisions have a common posterior limb (*black dotted line*)

Fig. 4.2 Burr hole placement and craniotomy cuts shown in the main figure. The cuts overlying dura are made with a craniotome attachment, while those overlying the sinus are made with a drilling burr (*2*). *Inset* shows the mastoidectomy which is performed subsequent to the craniotomy. The facial nerve (FC) and the semicircular canals (SC) are shown here for reference but are not exposed during the surgical approach in order to protect them. *TM* temporalis muscle, *SM* sternocleidomastoid muscle (Reproduced with permission from Al-Mefty [18])

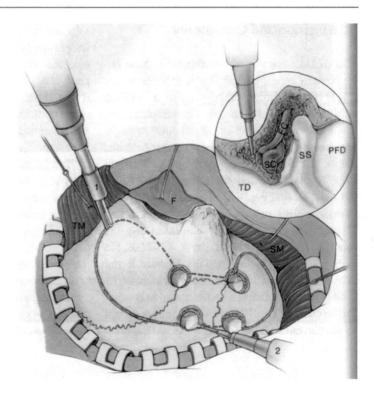

the jugular bulb and expose the presigmoid dura (Figs. 4.2 and 4.6). The mastoid cortex is removed en bloc prior to starting the mastoidectomy and saved along with the craniotomy flap for eventual reconstruction. The otic capsule and fallopian canal are left untouched in order to protect hearing and facial nerve function, respectively (Fig. 4.2, inset; Fig. 4.6b).

Dura opening proceeds by creating a linear incision along the floor of the middle cranial fossa and extending the opening back toward the tentorium, carefully preserving underlying venous anatomy (Fig. 4.3). Another dural opening is made in the presigmoid dura and expanded toward the tentorium; this step often results in sectioning of the endolymphatic sac. Once the tentorium is exposed from above and below, the superior petrosal sinus is controlled with coagulation, and the tentorium is incised with careful attention not to compromise any temporal lobe veins (Fig. 4.3, inset). Attention is given to the trochlear nerve at the medial tentorial edge, which often lies just above the level of the tentorium. In cases of tentorial meningiomas, the tentorium is excised instead of cut. Once the cut

reaches the incisura, the sigmoid sinus is liberated and may be retro-displaced which significantly increases the presigmoid working room afforded by the exposure (Figs. 4.4 and 4.6c) Microsurgical tumor resection may now proceed (Fig. 4.6d).

Combined Petrosal Approach

Patient Positioning

The patient is positioned in the same way as described for the posterior petrosal approach.

Skin Incision and Craniotomy

The skin incision is similar to that described for the posterior petrosal with slightly more anterior bias of the anterior-most limb to allow additional exposure of the middle fossa (Fig. 4.1).

A pedicled flap is elevated as described for the petrosal approach consisting of the temporalis fascia along with the attachment to the

Fig. 4.3 The dural opening are shown. Linear dural openings are made along the floor of the middle fossa (TD) as well as in the presigmoid dura (PFD). The *inset* demonstrated ligation and sectioning of the superior petrosal sinus (PS), which allows subsequent sectioning of the tentorium and mobilization of the sigmoid sinus (SS) (Reproduced with permission from Al-Mefty [18])

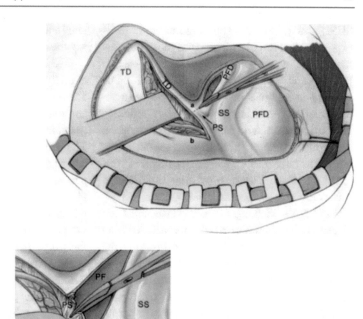

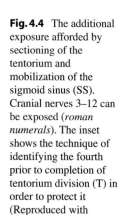

Fig. 4.4 The additional exposure afforded by sectioning of the tentorium and mobilization of the sigmoid sinus (SS). Cranial nerves 3–12 can be exposed (*roman numerals*). The inset shows the technique of identifying the fourth prior to completion of tentorium division (T) in order to protect it (Reproduced with permission from Al-Mefty [18])

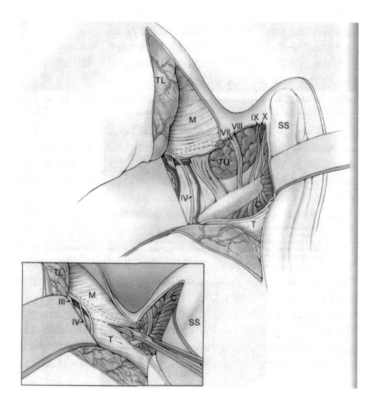

SCM and retracted. The zygomatic arch is exposed, and osteotomies are made along the root of the zygoma and as anterior as possible just behind the maxillary eminence. The zygoma is left in situ to preserve the attachments of the masseter muscles, but reflected inferiorly along with the temporalis muscle; this additional maneuver allows retraction of the temporalis muscle caudally into the infratemporal fossa, thus providing unhindered access to the middle cranial fossa floor.

Burr holes flanking the transverse sinus are placed similar to the petrosal approach, with an additional burr hole added anteriorly along the floor of the middle fossa near the temporal root of the zygoma. Burr holes are connected as previously described, and a bone flap is created that encompasses a larger component of the temporal squamosa. A mastoidectomy is performed as described in the previous section, skeletonizing the sigmoid sinus to the level of the jugular bulb and exposing the presigmoid dura.

Prior to elevating the temporal dura off the middle cranial fossa floor, a small dural opening is made in the presigmoid area and cerebrospinal fluid is released. The temporal lobe is elevated from the middle cranial fossa floor, proceeding in a posterior-to-anterior direction in order to more readily identify the greater superficial petrosal nerve (GSPN). During the dissection attention should be given to the presence of bony dehiscences; various structures including the geniculate ganglion of the facial nerve and the carotid artery may lack a roof and thus be at risk of iatrogenic injury. There is also frequently significant thinning or frank dehiscence in the tegmen tympani. The middle meningeal artery is identified at the foramen spinosum, cauterized and cut. The foramen spinosum is packed with bone wax. The extent of extradural dissection of the lateral wall of the cavernous sinus is tailored to the extent of sinus involvement with tumor. The inferior aspect of the third division of the trigeminal nerve is dissected and elevated, which aids in the subsequent mobilization of the trigeminal nerve and the Gasserian ganglion during the anterior petrosectomy.

The anatomical landmarks along the middle cranial fossa floor are identified including the arcuate eminence, trigeminal depression and trigeminal prominence, the second and third trigeminal divisions, and their respective foramina. The petrous carotid canal is unroofed in order to definitively locate the horizontal segment of the petrous carotid artery. A Fogarty balloon may be placed along the carotid artery within the canal, which can be inflated in the event of vascular injury in order to obtain proximal control [14]. At this point, anterior petrosectomy can proceed by drilling the bone of the petrous apex within Kawase's triangle from the internal auditory canal to the petroclival junction, taking care to avoid the cochlea which is located at the posterolateral aspect of the exposure.

Dural opening is similar to that described for the posterior petrosal approach except that the temporal dura opening can extend more anteriorly to take advantage of the additional space created by the anterior petrosectomy.

Tumor Resection

The main determinates of the extent of resection possible for lesions of the skull base include the presence of an arachnoid dissection plane, the consistency of the tumor, and the tumor's level of adherence to surrounding neurovascular structures; particularly fragile for this location are the basilar artery perforators. For meningiomas, by virtue of having performed a petrosectomy, the blood supply would have already been interrupted. Once reasonable devascularization is achieved, the tumor is incised and the tumor debulked using suction or an ultrasonic aspirator; significant debulking will allow dissection of the development of the intra-arachnoidal plane for dissection preserving neurovascular structures. Involved bone, either grossly or radiographically, should be removed using a high-speed drill.

Surgical resection of previously radiated tumors carries increased risk of neurovascular injury. At all times sharp dissection is preferred to blunt dissection in order to avoid unintended traction on neurovascular structures. The use of an ultrasonic aspiration device allows rapid debulking, but should be used carefully as large tumors can engulf cranial nerves and arteries. The tandem use of an endoscope and microscope has proven to be of tremendous value in increasing the extent of resection while minimizing complications [15].

Closure

Closing the dura following this approach often requires a duraplasty. After securing the graft in place, strips of the fat graft harvested from the abdomen are placed in the region of the cavernous sinus and used to obliterate any exposed air cells including the mastoid cavity. The previously preserved pedicled temporalis fascia is rotated such that it lies along the floor of the middle cranial fossa and covers the mastoid cavity and secured in place with sutures (Fig. 4.5). The mastoid cortex is plated in anatomical position using titanium plating along with the remainder of the craniotomy flap. Hydroxyapatite

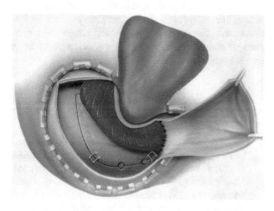

Fig. 4.5 Closure. The previously reserved pedicled temporalis fascia is placed along the floor of the middle fossa and secured with suture, clips and/or fibrin glue (Reproduced with permission from Al-Mefty [18])

is used to fill in any remaining defects and cover implanted hardware such that it would not be palpable by the patient. If osteotomies were made along the zygomatic arch, it is plated. The temporalis muscle is re-suspended in anatomic position using sutures. The galea and subsequently the skin are closed in layers in the usual fashion. A sterile dressing is applied, along with a head-wrap (Fig. 4.6).

Tricks and Pitfalls

There are a number of surgical precautions that should be followed for the safe execution of the posterior and combined petrosal approaches. The chief concern is the patient's particular variations of the venous anatomy surrounding the Labbe complex, petrosal complex, and basal temporal and occipital venous complexes. The point of insertion of the vein of Labbe, which may be multiple, should be well understood in advance of surgery such that the tentorial cut can be planned rostral to that location. Certain variants, such as the presence of a dominant venous channel within the tentorium, may absolutely contraindicate an approach involving cutting the tentorium. Others, such as the presence of a single sigmoid sinus ipsilateral to the tumor, require particular attention to avoid thrombosis or injury to the sinus.

With large musculocutaneous flaps, extensive bone drilling, and intradural exposure of multiple CSF cisterns comes increased risk for pseudomeningocele formation and spinal fluid leak. This risk is mitigated by conforming to a meticulous multilayered closure that takes advantage of a well-vascularized, pedicled temporalis flap. Dural closure frequently requires the use of a dural graft. Fat is used generously to obliterate exposed air cells, but the use of large uncut pieces is avoided in order to reduce the risk of fat necrosis [16]. Cranioplasty, by replacing all removed bone including the mastoid cortex, also reduces the risk of leak and improves cosmetic outcomes [17].

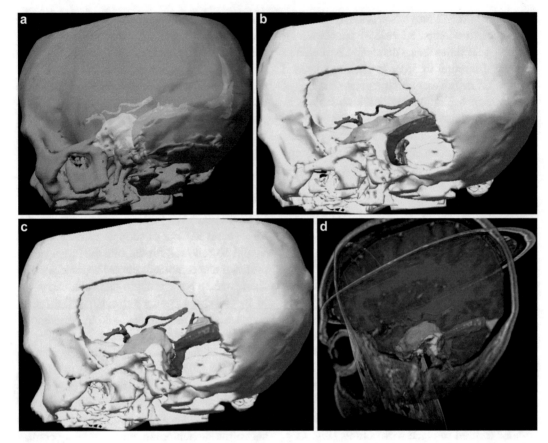

Fig. 4.6 3D reconstruction using segmentation of brain MRI for a patient who underwent a combined petrosal approach for resection of a petroclival meningioma. (**a**) A full 3D reconstruction prior to the craniotomy showing the location of the dural sinuses (*blue*), tumor (*green*), and the arterial system (*red*). (**b**) 3D reconstruction following the combined supratentorial and infratentorial craniotomy and mastoidectomy with the head in the surgical position. Tumor (*green*) presence in the posterior and middle cranial fossae is well demonstrated. Presigmoid (*blue*) access to the tumor is limited. The tentorium (*brown*) and the arterial vasculature (*red*) are also shown. (**c**) 3D reconstruction after the tentorium (*brown*) has been cut allowing the sinus (*blue*) to be mobilized. The maneuver allows full access to the tumor (*green*) without the need for retraction. The arterial vasculature (*red*) is also shown. (**d**) Volumetric 3D reconstruction of the tumor (*green*), dural venous sinuses (*blue*), and the arterial vasculature (*red*) is shown with the three orthogonal MRI planes in order to demonstrate their relationship to the surrounding brain parenchyma

Conclusion

The posterior petrosal and combined petrosal approaches are important neurosurgical routes that provide excellent access to lesions in the petroclival region, spanning the middle and lower clivus, petrous apex, cavernous sinus, and Meckel's cave. The approaches provide generous access while preserving function (including hearing) and allowing for multiple angles of attack for tumor resection and neurovascular preservation.

References

1. Hakuba A, Nishimura S, Tanaka K, Kishi H, Nakamura T. Clivus meningioma: six cases of total removal. Neurol Med Chir (Tokyo). The Japan Neurosurgical Society. 1977;17(1):63–77.
2. Gross BA, Tavanaiepour D, Du R, Al-Mefty O, Dunn IF. Evolution of the posterior petrosal approach. Neurosurg Focus. 2012;33(2):E7.
3. Al-Mefty O, Fox JL, Smith RR. Petrosal approach for petroclival meningiomas. Neurosurgery. LWW. 1988;22(3):510–7.
4. Al-Mefty O, Ayoubi S, Smith RR. The petrosal approach: indications, technique, and results. In: Acta

Neurochirurgica Supplementum (Wien). Austria. Springer Science + Business Media; 1991;53:166–70.

5. Kawase T, Shiobara R, Toya S. Anterior transpetrosal-transtentorial approach for sphenopetroclival meningiomas: surgical method and results in 10 patients. Neurosurgery. 1991;28(6):869–76.

6. Erkmen K, Pravdenkova S, Al-Mefty O. Surgical management of petroclival meningiomas: factors determining the choice of approach. Neurosurg Focus. Journal of Neurosurgery Publishing Group (JNSPG). 2005;19(2):1–12.

7. Abolfotoh M, Dunn IF, Al-Mefty O. Transmastoid retrosigmoid approach to the cerebellopontine angle: surgical technique. Neurosurgery [Internet]. 2013 Sep;73(1 Suppl Operative):ons16–23–discussionons23. Available from: http://content.wkhealth.com/linkback/openurl?sid=WKPTLP:landingpage&an=01787389-201309001-00004.

8. Al-Mefty O, Ayoubi S, Kadri PAS. The petrosal approach for the resection of retrochiasmatic craniopharyngiomas. Neurosurgery. 2008;62(5 Suppl 2):ONS331–5. –discussionONS335–6

9. Gross BA, Tavanaiepour D, Du R, Al-Mefty O, Dunn IF. Petrosal approaches to posterior circulation aneurysms. Neurosurg Focus. 2012;33(2):E9.

10. Gross BA, Dunn IF, Du R, Al-Mefty O. Petrosal approaches to brainstem cavernous malformations. Neurosurg Focus. 2012;33(2):E10.

11. Sakata K, Al-Mefty O, Yamamoto I. Venous consideration in petrosal approach: microsurgical anatomy of the temporal bridging vein. Neurosurgery. 2000;47(1):153–60. –discussion160–1

12. Topsakal C, Al-Mefty O, Bulsara KR, Williford VS. Intraoperative monitoring of lower cranial nerves in skull base surgery: technical report and review of 123 monitored cases. Neurosurg Rev. 2008;31(1):45–53.

13. Kadri PAS, Al-Mefty O. The anatomical basis for surgical preservation of temporal muscle. J Neurosurg. 2004;100(3):517–22.

14. Wascher TM, Spetzler RF, Zabramski JM. Improved transdural exposure and temporary occlusion of the petrous internal carotid artery for cavernous sinus surgery: technical note. J Neurosurg. Journal of Neurosurgery Publishing Group. 1993;78(5):834–7.

15. Abolfotoh M, Bi WL, Hong C-K, Almefty KK, Boskovitz A, Dunn IF, et al. The combined microscopic-endoscopic technique for radical resection of cerebellopontine angle tumors. J Neurosurg. 2015;123(5):1301–11.

16. Taha ANM, Almefty R, Pravdenkova S, Al-Mefty O. Sequelae of autologous fat graft used for reconstruction in skull base surgery. World Neurosurg. 2011;75(5–6):692–5.

17. Arriaga MA, Chen DA. Hydroxyapatite cement cranioplasty in translabyrinthine acoustic neuroma surgery. Otolaryngol Head Neck Surg.; Sage Publication. 2002;126(5):512–7.

18. Al-Mefty O. Meningiomas of the posterior cranial base. In: Operative atlas of meningiomas. Lippincott-Raven (Philadelphia); 1998.

Far Lateral Approach and Its Variants

5

Karolyn Au, Angela M. Richardson,
and Jacques Morcos

Introduction

A general surgical principle is worth stating at the outset of this chapter: choice of surgical approach is entirely determined by the nature and extent of the pathology. A large, soft, avascular tumor of the craniovertebral junction such as a schwannoma, paradoxically, may require a *smaller* exposure than a small ruptured but high PICA/VA aneurysm. Tumors displace the surrounding anatomy and in the process provide a surgical path to their own resection; one may call this a "trans-tumor" corridor. Vascular lesions such as aneurysms, AVMs, and cavernomas do not do this, and choosing the exactly appropriate approach in these instances is perhaps more important. A rote approach to neurosurgery is inappropriate and counterproductive, and in the decision-making process, the surgeon must integrate considerations of the anatomy, location, and texture of the pathology.

Having said that, there are general principles that apply, particularly regarding the surgical approaches to the foramen magnum/craniovertebral junction region. Accessing the anterior and anterolateral foramen magnum is a challenge due to the numerous neurologic, vascular, and ligamento-osseous structures that must be traversed along a deep corridor. A direct anterior trajectory is limited by vital structures laterally, so a posterolateral approach is commonly employed. The far lateral technique thus creates an exposure via a suboccipital craniotomy and removal of the foramen magnum rim to the occipital condyle, along with removal of the posterior arch of C1 to the lateral mass of C1. Its supracondylar, transcondylar, and paracondylar variants incorporate additional removal of lateral structures such as the occipital condyle, C1 lateral mass, jugular tubercle, and jugular process. The successive gains in anterolateral exposure and widened working corridor must be balanced against increased risk of injury to the vertebral artery, jugular bulb, and lower cranial nerves, as well as destabilization of the atlanto-occipital junction.

Anesthetic Technique and Positioning

Optimizing safety of surgery around the lower brainstem requires particular consideration and communication between the surgical and anesthetic teams. To minimize the need for brain retraction, standard anesthetic measures to facilitate brain relaxation are employed including hyperventilation and mannitol administration.

K. Au, MD, MSc • A.M. Richardson, MD, PhD
J. Morcos, MD, FRCS(Eng), FRCS(Ed), FAANS (✉)
Department of Neurological Surgery, University of Miami/Jackson Memorial Hospital, Miami, FL, USA
e-mail: jmorcos@med.miami.edu

© Springer International Publishing AG 2018
W.T. Couldwell (ed.), *Skull Base Surgery of the Posterior Fossa*,
https://doi.org/10.1007/978-3-319-67038-6_5

Early warning of neurologic compression, retraction, or ischemic injury can be provided by electrophysiologic monitoring of somatosensory, motor, and brainstem auditory evoked potentials. Free running and stimulated electromyographic monitoring of lower cranial nerve function may be also useful, especially in the setting of a mass lesion causing displacement of normal structures.

The patient is placed in the three-quarter prone position, the side of the lesion uppermost, which preserves alignment of the craniocervical junction, allows the cerebellar hemisphere to fall away, and maintains a low risk for venous air embolism. A gel roll is placed below the axilla and a cushion between the legs, and the dependent arm is supported in a sling beyond the end of the operating table.

The Mayfield clamp is placed with the single pin 2 cm superior and anterior to the ipsilateral pinna and the paired pins 2 cm superior to the contralateral pinna, all points maintaining a low profile. Placement of the pins is critical should the procedure require access to the occipital artery for a bypass graft. The head is fixed with incorporation of four movements (Fig. 5.1): (1) anteroposterior flexion to uncover the suboccipital region and rostral clivus, (2) contralateral flexion to increase working space beside the ipsilateral shoulder, (3) contralateral rotation to bring the suboccipital surface uppermost in the field, and (4) upward translation to partially sublux the ipsilateral atlanto-occipital joint and facilitate drilling of the condyle if needed. The ipsilateral shoulder is gently pulled toward the patient's feet while avoiding excessive traction on the brachial plexus, and the entire body secured with adhesive tape to allow for side-to-side rotation of the table. The table is placed in reverse Trendelenburg, elevating the head slightly above the heart, to decrease cerebral venous congestion.

Incision and Muscle Dissection

A hockey stick incision is started in the midline at the level of the C2 spinous process, and extended superiorly to 2 cm above the inion (Fig. 5.2a, b).

It is continued laterally above the superior nuchal line to a point directly superior to the mastoid process and then turned inferiorly to end at the mastoid tip. The occipital artery is preserved if required later in the procedure, as is pericranium for potential duraplasty. Dissection through the midline aponeurosis decreases muscle trauma and allows for early identification of the C1 lamina at a distance from the vertebral artery (Fig. 5.2c). The trapezius and sternocleidomastoid muscles overlie the semispinalis capitis and splenius capitis, which together conceal the suboccipital triangle. The superficial muscles are reflected as a single flap, maintaining a cuff along the superior nuchal line for a tight closure to decrease risk of cerebrospinal fluid leak (Fig. 5.2d). The muscle mass is elevated in the subperiosteal plane and swept laterally to expose the mastoid process and digastric groove (Fig. 5.2e). The attachments of longissimus capitis and posterior belly of digastric muscle are then released. As the technique aims to approach the ventral brainstem from a lateral trajectory, adequate inferolateral retraction is necessary to prevent encroachment upon the exposure by muscle bulk; hooked retractors on elastics serve this function better than hinged self-retaining retractors.

Incisions including the linear/curvilinear retromastoid incision and the S-shaped incision, beginning in the retromastoid region and extending medially to the midline, reduce the lateral bulk by directing the exposure through the musculature. However, these approaches increase muscle trauma and likelihood of sectioning the occipital artery and nerve, and place the vertebral artery at greater risk of injury as bony landmarks are not readily identified. Alternatively, the lateral muscle bulk can be decreased by individually identifying and dividing the sternocleidomastoid, splenius capitis, and semispinalis capitis and reflecting the muscles medially, although this approach increases the risk of wound dehiscence.

As the subperiosteal dissection continues inferiorly, the occipital attachments of the rectus capitis posterior minor, rectus capitis posterior major, and obliquus capitis supe-

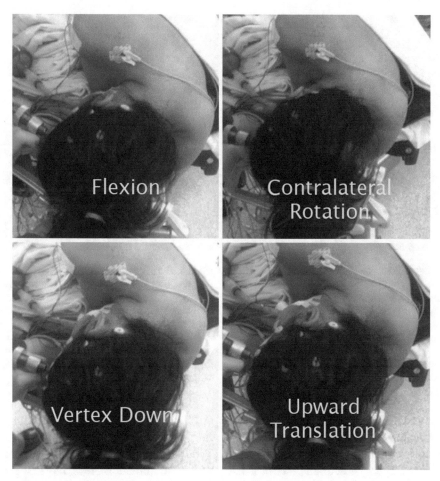

Fig. 5.1 Head positioning incorporates four movements: anteroposterior flexion to expose the suboccipital region; contralateral flexion to bring the vertex away from the shoulder; contralateral rotation to make the suboccipital region highest in the field; and upward translation to partially sublux the atlanto-occipital joint

rior are released. These latter two muscles, along with the obliquus capitis inferior, form the suboccipital triangle, which overlies the V3 segment of the vertebral artery and the C1 nerve root. The rectus capitis posterior major arises from the spinous process of C2 and forms the medial border of the suboccipital triangle. The obliquus capitis superior arises from the transverse process of C1 and forms the superior border, and the obliquus capitis inferior arises from the spinous process of C2 and inserts on the transverse process of C1, forming the inferior border. Elevation of the muscles laterally exposes the foramen magnum rim and lamina of C1, and the vertebral artery.

After the vertebral artery ascends through the C1 transverse foramen, it turns medially behind the atlanto-occipital joint and crosses the sulcus arteriosus of C1 in the depths of the suboccipital triangle. It then passes under the inferior border of the posterior atlanto-occipital membrane, and finally penetrates the dura (Fig. 5.2f). A rich venous plexus surrounds the artery and can cause brisk bleeding; coagulation and packing with hemostatic agents generally suffice to control it, although in some instances it may need to be resected. This segment of the artery is particularly vulnerable, as an aberrant loop toward the occipital bone may be injured during muscle dissection, or it may be compressed or avulsed against an ossified atlanto-occipital membrane

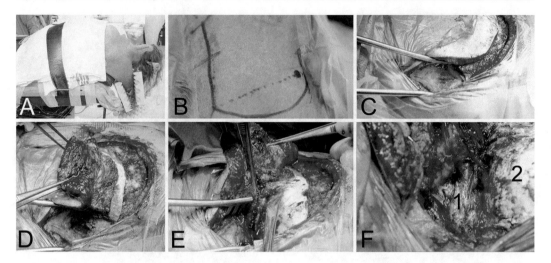

Fig. 5.2 Muscle dissection of the far lateral approach. (**a**) The final position maintains alignment of the craniocervical junction to facilitate orientation during dissection. (**b**) The hockey stick incision begins at C2, extends above the inion, then continues laterally and inferiorly to end at the mastoid tip. (**c**) Below the inion, a midline dissection decreases muscle trauma and allows for exposure of C1 a safe distance from the vertebral artery. (**d**) Preservation of a muscle cuff along the superior nuchal line facilitates a tight closure to decrease CSF leak. The skin is retained on the muscle surface to reduce postoperative pseudomeningocele formation. (**e**) A single muscle flap is elevated laterally and caudally. (**f**) Completed muscle dissection has exposed the lamina of C1 (*1*) and the suboccipital bone (*2*) to the foramen magnum. Laterally, the digastric groove and mastoid tip are seen. The V3 horizontal segment of the vertebral artery is seen passing over the sulcus arteriosus and penetrating the dura

arch. Electrocautery should be avoided when dissecting in the lower suboccipital area, as a sharp inadvertent arteriotomy is more readily repaired than a thermal injury. In addition, the muscular and posterior meningeal branches that arise in this segment may need to be divided in order to mobilize the artery. However, the posterior spinal artery or posterior inferior cerebellar artery (PICA) may have an extradural origin [1] and must be distinguished from muscular branches. Thorough preoperative imaging investigations provide forewarning about such variations and can guide decisions about repair or sacrifice of an injured vessel.

Extradural Exposure

The suboccipital craniotomy extends superolaterally from the rostral extent of the pathology to inferomedially across the midline at the foramen magnum (Fig. 5.3a). The posterior arch of C1 is likewise removed from beyond the midline to the sulcus arteriosus near the lateral mass of C1, approximately 1 cm lateral to the dural ring surrounding the vertebral artery (Fig. 5.3b). Variations in anatomy such as an incomplete C1 arch or assimilation of C1 must be recognized and are ideally anticipated on preoperative imaging. Removal of bone around the foramen magnum continues to the occipital condyle (Fig. 5.3c). This extensive lateral exposure forms the crux of the far lateral approach, allowing for an inferolateral approach to the anterior brainstem while avoiding retraction; the lateral lip of the foramen magnum is thus analogous to the greater sphenoid wing in the pterional craniotomy. As the foramen edge becomes more vertical, further bone removal is facilitated by use of a high-speed drill while the surgical assistant retracts and protects the vertebral artery and its venous plexus (Fig. 5.3d). At the posterior aspect of the condyle, bleeding may be encountered from the posterior condylar emissary vein, which communicates the vertebral venous plexus with the sigmoid sinus. It traverses the condylar canal, the extracranial opening of which lies at the base of a depression, the con-

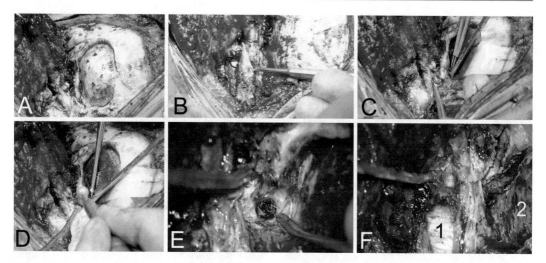

Fig. 5.3 Bone removal of the far lateral approach. (**a**) The teardrop-shaped suboccipital craniotomy extends across the rim of foramen magnum. (**b**) Soft tissue attachments are stripped from the ventral surface of the C1 lamina prior to its removal. (**c**) The dura is stripped from the rim of foramen magnum to allow for further lateral bone removal. (**d**) A high-speed diamond burr is used to remove bone of the foramen magnum toward the occipital condyle. (**e**) Exposure of the posterior condylar emissary vein (particularly large in this specimen) within the condylar canal denotes the lateral limit of the far lateral approach. (**f**) Removal of the foramen magnum rim to the base of the condyle and of C1 to the lateral mass completes the far lateral approach. The dura previously underlying the C1 arch (*1*) and suboccipital bone (*2*) is fully exposed

dylar fossa (Fig. 5.3e). Exposure of the emissary vein denotes the lateral limit of the basic far lateral approach (Figs. 5.3f and 5.4).

changes from condylar cortex, to cancellous bone within the condyle, to the posterior cortex of the canal.

Transcondylar Variants

Increased anterior exposure of the lower clivus, basilar artery, and anterior medulla may be gained with removal of the occipital condyle in part or whole. The condyles lie in a posterolateral to anteromedial orientation at the anterolateral aspect of the foramen magnum. Their articular surfaces are convex and are oriented inferolaterally toward the superior facets of C1, which are oriented superomedially. The intracranial opening of the hypoglossal canal is situated approximately 5 mm superior to the condyle, one-third of the distance from its posterior edge, typically 6–10 mm [2]. The canal courses anterolaterally, exiting one-third of the distance behind the anterior edge of the condyle, medial to the jugular foramen. As it carries the hypoglossal nerve within a channel fully surrounded by cortical bone, removal of the condyle is guided by the

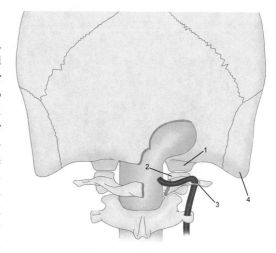

Fig. 5.4 Schematic diagram of the basic far lateral exposure. The suboccipital craniotomy and bone removal of foramen magnum extends from midline to occipital condyle. The laminectomy of C1 extends from midline to the lateral mass. Occipital condyle (*1*), lateral mass of C1 (*2*), transverse foramen of C1 (*3*), mastoid tip (*4*)

The occipito-transcondylar variant is readily incorporated into the basic far lateral approach, extending the removal of bone to the hypoglossal canal (Fig. 5.5a). The posterior third of the condyle is drilled away, limited at its medial aspect by the cortex of the hypoglossal canal. The condylar emissary vein may be encountered, its bleeding controlled with bone wax, and should not be confused for the venous plexus within the hypoglossal canal. Although the posterior two-thirds of the condyle may be drilled while remaining lateral to the hypoglossal canal, such extensive removal may cause instability of the atlanto-occipital joint.

Circumferential access to the dural ring surrounding the entrance of the vertebral artery is obtained using the atlanto-occipital variant, by removing the posterior aspect of both the occipital condyle and C1 lateral mass. Further access to the atlanto-occipital articular pillar is gained in the complete transcondylar variant by transposing the vertebral artery (Fig. 5.5b); the obliquus capitis superior and inferior muscles are detached from the C1 transverse foramen, which is then opened posteriorly, allowing for medial and inferior displacement of the vessel. The posterior

condyle and C1 lateral mass can then be drilled anteriorly to the level of the hypoglossal canal. An unrecognized tortuous vertebral artery may be injured if it loops posteriorly between the C2 and C1 transverse processes. Complete removal of the condyle requires skeletonization of the hypoglossal nerve and stabilization of the craniovertebral junction, and is reserved for extradural pathology involving the condyle [3].

Supracondylar Variants

Increased rostral exposure may be achieved by removing bone superior to the occipital condyle. The supracondylar approach can be directed superiorly to expose the hypoglossal canal above the condyle, or both below and above the hypoglossal canal toward the lateral clivus, while preserving the articular surface (Fig. 5.6a). The cortical bone of the hypoglossal canal can also be preserved to decrease likelihood of injury to the nerve.

Approximately 5 mm superior to the intracranial opening of the hypoglossal canal, medial to the lower edge of the jugular foramen, arises the rounded prominence of the jugular tubercle. The

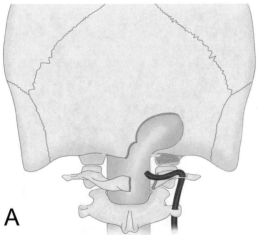
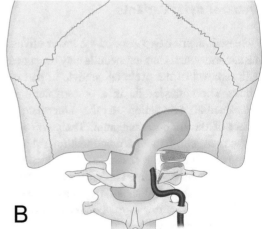

A   B

Fig. 5.5 The transcondylar variants. (**a**) The occipito-transcondylar variant incorporates removal of the posterior third of the condyle, to the hypoglossal canal. The shaded area denotes exposed cancellous bone, deep to the articular surface of the condyle and caudal to the hypoglossal canal. (**b**) The complete transcondylar variant requires removal of the posterior aspect of the C1 lateral mass to open the transverse foramen. This allows for inferomedial displacement of the vertebral artery. The condyle and C1 lateral mass are then both drilled to the depth of the medial hypoglossal canal

protrusion of the jugular tubercle may limit anterior exposure, and in the manner that removal of the occipital condyle prominence provides an opening to the pre-medullary region, so removal of the jugular tubercle prominence gains access to the pre-pontomedullary space (Fig. 5.6b). As the glossopharyngeal, vagus, and accessory nerves cross the posterior surface of the jugular tubercle intradurally, performing the transtubercular approach requires the removal of the tubercle without causing cranial nerve injury by traction or heat. The drilling is most safely done through an intradural approach, with direct visualization of the lower cranial nerves. Caution must be also be exercised when drilling the lateral aspect of the jugular tubercle, which abuts the medial edge of the jugular bulb.

The transtubercular approach can be appreciated by drawing parallels with the familiar cranio-orbital approach (Table 5.1); each involves stepwise removal of bone to gain exposure of a deep target while preserving critical adjacent neural and vascular structures.

Paracondylar Variants

Further lateral exposure, or access to the posterior aspect of the jugular foramen, can be obtained with the transjugular variant. Lateral to the posterior part of the occipital condyle is a quadrilateral prominence extending toward the squamous occipital bone, the jugular process. The rectus capitis lateralis extends upward from the transverse process of C1 to insert on the jugular process, and detaching this muscle reveals the extracranial aspect of the jugular foramen immediately anterior. Removal of the jugular process exposes the transition between the sigmoid sinus and jugular bulb (Fig. 5.7a). Further lateral exposure of the jugular bulb can be better achieved using a lateral technique, such as a transtemporal approach.

Lateral to the jugular foramen, at the anteroinferior end of the digastric groove, is the stylomastoid foramen bearing the facial nerve. To gain access to the mastoid segment of the facial nerve and the presigmoid dura in the transmastoid variant, the posterior mastoid is removed up to the facial canal (Fig. 5.7b). The sigmoid sinus can then be retracted laterally.

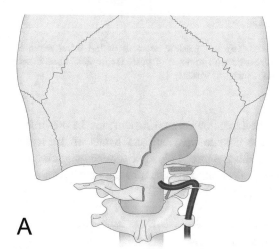

A

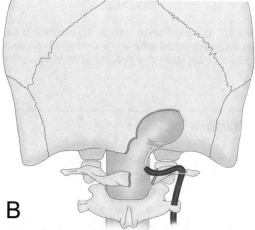

B

Fig. 5.6 The supracondylar variants. (**a**) The supracondylar variant increases rostral exposure while preserving the articular surface of the condyle. The shaded region denotes exposed cancellous bone below the hypoglossal canal. (**b**) Removal of the jugular tubercle in the transtubercular variant provides access to the pre-pontomedullary region. The edge of bone that is removed is depicted by the *dotted line*, and the intradural course of the cranial nerves exiting the jugular foramen is shown in *yellow*

Table 5.1 Comparison of the cranio-orbital and transtubercular approaches

	Cranio-orbital	Transtubercular
Craniotomy	Frontotemporal	Far lateral
Blood supply	Superficial temporal artery	Occipital artery
Muscle	Temporalis	Suboccipital muscle group
Bony obstacle (outer)	Greater sphenoid wing	Foramen magnum
Bony obstacle (middle)	Lesser sphenoid wing	Occipital condyle
Bony obstacle (inner)	Anterior clinoid process	Jugular tubercle
"Buried" nerve	Optic nerve	Hypoglossal nerve
Nerves at risk	Superior orbital fissure contents	Jugular foramen contents
Nearby artery	ICA (clinoidal and supraclinoid segments)	VA (V3 and V4 segments)
Nearby venous lake	Cavernous sinus	Jugular bulb
Connecting venous channel	Clinoidal space	Condylar emissary vein

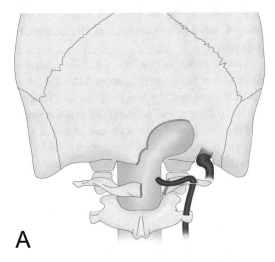

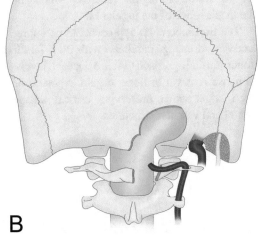

A

B

Fig. 5.7 The paracondylar variants. (**a**) Removal of the jugular process lateral to the occipital condyle in the transjugular variant exposes the posterior aspect of the jugular bulb. (**b**) The mastoid segment of the facial nerve is exposed with removal of posterior mastoid bone in the transmastoid variant

Intradural Exposure

The dura is opened as an inverted-U with the medial limb extending inferiorly across the foramen magnum opening, and retracted laterally (Fig. 5.8a). Variations such as a low or medial sigmoid sinus or transdural PICA must be recognized. Brisk bleeding may arise from a prominent marginal sinus. If the vertebral artery has been mobilized medially, the dura is opened while maintaining a circumferential cuff at its penetration; the posterior spinal artery may be incorpo-

rated into this fibrous ring and must be preserved. The dentate ligament and bands of arachnoid membrane are divided to create windows for visualization and access to the target pathology (Fig. 5.8b).

Conclusions

The modifications of the far lateral technique that are incorporated into any procedure are determined by the location and extent of pathology and the specific anatomy of each patient

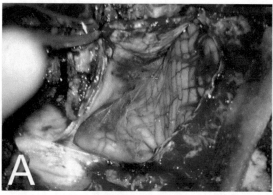
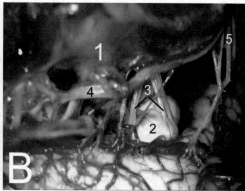

Fig. 5.8 Intradural exposure achieved with the far lateral approach. (**a**) The dural flap is retracted laterally to ensure the widest exposure is maintained. Note the low profile of the dural base achieved by the extradural bone removal.

(**b**) The far lateral approach provides access to pathology such as a VA-PICA aneurysm. Dural penetration of vertebral artery (*1*), upper rootlets of hypoglossal nerve (*2*), spinal accessory nerve (*3*), aneurysm at PICA origin (*4*)

Table 5.2 Summary of the exposure obtained with variants of the far lateral approach

Approach	Indications
Basic far lateral	Lateral/anterolateral foramen magnum
Transcondylar	
Occipito-transcondylar	Lower clivus, pre-medullary space
Atlanto-occipital	Vertebral artery at dural ring
Complete transcondylar	Anterior foramen magnum
Supracondylar	
Hypoglossal canal	Lateral lower clivus
Transtubercular	Pre-pontomedullary space, high PICA origin
Paracondylar	
Transjugular	Posterior jugular bulb
Transmastoid	Presigmoid dura, mastoid segment of facial nerve

(Table 5.2). The basic far lateral exposure may often be sufficient to access lesions along the anterolateral margin of the foramen magnum. The greatest gain in visualization is obtained with removal of the jugular tubercle [4], and the risk of injury to cranial nerves and the jugular bulb in carrying out this step may be justified in some cases. Posterior partial condylectomy increases visualization to only a small extent, but provides much improved freedom for surgical manipulation; this step can be performed with relatively low morbidity [5].

References

1. Fine AD, Cardoso A, Rhoton AL Jr. Microsurgical anatomy of the extracranial-extradural origin of the posterior inferior cerebellar artery. J Neurosurg. 1999;91(4):645–52.
2. Wen HT, Rhoton AL Jr, Katsuta T, de Oliveira E. Microsurgical anatomy of the transcondylar, supracondylar, and paracondylar extensions of the far-lateral approach. J Neurosurg. 1997;87(4):555–85.
3. Vishteh AG, Crawford NR, Melton MS, Spetzler RF, Sonntag VK, Dickman CA. Stability of the craniovertebral junction after unilateral occipital condyle resection: a biomechanical study. J Neurosurg. 1999;90(1 Suppl):91–8.
4. Spektor S, Anderson GJ, McMenomey SO, Horgan MA, Kellogg JX, Delashaw JB Jr. Quantitative description of the far-lateral transcondylar transtubercular approach to the foramen magnum and clivus. J Neurosurg. 2000;92(5):824–31.
5. Bertalanffy H, Seeger W. The dorsolateral, suboccipital, transcondylar approach to the lower clivus and anterior portion of the craniocervical junction. Neurosurgery. 1991;29(6):815–21.

Endoscopic Endonasal Approach for Posterior Fossa Tumors

6

André Beer-Furlan, Alexandre B. Todeschini, Ricardo L. Carrau, and Daniel M. Prevedello

Introduction

Driven by the revolution of endoscopic pituitary surgery, the development of the expanded endoscopic endonasal approach (EEA) and the associated surgical tools have pushed the limits of transnasal access to the ventral skull base. The EEA rapidly became a safe alternative in the armamentarium of skull base approaches, and it has been increasingly used in the management of ventral extradural and intradural posterior fossa tumors. It provides the advantage of direct access to pathologies with near-field magnification while minimizing manipulation of neurovascular structures and avoiding brain retraction, ultimately decreasing morbidity [1–5].

A. Beer-Furlan
Neurological Surgery, Rush University Medical Center, 1725 W. Harrison St. Suite 855, Chicago, IL 60612, USA
e-mail: andre_beerfurlan@rush.edu

A.B. Todeschini • D.M. Prevedello (✉)
Neurological Surgery, The Ohio State University, 410 West 10th Avenue, Columbus, OH 43210, USA
e-mail: abtodeschini@gmail.com;
Daniel.Prevedello@osumc.edu

R.L. Carrau
Department of Otolaryngology, The Ohio State University Wexner Medical Center, 320 West 10th Avenue, B221, Columbus, OH 43210, USA
e-mail: Ricardo.Carrau@osumc.edu

In this chapter, the ventral posterior cranial fossa tumors are divided in "extradural" and "intradural" due to the differences in approach selection, surgical strategy, complexity of the surgery and microsurgical dissection, and skull base reconstruction depending of the site of origin and type of tumor.

The "extradural" posterior fossa tumor group is represented by chordomas and chondrosarcomas. Although sometimes there is intradural tumor extension (Figs. 6.1 and 6.2), chordomas and chondrosarcomas are mainly located extradurally within the skull base bone. Hence, a significant part of the tumor resection is done during the bone work of the approach. In addition, the tumor resection is often completed without a cerebrospinal fluid leak facilitating skull base reconstruction and reducing postoperative complications.

The "intradural" posterior fossa tumors that are suitable to EEA resection are represented mainly by meningiomas (Fig. 6.3). In general, EEA for intradural tumors involves more challenging microsurgical dissection and skull base reconstruction. Ventral posterior fossa intradural epidermoid and dermoid cysts may be resected through EEA, but our previous experience suggests that the transnasal corridor may increase the risk of infection and abscess occurrence within the residual tumor, so we do not recommend it. Schwannomas are also another common type of intradural posterior fossa tumor.

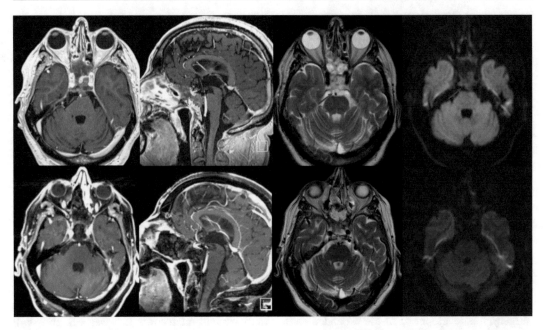

Fig. 6.1 Recurrent chordoma in a 61-year-old male patient. Patient underwent an upper and middle transclival EEA to remove the tumor (*red arrows*). A small dural invasion and opening into the posterior fossa was observed in the preoperative images. The postoperative MRI shows Duragen occluding the opening and protecting the basilar artery and brainstem (*first layer*), covered with a free fat graft (*second layer*) and the nasoseptal flap on top (*third layer*). Notice in the DWI image pre (*upper row*)- and post (*lower row*)-operative that the hyperintensity suggesting a high cellular density is no longer present in the postoperative image

Nevertheless, the EEA cannot be used to treat the most common posterior fossa schwannomas that arise from CN VIII based on the fact that the cranial nerve VII is anteriorly located and would prevent a ventral approach. Likewise, the EEA is not an adequate approach to less common schwannomas (CN VII, IX, X, XI) since they arise at the lateral aspect of the brainstem with the inferior cranial nerves pushed ventrally. Anatomically, there is a potential application of this approach in the treatment of schwannomas of CN VI and CNXII, but these are extremely rare tumors that even when diagnosed may be managed conservatively.

Endoscopic Endonasal Transclival Approach

The endoscopic transnasal access to the posterior fossa is done through a transclival approach. It may be expanded laterally on the petrous bone depending on the tumor extent and required exposure. The clivus separates the nasopharynx from the posterior cranial fossa. It is composed of the posterior portion of the sphenoid body (basisphenoid) and the basilar part of the occipital bone (basiocciput), and it is further subdivided into upper, middle, and lower thirds:

- Upper clivus is at the level of the sphenoid sinus and is formed by the basisphenoid bone including the dorsum sella.
- Middle clivus corresponds to the rostral part of the basiocciput, and it is located above a line connecting the caudal ends of the petroclival fissures.
- Lower clivus is formed by the caudal part of the basiocciput.

Approaching the posterior fossa through the upper two thirds of the clivus requires wide opening of the sphenoid sinus. When the posterior fossa was approached at the lower clivus, the bone removal may be done solely below the sphenoid rostrum.

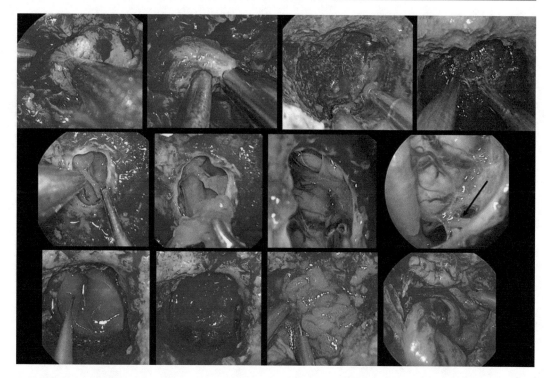

Fig. 6.2 Recurrent chordoma in a 61-year-old male. (**a, b**) Tumor and scar tissue in front of the clivus being removed. (**c**) Clivus drilling. (**d**) Dural opening and posterior fossa invasion. (**e**) Microsurgical dissection and removal of the tumor from the basilar artery. (**f, g**) Cranial nerves no longer covered by the tumor. (**h, i**) Duragen "plug." (**j**) Fat-free graft. (**k**) Nasoseptal flap being placed

The intracranial surface of the upper two thirds of the clivus faces the pons and is concave from side to side. The extracranial surface of the clivus gives rise to the pharyngeal tubercle at the junction of the middle and lower clivus. The upper clivus faces the roof of the nasopharynx that extends downward in the midline to the level of the pharyngeal tubercle.

The upper and middle clivus are separated from the petrous portion of the temporal bone on each side by the petroclival fissure. The basilar venous plexus is situated between the two layers of the dura of the upper clivus and is related to the dorsum sella and the posterior wall of the sphenoid sinus. It forms interconnecting venous channels between the inferior petrosal sinuses laterally, the cavernous sinuses superiorly, and the marginal sinus and epidural venous plexus inferiorly. The basilar sinus is the largest communicating channel between the paired cavernous sinuses [6].

Extradural Posterior Fossa Tumors

Chondrosarcomas and Chordomas

Chondrosarcomas are rare slow-growing malignant bone tumor of chondroid origin cells throughout the axial and appendicular skeleton (Fig. 6.4) [7–9]. They often arise from the lateral aspects of the skull base that house cartilage, including the temporo-occipital synchondrosis, the spheno-occiput, and the sphenoethmoid complex [10]. Most skull base chondrosarcomas involve the clivus (32%), followed by other synchondroses [11]. They can also involve the cavernous sinus, petrous bone, and sphenoid bone. In the skull base, 64% arise in the middle fossa, 14% involve both middle and posterior fossa, 14% occur in the anterior fossa, and 7% originate in the posterior fossa [7].

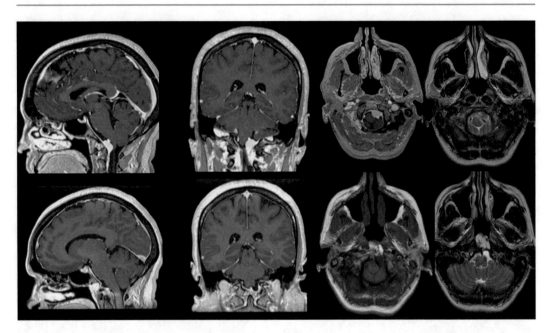

Fig. 6.3 Ventral foramen magnum meningioma in a 47-year-old female patient. Patient underwent a lower transclival EEA for removal of the lesion (*red arrows*). Postoperative MRI shows a gross total resection with the multilayered reconstructions of the small clival opening

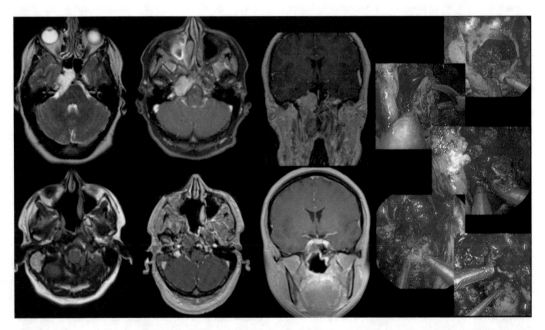

Fig. 6.4 Right side chondrosarcoma in a 32-year-old female patient (*red arrows*). Patient underwent an EEA for total resection. Notice in the surgical images the access is limited by the Eustachian tube that is then removed allowing an adequate access to the tumor and gross total resection

Chordomas are rare primary bone tumor thought to arise from transformed notochord remnants with an estimated incidence rate of 0.08–0.09 per 100,000. It occurs most commonly in males with a peak incidence in their fourth to fifth decades of life and rarely affects children and adolescents. Skull base chordomas are essentially midline lesions that occur at the vicinity of the clivus (spheno-occipital bones) and represent only 0.15% of all intracranial tumors [8]. They are considered a low-malignancy neoplasm with slow-growing pattern that rarely metastasizes. However, chordomas have a local aggressive behavior and high recurrence rates [11–13].

The slow-growing nature of most skull base chordomas and chondrosarcomas often leads to variable presentation of clinical signs and symptoms based on the location of the tumor. Treatment goals should involve complete surgical resection that should be tempered with a judicious effort to avoid neurological compromise. The extent of surgical resection correlates directly with recurrence rates. Among all chordoma patients, median survival is 6.29 years with 5-, 10-, and 20-year survival rates precipitously dropping to 67.6%, 39.9%, and 13.1% across all races and genders underscoring the dismal prognosis of this disease. Nonsurgical management or observation may be reserved for some patients who are high-risk surgical candidates. Chondrosarcomas tend to have a slightly better prognosis and are regarded to be less aggressive with higher recurrence-free survival rates when compared to chordoma. In one study, recurrence-free survival at 5 years was as high as 90%. Surgical and postoperative management goals of chordomas and chondrosarcomas are often very similar, and case series often report results for both these pathologies together because of the rarity of the diseases.

While aggressive gross total resection may be achieved through a variety of skull base approaches including EEA (Fig. 6.4), en bloc resection may not be feasible in the skull base as has been described in the spine due to involvement of critical neurovascular structures, with surgeons most often resorting to piecemeal removal of the tumor. Based on available clinical case series from experienced skull base surgeons, aggressive surgical resection is only possible 48–61% of the time underscoring the technical challenge that surgeons have with treatment of tumors in this location. As a result, radiation treatment has played an important role in the postoperative management of these patients.

Preoperative Radiological Assessment

Radiologic investigation and preoperative planning for skull base approaches of chordomas and chondrosarcomas have greatly improved because of rapidly evolving imaging methods. Computed tomography (CT) and magnetic resonance imaging (MRI) should always be performed in cases of suspected skull base bone lesion for bone and soft tissue assessment, respectively. The combination of these two radiologic modalities permits the definition of important diagnostic and therapeutic characteristics of skull base tumors: radiologic appearance, location, extension, and relation to critical neurovascular structures.

Chordomas and chondrosarcomas have an overall similar appearance on MRI, and sometimes it is impossible to differentiate them without histopathology. In general, chordomas typically present as midline extradural masses originating within bone and tend to expand posteriorly and laterally. They usually present as well-delineated soft tissue masses that may displace and compress adjacent structures. More advanced tumors show local invasiveness and characteristic bone destruction.

The CT scans demonstrate best bone erosion, osteolysis, and intratumoral calcifications. There is typically no surrounding sclerosis. Moderate to marked heterogeneous enhancement following administration of iodinated contrast material can also be depicted. Most chordomas are hypointense or isointense on T1-weighted images. High signal correlates with hemorrhage or mucinous collection. T2-weighted images characteristically demonstrate a high signal. Gadolinium enhancement is mostly heterogeneous and often presents a "honeycomb" appearance [14].

Chondroid chordomas represent 5–15% of all chordomas and are characterized by the partial replacement of their gelatinous matrix by cartilaginous tissue. Compared with typical chordomas, they normally present in a more lateral position, and intratumoral calcifications are more often evidenced on CT scans. Because of the differences in composition, chondroid chordomas may not appear as bright as typical chordomas on T2-weighted MRIs. These findings are important prognostic factors because of significantly better survival rates of patients with chondroid chordomas.

In chondrosarcomas, CT scan demonstrates bony destruction of the skull base lateral to the midline; the typical appearance is a destructive lesion with scalloped erosive borders. Like in chordomas, the tumor has a low to intermediate signal intensity on T1-weighted images and high signal intensity on T2-weighted images. The enhancement is usually marked, and signal heterogeneity post-contrast is observed frequently because of matrix mineralization and prominent fibrocartilaginous elements within the tumor.

Imaging studies have an important role in defining diagnosis and planning the surgical approach. Angiographic studies (CTA, MRA, or conventional) are important whenever vascular compromise is suspected. The presence of arterial displacement or encasement must be assessed before surgery, so the dissection and debulking of the tumor can proceed safely. Arterial narrowing is highly suggestive of adventitia invasion, which hinders a total resection when the encased artery cannot be sacrificed. Despite not being routinely performed for skull base bone lesions, conventional angiography studies may help to define whether sacrifice of an encased artery is possible or not by defining the patient's tolerance and collateral flow on balloon test occlusion.

The location and extension of the skull base lesion determines the pattern of CN displacement and involvement, hence the surgical corridors available for tumor resection. New MRI technologies (fast imaging with steady-state precession and fast imaging using steady-state acquisition) now permit clear identification of the CN and its relationship to the skull base lesion, instead of simply assuming it based on the extension and position of the tumor [14].

Approach Selection

The main approaches to the skull base are divided into anterior (transbasal, transsphenoidal, transoral, and EEA), anterolateral (pterional and orbitozygomatic), lateral (subtemporal and anterior petrosal), and posterolateral approaches (posterior petrosal, suboccipital retrosigmoid, and transcondylar). In the past decades, the microsurgical anterior approaches were gradually replaced by the expanded EEA.

Because of the midline origin of the skull base chordomas, the endoscopic endonasal transclival approach is frequently the first and best option when defining the surgical route. As a general rule, a second approach should always be considered in chordomas with lateral extension. Exceptions for not choosing the EEA as the first surgical route are inability to resolve the patient's main neurologic signs and symptoms through the EEA, need for cranio-cervical junction stabilization/fusion, and impossibility to adequately reconstruct the resulting skull base defect.

Chondrosarcomas tend to have a paramedian origin at petroclival synchondrosis, and the approach selection is based on tumor extension (midline vs. lateral vs. superior) and patient's symptoms. Since the majority of these tumors start on the petroclival synchondrosis, there is a major advantage on using the EEA route to reach these tumors primarily. The midline location of the tumor extension further facilitates an EEA. The lateral extensions of these tumors are followed from a midline to lateral approach behind the ICA and frequently can be completely resected via EEA (Fig. 6.4).

The first and the best surgical approach for chondrosarcomas is the one that will provide maximal tumor resection and/or improvement of the patient's symptoms. Most of the time, the EEA is the initial and ideal surgical approach that may be combined to a lateral or posterolateral approach when lateral residual tumor cannot be reached.

The Role of EEA

Endoscopic endonasal approaches provide the most direct access to the ventral skull base. Chondrosarcomas (usually originated at the petroclival region) and chordomas (originated at midline clivus) tend to displace neurovascular elements laterally, superiorly, and posteriorly. For that reason we advocate the use of EEA as the initial surgical corridor. In a single procedure, EEA allows access to multiple skull base compartments avoiding extensive retraction of neurovascular structures. It also allows extensive drilling of the clivus, sphenoid bone, and petrous portions of the temporal bone, which are frequently invaded by tumor.

For lesions located in the upper petroclival region, cavernous sinus, and middle cranial fossa, the transsphenoidal approach with removal of the sphenoid and temporal bony encasement is indicated. Tumors extending in the middle third of the clivus can be approached through a transsphenoidal approach associated to clivectomy and petrosectomy. Lesions in the lower clivus and infratemporal fossa extension require a transpterygoid approach.

Depending on the location of the tumor, some other following steps may be necessary. Tumors located inferior to the petrous apex may require removal or mobilization of the Eustachian tube (Fig. 6.4). Removing the pterygoid processes and adjacent musculature can provide access to the infratemporal fossa. In order to gain access to the anterior portion of Meckel's cave and medial middle cranial fossa, the lateral sphenoid recess must be accessed [15].

Chondrosarcomas and chordomas are often soft; however, it sometimes can be hard and very calcified. Usually, extensive bone removal to expose the whole tumor is done before soft tumor resection. Lateralization of the ICA allows the removal of the paramedian tumor located on the petroclival synchondrosis. Dissection within the cavernous sinus, jugular foramen, infratemporal fossa, and high cervical region is performed using stimulating dissectors to prevent cranial nerve injuries.

Intradural Posterior Fossa Tumors

Meningiomas

The role of the expanded EEA in the management of ventral posterior fossa meningiomas is still restricted due to limited surgical indications in selected cases [16]. However, when surgery is well indicated, the surgeon may benefit from the advantages of EEA such as direct access to ventral skull base pathologies avoiding brain and brainstem retraction, near-field magnification, better surgical field illumination, and minimal manipulation of neurovascular structures [1–5].

Nevertheless, unlike the EEA to sellar pathology, there is a relative paucity of literature regarding endoscopic management of posterior fossa meningiomas. The probable reason is the combination of limiting factors including rarity of the pathology and the indication of approaching it through an EEA, technical challenges in tumor resection and skull base reconstruction, expertise of the surgical team, and available resources [16].

The current literature involving the endoscopic management of posterior fossa meningiomas consists in the collective experience of an approach rather than experience with the particular type of tumor [16–25].

Ventral posterior fossa meningiomas are challenging lesions to manage independently of the selected surgical approach and are unique tumors in the type of pathological displacement of the surrounding anatomy. Despite the recent reports demonstrating the role of radiation therapy on their management, surgical resection continues to be the first and best treatment method aiming the permanent tumor eradication [26, 27].

The surgical outcomes for petroclival meningiomas, regardless of the approach used, have greatly improved over the past decades with the development of better microsurgical technique, intraoperative monitoring, and radiological imaging. Nevertheless, it is still associated with significant morbidity specially regarding new cranial nerve palsies or persisting/worsening of preexisting palsies that range from 39% to 76% of the patients [28–31].

Preoperative Radiological Assessment

The evolution of imaging studies improved the preoperative information on the pathological anatomy of the tumors, enabling surgeons to plan the best approach or combination of approaches to resect the tumor safely. The radiological preoperative investigation for a meningioma should always include a computed tomography angiography (CTA) and a magnetic resonance imaging (MRI) for bone, vascular, and soft tissue assessment, respectively [32–35].

It is essential to identify the primary base of the meningioma and understand the growth pattern of the tumor and displacement of surrounding neurovascular structures. It may help predict intraoperative difficulties due to pathological anatomy, and it is crucial on the approach selection [36–39].

The T1-weighted with gadolinium-enhanced contrast imaging is the best MRI sequence to define the dural attachment site ("dural tail") of the meningioma. Although MRI provides superior soft tissue assessment, the CT scan with bone window remains the tool of choice for identifying calcification, hyperostosis, and osseous anatomy. Frequently, a hyperostotic bone is found at the primary base of the tumor. Additionally, the CT scan bone assessment provides a better idea of the surgical corridor available and allows planning of the extent of bone removal necessary for tumor resection [16].

The vascular relationships to the petroclival meningiomas may be evaluated through angiographic studies (CTA, MRA, or conventional angiography). The presence of arterial encasement must be assessed before surgery so the internal debulking of the tumor can proceed safely. The arterial narrowing is highly suggestive of adventitia invasion, which hinders a total resection when the encased artery cannot be sacrificed. The conventional angiography may also help to define whether sacrifice of the encased artery is possible by defining collateral flow and the patient's tolerance to balloon occlusion test.

The cranial nerve positioning is crucial to define the limit of the surgical corridors available for tumor resection. As mentioned previously, the primary base of the meningioma determines the pattern of cranial nerve displacement. The evolution of MRI (steady-state free precession imaging and diffusion tension imaging improvements) permitted clear identification of the cranial nerves, instead of assuming its position based on the origin of the tumor [40, 41]. With a better understanding of the cranial nerve positioning in relation to the tumor, one can define if an EEA, a craniotomy, or a combination of both is the best approach. In general, it is the position of the VI cranial nerve and the XII cranial nerves that will determine if the ideal approach is anteromedial (EEA) or posterolateral (eg, petrosectomy, far lateral).

Once the choice of an EEA is made, the preoperative radiological assessment of the nasosinusal region is imperative. A CT scan with fine imaging cuts provides information on the patient anatomy such as nasal septum deviations, integrity and degree of aeration of the paranasal sinuses (particularly the sphenoid sinus), location and presence of intersinus septa, presence of an Onodi cell, presence and extent of bone erosions, dehiscence or hyperostosis of the skull base, position of the internal carotid arteries, and thickness and incline of the clivus (basal angle) [16].

Pathological Anatomy

Petroclival Meningiomas

The petroclival meningiomas have its primary base at the petroclival fissure and have a particular displacement pattern of surrounding structures. They tend to dislocate the cranial nerves V, VII, VIII, IX, X, and XI posteriorly. The cranial nerve VI most times it is displaced medially, however a careful analysis of MRI is necessary to confirm that. The brainstem is medially and posteriorly dislocated.

The main advantage of approaching these tumors through an anterior route is the posterior displacement of the majority of the cranial nerves. However, the medial displacement of CN VI may pose a significant surgical difficulty, and its injury risk must be weighted in the case selection. Situations where the tumor is more superiorly positioned (e.g., lateral *dorsum sellae* origin), CN VI is pushed inferiorly allowing an EEA to be performed. Similarly, when the tumor has a more inferior origin, as it occurs when centered on the *tuberculum jugulare*, the CN VI may be pushed superiorly allowing an EEA to be performed safely as well.

There are situations that CN VI is simply traveling through the tumor and a combination of approaches may be the more adequate solution. The midline component of these tumors is prone for an EEA resection, whereas the lateral component can be accessed by a retrosigmoid, presigmoid, or anterior petrosectomy approach.

Nevertheless, petroclival meningiomas are unlikely to be completely removed through an endoscopic transclival approach due to its paramedian origin. The exception is for the rare retroclival tumors, where the entire tumor is medial to the CN VI as explained below. In general, petroclival meningiomas should be considered in combination with a posterior or lateral surgical routes or when the surgical goal is brainstem decompression.

Clival Meningiomas

Clival meningiomas have their primary base at the midline. They tend to displace CN V laterally and superiorly; CN VI laterally and posteriorly; CNs VII, VIII, IX, X, and XI posteriorly; CN XII posteriorly and inferiorly; and the brainstem posteriorly. The primary base and pattern of displacement make clival meningiomas ideal for the EEA.

Foramen Magnum Meningiomas

The foramen magnum meningiomas may be cranial or spinocranial lesions. The spinocranial meningiomas have its origin below the foramen magnum and thereby displace the cranial nerves and the vertebral arteries to the superior pole of the tumor. On the other hand, the cranial lesions may have its origin anywhere at the foramen magnum with different patterns of structure dislocation.

Tumors with primary base at the poster border of the foramen magnum are easily accessed through a posterior surgical route. If the origin is at the lateral border of the foramen magnum, between the jugular and hypoglossal foramina, CN XII will be found medial and CNs IX, X, and XI laterally.

These tumors are also better approached through a posterior or lateral surgical route.

The anterior cranial lesions originating at the anterior border of the foramen magnum are suited for the EEA (Fig. 6.3). Its origin is medial to the hypoglossal and jugular foramen, so the displacements pattern of all the cranial nerves is posteriorly and laterally. However, the cervical extension of these tumors may pose a limitation for the EEA because of the cranio-cervical instability associated with the removal of anterior arch of C1, C2 odontoid process, and its ligamentous complex. Therefore, a posterior approach is usually the choice for a single- or first-stage surgery for ventral foramen magnum meningiomas that extend inferiorly to C1 and C2 levels.

EEA Indications in Posterior Fossa Meningiomas

The general surgical indications for any posterior fossa meningiomas are symptomatic lesions, asymptomatic large volume lesion, and tumor growth on radiological follow-up.

The tumors with major portion of its dural base located at the midline of the clival region are the ones favorable for resection through an expanded EEA.

Contraindications for EEA in petroclival and clival meningiomas include patient comorbidities precluding those from prolonged general anesthesia, major dural attachment located laterally, vascular encasement, unfavorable anatomy for transsphenoidal surgery, and lack of specialized equipment/instruments.

Advantages and Limitations

The main advantages of approaching the ventral posterior fossa through an endoscopic transclival approach include the ability to avoid any cerebral retraction and decrease the incidence of injury to the cranial nerves. It enables the tumor resection without crossing the cranial nerves [4, 13, 42, 43].

In addition, the approach utilizes a natural corridor providing direct and relatively quick access to the tumor. The early access to the meningioma vascular supply (cranial base dura) can greatly reduce intraoperative blood loss and facilitate removal. Further advantages of this approach include removal of involved bone and dura as a part of the approach, which allows a Simpson Grade I resection. The surgeons must be very careful when indicating an EEA for a petroclival meningioma as the cranial nerve VI may be pushed medially blocking the safe access. The cases where CN VI is pushed inferiorly (dorsum sellae meningiomas) or superiorly (tuberculum jugulare meningioma) are potential good indications for EEA. For the situations where the CN VI is inside the tumor, we believe that a combination of approaches is more appropriate for safe management of the tumor. We usually start with the approach that will give us access to most of the base of the tumor in order to provide better devascularization. In these cases a retrosigmoid approach would be indicated if most of the tumor is based on the petrous surface and a second-stage EEA would address the medial component. On the other hand, a tumor with a wide clival base would be approached with an EEA transclival approach primarily followed by a retrosigmoid, far lateral, presigmoid, or anterior petrosectomy to complement the resection depending on the position of the residual tumor.

Although endoscopes do not allow a three-dimensional perspective, they do provide a close and wide view of the operative field from different angles. However, endoscopes only allow for a narrow operative field, which is surrounded by critical neurovascular structures making the risks of major intradural bleeding, CSF leakage, and neural damage still possible [20].

The main disadvantages of EEA are related to the resection of lateral extension of tumors and the reconstruction of large dural and bone defects of the posterior fossa, being CSF leak rates quite high (ranging between 4% and 33.3%) [18, 42, 44].

The expanded EEA, in its current form, is not a substitute of the posterior skull base approaches in the treatment of ventral posterior fossa meningiomas. It is a safe alternative for the rare cases of meningiomas with most part of its dural base at the midline clival region, and it may be used as solely or combination of other approaches. Thus, appropriate case selection may optimize the advantages of the approach and reduce morbidity of this complex pathology.

Skull Base Reconstruction

Skull base defects can be divided into extradural and intradural. Intradural defects are further subdivided into low- or high-flow leaks. A high-flow CSF leak is defined by the communication of multiple subarachnoid cisterns or a ventricle with the dural defect. Extradural defects are defined by the resection of the skull base bone with an intact dura and, therefore, no CSF leak. Reconstruction following resection of ventral posterior fossa lesions is particularly challenging due to the lack of gravity effect given the vertical position of the brainstem, which limits the support available for the reconstruction provided by the weight of the brain and supporting bony structures to stabilize inlay grafts, in addition to the associated large dural defects with the risk for high-flow CSF leaks [45].

Regardless of the approach, the goals of reconstruction of skull base defects are the same and include:

- Water and airtight closure to prevent CSF leak, pneumocephalus, meningitis, and other intracranial infections.
- Complete separation of the cranial cavity and the brain from the sinonasal tract.
- Protection of the brain, cranial nerves, and intracranial vessels from desiccation and infection.
- Accelerate the healing process especially if the patient is scheduled to undergo postoperative external beam irradiation.
- Preservation and rehabilitation of function.
- Preservation or restoration of cosmesis.
- Avoidance of dead spaces that may contribute to hematomas and infection.

Critical factors to be considered when reconstructing defects following the resection of skull base lesions are the size and location of the bony and dural defect, high- versus low-flow CSF leaks, prior radiation therapy or scheduled postoperative radiotherapy, previous sinonasal or skull base surgery, extent of invasion of sinonasal structures, morbid obesity and obstructive sleep apnea (requiring CPAP), and possibility of increased CSF pressure as suggested by imaging findings (e.g., dilated ventricles, empty sella, dilated optic nerves). Finally, the route for tumor resection should be adequate to reconstruct the skull base, thus avoiding the morbidity of a second approach.

The authors favor reconstruction of skull base defects using pedicled vascular flaps, multilayer reconstruction techniques, and the aforementioned principles, especially for central skull base defects. However, multiple options are available to reconstruct the skull base bone and dura and can be divided in free grafts, synthetic/heterologous materials, and vascularized flaps.

Free autografts imply the harvesting of tissue from a donor site that is then transferred and implanted in a recipient site. They lack their own vascularization as there is no attachment to the donor site; therefore, they require a well-vascularized recipient bed to optimize the take of the graft. Commonly used free autografts include the following: free mucoperiosteal/ mucoperichondrial autograft, autologous fascia lata graft, free fat autograft, free cartilage autograft, and free bone autograft. The synthetic and heterologous materials most commonly used are collagen matrix and acellular dermal matrix processed from banked human cadaver skin [45].

There are numerous vascularized flaps that can be used to reconstruct the ventral skull base, and they are divided into intranasal or local and extranasal or regional. The main intranasal flaps that are suitable for reconstruction of petroclival defects include the nasoseptal flap, the posteriorly based lateral nasal wall flap, and the inferior turbinate flap. The main extranasal flaps are the temporoparietal fascia flap and the pericranial flap. Lumbar drain is not used routinely, but may be considered in large posterior fossa dural defects [45].

References

1. Jho HD, Carrau RL. Endoscopic endonasal transsphenoidal surgery: experience with 50 patients. J Neurosurg. 1997;87(1):44–51.
2. Cavallo LM, Messina A, Cappabianca P, Esposito F, de Divitiis E, Gardner P, Tschabitscher M. Endoscopic endonasal surgery of the midline skull base: anatomical study and clinical considerations. Neurosurg Focus. 2005;19(1):1–4.
3. Kassam A, Snyderman CH, Mintz A, Gardner P, Carrau RL. Expanded endonasal approach: the rostrocaudal axis. Part I. Crista galli to the sella turcica. Neurosurg Focus. 2005;19(1):1–2.
4. Kassam A, Snyderman CH, Mintz A, Gardner P, Carrau RL. Expanded endonasal approach: the rostrocaudal axis. Part II. Posterior clinoids to the foramen magnum. Neurosurg Focus. 2005;19(1):1–7.
5. Beer-Furlan A, Evins AI, Rigante L, Anichini G, Stieg PE, Bernardo A. Dual-port 2D and 3D endoscopy: expanding the limits of the endonasal approaches to midline skull base lesions with lateral extension. J Neurol Surg Part B: Skull Base. 2014;75(03):187–97.
6. Bailey BJ, Johnson JT, Newlands SD, editors. Head & neck surgery – otolaryngology. Philadelphia: Lippincott Williams & Wilkins; 2006. p. 3855–76.
7. Bloch O, Parsa AT. Skull base chondrosarcoma: evidence-based treatment paradigms. Neurosurg Clin N Am. 2013;24(1):89–96.
8. Brackmann DE, Teufert KB. Chondrosarcoma of the skull base: long-term follow-up. Otol Neurotol. 2006;27(7):981–91.
9. Uhl M, Mattke M, Welzel T, Oelmann J, Habl G, Jensen AD, Ellerbrock M, Haberer T, Herfarth KK, Debus J. High control rate in patients with chondrosarcoma of the skull base after carbon ion therapy: first report of long-term results. Cancer. 2014;120(10):1579–85.
10. Jones PS, Aghi MK, Muzikansky A, Shih HA, Barker FG, Curry WT. Outcomes and patterns of care in adult skull base chondrosarcomas from the SEER database. J Clin Neurosci. 2014;21(9):1497–502.
11. Frassanito P, Massimi L, Rigante M, Tamburrini G, Conforti G, Di Rocco C, Caldarelli M. Recurrent and self-remitting sixth cranial nerve palsy: pathophysiological insight from skull base chondrosarcoma: report of 2 cases. J Neurosurg Pediatr. 2013;12(6):633–6.
12. Bailey BJ, Johnson JT, Newlands SD, editors. Head & neck surgery – otolaryngology. Philadelphia: Lippincott Williams & Wilkins; 2006. p. 1725–44.
13. Frank G, Sciarretta V, Calbucci F, Farneti G, Mazzatenta D, Pasquini E. The endoscopic transnasal transsphenoidal approach for the treatment of cranial base chordomas and chondrosarcomas. Neurosurgery. 2006;59(1):ONS-50.
14. Mangussi-Gomes J, Beer-Furlan A, Balsalobre L, Vellutini EA, Stamm AC. Endoscopic endonasal management of skull base chordomas: surgical technique, nuances, and pitfalls. Otolaryngol Clin N Am. 2016;49(1):167–82.
15. Qiu QH, Liang MZ, Liu H, Chen SH, Zhang HB, Zhang QH. Nasal endoscopic surgical treatment for chondrosarcoma of paranasal sinus and the skull base. Zhonghua er bi yan hou tou jing wai ke za zhi Chin J Otorhinolaryngol Head Neck Surg. 2010;45(7):551–4.

16. Beer-Furlan A, Vellutini EA, Balsalobre L, Stamm AC. Endoscopic endonasal approach to ventral posterior fossa meningiomas: from case selection to surgical management. Neurosurg Clin N Am. 2015;26(3):413–26.

17. Gardner PA, Kassam AB, Thomas A, Snyderman CH, Carrau RL, Mintz AH, Prevedello DM. Endoscopic endonasal resection of anterior cranial base meningiomas. Neurosurgery. 2008;63(1):36–54.

18. Fraser JF, Nyquist GG, Moore N, Anand VK, Schwartz TH. Endoscopic endonasal minimal access approach to the clivus: case series and technical nuances. Oper Neurosurg. 2010;67(3):ons150–8.

19. Alexander H, Robinson S, Wickremesekera A, Wormald PJ. Endoscopic transsphenoidal resection of a mid-clival meningioma. J Clin Neurosci. 2010;17(3):374–6.

20. Prosser JD, Vender JR, Alleyne CH, Solares CA. Expanded endoscopic endonasal approaches to skull base meningiomas. J Neurol Surg Part B: Skull Base. 2012;73(03):147–56.

21. Fernandez-Miranda JC, Gardner PA, Rastelli MM Jr, Peris-Celda M, Koutourousiou M, Peace D, Snyderman CH, Rhoton AL Jr. Endoscopic endonasal transcavernous posterior clinoidectomy with interdural pituitary transposition: technical note. J Neurosurg. 2014;121(1):91–9.

22. Julian JA, Álvarez PS, Lloret PM, Ramirez EP, Borreda PP, Asunción CB. Full endoscopic endonasal transclival approach: meningioma attached to the ventral surface of the brainstem. Neurocirugia. 2014;25(3):140–4.

23. Iacoangeli M, Di Rienzo A, di Somma LG, Moriconi E, Alvaro L, Re M, Salvinelli F, Carassiti M, Scerrati M. Improving the endoscopic endonasal transclival approach: the importance of a precise layer by layer reconstruction. Br J Neurosurg. 2014;28(2):241–6.

24. Muto J, Prevedello DM, Ditzel Filho LF, Tang IP, Oyama K, Kerr EE, Otto BA, Kawase T, Yoshida K, Carrau RL. Comparative analysis of the anterior transpetrosal approach with the endoscopic endonasal approach to the petroclival region. J Neurosurg. 2016;125(5):1171–86.

25. Beer-Furlan A, Abi-Hachem R, Jamshidi AO, Carrau RL, Prevedello DM. Endoscopic trans-sphenoidal surgery for petroclival and clival meningiomas. J Neurosurg Sci. 2016;60(4):495–502.

26. Maclean J, Fersht N, Short S. Controversies in radiotherapy for meningioma. Clin Oncol. 2014;26(1):51–64.

27. Rogers L, Barani I, Chamberlain M, Kaley TJ, McDermott M, Raizer J, Schiff D, Weber DC, Wen PY, Vogelbaum MA. Meningiomas: knowledge base, treatment outcomes, and uncertainties. A RANO Rev J Neurosurg. 2015;122(1):4–23.

28. Campbell E, Whitfield RD. Posterior fossa meningiomas. J Neurosurg. 1948;5(2):131–53.

29. Bricolo AP, Turazzi S, Talacchi A, Cristofori L. Microsurgical removal of petroclival menin-

giomas: a report of 33 patients. Neurosurgery. 1992;31(5):813–28.

30. Natarajan SK, Sekhar LN, Schessel D, Morita A. Petroclival meningiomas: multimodality treatment and outcomes at long-term follow-up. Neurosurgery. 2007;60(6):965–81.

31. Almefty R, Dunn IF, Pravdenkova S, Abolfotoh M, Al-Mefty O. True petroclival meningiomas: results of surgical management: clinical article. J Neurosurg. 2014;120(1):40–51.

32. Buetow MP, Buetow PC, Smirniotopoulos JG. Typical, atypical, and misleading features in meningioma. Radiographics. 1991;11(6):1087–106.

33. Osborn AG, Salzman KL, Jhaveri MD, Barkovich AJ. Diagnostic imaging: brain. Elsevier Health Sci. 2015;24:72–81.

34. Ojemann RG. Management of cranial and spinal meningiomas (honored guest presentation). Clin Neurosurg. 1993;40:321.

35. Hallinan JT, Hegde AN, Lim WE. Dilemmas and diagnostic difficulties in meningioma. Clin Radiol. 2013;68(8):837–44.

36. Cushing H, Eisenhardt L. Meningiomas. Their classification, regional behaviour, life history, and surgical end results. Bull. Med. Libr. Assoc. 1938;27(2):185.

37. Castellano F, Ruggiero G. Meningiomas of the posterior fossa. Acta Radiol Suppl. 1953;104:1–77.

38. Sekhar LN, Wright DC, Richardson R, Monacci W. Petroclival and foramen magnum meningiomas: surgical approaches and pitfalls. J Neuro-Oncol. 1996;29(3):249–59.

39. Al-Rodhan RF, Laws ER. The history of intracranial meningiomas. Meningiomas. New York: Raven Press, Ltd; 1991. p. 1–6.

40. Schmitz B, Hagen T, Reith W. Three-dimensional true FISP for high-resolution imaging of the whole brain. Eur Radiol. 2003;13(7):1577–82.

41. Mikami T, Minamida Y, Yamaki T, Koyanagi I, Nonaka T, Houkin K. Cranial nerve assessment in posterior fossa tumors with fast imaging employing steady-state acquisition (FIESTA). Neurosurg Rev. 2005;28(4):261–6.

42. Dehdashti AR, Karabatsou K, Ganna A, Witterick I, Gentili F. Expanded endoscopic endonasal approach for treatment of clival chordomas: early results in 12 patients. Neurosurgery. 2008;63(2):299–309.

43. Stippler M, Gardner PA, Snyderman CH, Carrau RL, Prevedello DM, Kassam AB. Endoscopic endonasal approach for clival chordomas. Neurosurgery. 2009;64(2):268–78.

44. Shiley SG, Limonadi F, Delashaw JB, Barnwell SL, Andersen PE, Hwang PH, Wax MK. Incidence, etiology, and management of cerebrospinal fluid leaks following trans-sphenoidal surgery. Laryngoscope. 2003;113(8):1283–8.

45. Hachem RA, Elkhatib A, Beer-Furlan A, Prevedello D, Carrau R. Reconstructive techniques in skull base surgery after resection of malignant lesions: a wide array of choices. Curr Opin Otolaryngol Head Neck Surg. 2016;24(2):91–7.

Part III

Specific Diseases

Petroclival Meningiomas

7

Amol Raheja and William T. Couldwell

Introduction

Petroclival (PC) meningiomas are skull base lesions with primary dural attachment along the PC synchondrosis, typically near the upper two thirds of the clivus [1–4]. The origins of these lesions are anatomically situated medial to cranial nerves V and VII–XI than posterior petrous meningiomas, in which the origin of the tumors is located laterally to these nerve complexes. Clival meningiomas in the lower third of the clivus are often categorized separately as foramen magnum meningiomas, and they are accessed via entirely different surgical approaches than their PC counterparts and are covered elsewhere in this text [1–4]. Although Hallopeau first described PC meningioma in 1874 [2], Olivecrona and Tonnis [5] described the first attempt at surgical resection in 1927. Surgery for these tumors was associated with dismal outcomes and mortality rates exceeding 50% [6, 7]

until the microneurosurgical era [8]. Since the original classification of PC meningiomas by Castellano and Ruggiero in 1954 [9], multiple classification schemes have been proposed for these tumors based on anatomical locations, tumor extensions, and tumor dimensions. PC meningiomas are notorious for having tumor extensions along the cavernous sinus (CS) , Meckel's cave, jugular foramen, sella, parasellar region, and foramen magnum, making aggressive surgical resection without iatrogenic neurological deficits technically challenging. The interposition of cranial nerves between the surgeon and the tumor and the intimate relation of the tumor and the brainstem vascular supply limit the safe and aggressive resectability.

The management of PC meningiomas has undergone paradigm shifts over the past few decades from radical resection to more tailored surgical decompression that offers deficit-free survival. These changes have been enabled by the advent of modern microneurosurgical skull base techniques, better understanding of the surgical anatomy, and availability of intraoperative neurophysiological monitoring and efficacious adjuvant therapy option such as stereotactic radiosurgery (SRS) in the armamentarium of modern skull base neurosurgeon. This chapter reviews the natural history, clinical presentation, preoperative evaluation, decision-making, surgical approaches, role of SRS, and treatment outcomes in the era of multimodality management of PC meningiomas.

A. Raheja, MBBS, MCh (✉)
Department of Neurosurgery, All India Institute of Medical Sciences, New Delhi, India
e-mail: dramolraheja@gmail.com

W.T. Couldwell, MD, PhD
Department of Neurosurgery, Clinical Neurosciences Center, University of Utah, Salt Lake City, UT, USA
e-mail: neuropub@hsc.utah.edu

© Springer International Publishing AG 2018
W.T. Couldwell (ed.), *Skull Base Surgery of the Posterior Fossa*,
https://doi.org/10.1007/978-3-319-67038-6_7

Natural History and Clinical Presentation

PC meningiomas account for approximately 2% of all intracranial meningiomas and 0.15–0.4% of all intracranial tumors [2]. They occur predominantly in middle-aged and older women, with three times the incidence as compared with men [2]. The natural history of PC meningiomas demonstrates insidious and progressive growth leading to neurological decline from cerebellar dysfunction, cranial neuropathy, and brainstem compression, leading to death if left untreated [3]. In a cohort of patients who were managed conservatively (i.e., no neurosurgical or radiosurgical treatment) and monitored for a minimum of 4 years, up to 50% of asymptomatic patients developed cranial nerve (CN) palsy, and 20% of patients with preexisting CN palsies developed new CN deficits [10]. Even within the same histological tumor grade, there was a wide variation in growth rates. Overall, the average growth rate was 0.81 mm/year in diameter or 0.81 cm^3/year in volume [10]. Havenbergh et al. [10] also found a statistically significant correlation between infratentorial growth and moderate/severe functional deterioration and between tumor growth index and the severity of functional deterioration. They also observed that brainstem compression/displacement influenced functional outcome, and an increase in tumor growth index correlated with functional or clinical deterioration. In other words, an increase in the tumor growth rate often precedes neurological decline, thereby highlighting the importance of close radiological surveillance in patients with smaller asymptomatic lesions.

Petroclival meningiomas often reach sizeable dimensions (usually >2–3 cm) before they become clinically symptomatic from cranial nerve or brainstem compression. These benign tumors commonly present with a varied constellation of symptoms, including headache, facial numbness, chewing difficulties, dizziness, gait disturbances, facial weakness, hearing impairment, and diplopia. If there is further extension of the lesion, patients may have visual disturbances, ptosis, hormonal imbalance, swallowing difficulties, nasal regurgitation, hoarseness of voice, and tongue deviation. Out of this wide range of symptomatology, headache, gait disturbance, and trigeminal neuropathy are the most common presenting complaints, occurring in approximately 90% of patients [11].

Preoperative Assessment and Planning

Radiological Imaging

The radiological imaging of choice for patients with PC meningiomas is gadolinium-enhanced magnetic resonance imaging (MRI) to assess the site, size, and extent of the tumor [1, 2, 4]. Of particular importance is to understand where the epicenter of tumor is located. If the bulk of the tumor is located in the supratentorial compartment, then anterior and anterolateral approaches like the transbasal, pterional, orbitozygomatic, and transzygomatic subtemporal/pretemporal approaches are preferred. For tumors with the epicenter lying in the infratentorial compartment, lateral and posterolateral approaches such as the anterior/posterior/combined transpetrosal and retrosigmoid/far lateral approaches are more suitable for safe tumor resection [1–4]. In addition, T2/FLAIR MRI needs to be carefully examined to ascertain whether there is encasement of the basilar and internal carotid arteries (ICA) along with their major branches and to assess the presence of brainstem edema, which may be a surrogate for tumor invasion into the brainstem pia mater [1–4]. Both of these parameters have implications for the safety of radical tumor resection. To assess the bony anatomy and presence of any associated bony hyperostosis, thin-slice computed tomography (CT) of head is essential. Pneumatization of skull base should also be examined before performing any skull base approach to preemptively plan the reconstruction measures necessary to prevent postoperative cerebrospinal fluid (CSF) leak. Statistically, the most commonly utilized approach by the senior author for removal of petroclival tumors is the retrosigmoid approach, used in approximately 60% of cases (Fig. 7.1) [11, 12].

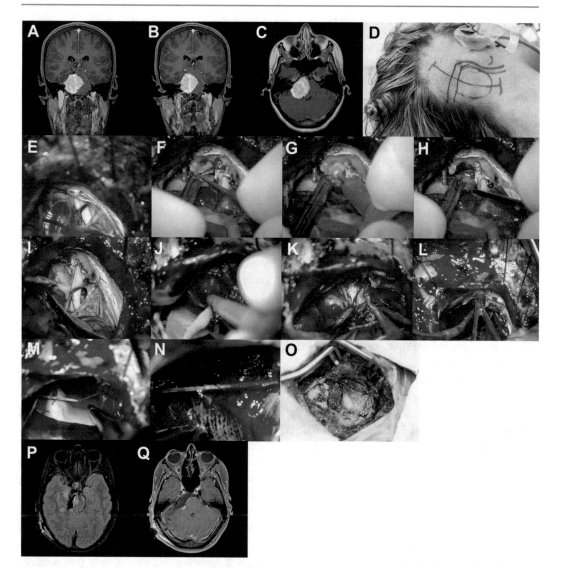

Fig. 7.1 Case illustration of removal of petroclival tumor via the retrosigmoid approach. (**a, b**) Coronal T1-weighted MRI with gadolinium demonstrating large petrotentorial tumor. (**c**) Axial T1-weighted MRI with gadolinium demonstrating large petroclival tumor with brainstem compression. (**d**) Surgical incision demonstrated in relationship to transverse and sigmoid sinus. (**e**) Upon exposure of the tumor, the VII and VIII nerve complex is noted lateral to the tumor. (**f**) The posterior lip of the IAC is drilled to assess the relationship between the tumor attachment and the IAC. (**g, h**) The suprameatal protuberance is drilled to afford exposure to the region of the tumor attachment. (**i**) The trigeminal nerve is noted adjacent to the attachment of the tumor. (**j**) The tumor is debulked using the ultrasonic aspirator. (**k**) The capsule of the tumor is then dissected free of the cerebellum and brainstem. (**l**) The remaining tumor is removed from the attachment to the petroclival-tentorial junction. (**m, n**) The trochlear nerve is repaired using end-to-end suture technique. A 9-0 filament suture is used. (**o**) After tumor removal is complete, the dura is closed in a watertight fashion. Here, the authors have used autologous fascia as a dural substitute. Note that the mastoid air cells have been occluded with bone wax. (**p, q**) Axial FLAIR image (**p**) and T1-weighted image with gadolinium (**q**) demonstrating complete removal of the tumor

The venous drainage system must be carefully evaluated before planning any skull base approach to the PC region. In particular, the variations in drainage patterns of the superficial middle cerebral venous and superior petrosal sinus systems need to be appropriately assessed using either CT or MR venography [13]. This is especially relevant for transpetrosal approaches in dominant hemispheres [13]. Apart from the venous anatomy, the arterial supply and its relation to the tumor can be assessed using MR angiography. If the cavernous segment of carotid artery is encased by the cavernous sinus extension of the PC meningioma, a digital subtraction angiogram may be warranted to assess the cross-flow from the contralateral circulation and ipsilateral posterior circulation. This can be performed using balloon occlusion test or carotid compression test [11]. Similarly, the dominance and cross-flow of blood across the posterior circulation need to be assessed in tumors encasing the basilar, posterior cerebral, and superior cerebral arteries if radical resection is planned. Tumor embolization may also be tried preoperatively if a particularly large arterial feeder is identified on angiogram, although in most cases, there are multiple small-caliber feeders (tumor blush), which cannot be embolized. The senior author rarely utilizes preoperative embolization for meningiomas in this location, as the primary supply often arises from internal carotid artery branches and the risk-benefit ratio is not in favor of embolization.

Preoperative Hearing Status

Hearing status is one of the primary factors to consider when choosing the appropriate skull base approach for PC meningiomas. Assessment via pure tone audiogram and speech discrimination score helps classify the hearing as serviceable or nonserviceable. Serviceable hearing (<50 dB hearing loss or >50% speech discrimination score) corresponds to American Academy of Otolaryngology – Head and Neck Surgery class A/B and Gardner-Robertson class I/II and warrants choosing a skull base approach that preserves hearing [1, 3, 4]. It is especially relevant for transpetrosal approaches, which put the vestibulocochlear apparatus and cochlear nerve at risk of iatrogenic injury. The anterior transpetrosal approach carries a lower risk of hearing deterioration than the posterior transpetrosal approaches. Among the various posterior trans-

petrosal approaches, the retrolabyrinthine and transcrusal approaches may enable hearing preservation in contrast to the more extensive translabyrinthine, transotic, and transcochlear approaches [1, 3, 4].

Preparation for Cerebral Revascularization

It is vital to anticipate and prepare for a cerebral revascularization procedure in PC meningioma surgery where the intent of surgery is radical resection, especially in younger patients with recurrent and more aggressive tumors (WHO grade II/III) with a poor cerebrovascular reserve [14, 15]. In general, the approach to these tumors is subtotal with adjuvant radiation therapy if the cavernous cranial nerves are functionally intact. However, at recurrence following radiation therapy in the central skull base, aggressive surgical resection is considered. The common indications for a high-flow or high-capacitance extracranial-to-intracranial bypass include (1) acute vascular injury during the surgical procedure along with preoperative evidence of intolerance to sacrifice; (2) the desire to preserve cerebrovascular reserve in a young patient with long life expectancy; (3) the invasion of tumor into major intracranial arteries requiring sacrifice of the pivotal vessel to achieve radical resection, especially for malignant or aggressive tumors; (4) poor preoperative vascular reserve with symptoms of preoperative ischemia; and (5) high risk of intraoperative vessel injury due to tumor encasement or invasion, especially in cases with prior radiation or surgical treatments [14, 15]. Although the primary assessment tool for cerebrovascular reserve is the balloon occlusion test, the false-negative rate means up to 8% of patients can still be missed [14, 15]. Given this risk, the senior author prefers to augment cerebrovascular reserve via a revascularization procedure in younger patients with longer life expectancy after radical surgical resection. The risk of surgical complications in this subset of patients is relatively low (<5%).

The Role of Intraoperative Electrophysiological Neuromonitoring and Safe Anesthetic Techniques

The intricate relation of PC meningiomas with multiple cranial nerves and brainstem puts these vital neural structures at risk during surgical resection. Recently, strong evidence has emerged supporting the use of intraoperative electrophysiological monitoring for safe surgical resection and optimal functional outcome [16]. The senior author has made it a practice to utilize at least motor evoked potentials, somatosensory evoked potentials, brainstem auditory evoked response, and facial nerve monitoring in all cases of PC meningioma resection. Lower cranial nerve monitoring to assess the vagus, spinal accessory, and hypoglossal nerves is also employed when indicated. Finally, electroencephalography is used to assess the depth of anesthesia in cases where burst suppression is indicated while performing cerebral revascularization procedures. Carefully titrated and judicious use of safe anesthetic agents and muscle relaxants is essential to optimize the interpretation of electrophysiological monitoring and keep the intracranial pressure within a desirable range. Baseline potentials should always be obtained before and after patient positioning to assess the baseline neurological deficits and any iatrogenic deficits arising from patient positioning, which can be rectified appropriately [11].

Decision-Making and Treatment Strategies

The primary factors influencing the decision-making process in choosing an appropriate treatment strategy for patients with PC meningioma include age of the patient, functional status of the patient, whether the patient is symptomatic or asymptomatic, baseline hearing status, and radiological parameters such as tumor size, pattern of tumor extension and its epicenter, cavernous sinus involvement, and tumor-brainstem interface. Treatment strategies include the options of conser-

vative management with close radiological surveillance, SRS, and surgical resection [1, 3, 4]. Because studies assessing the natural history of PC meningiomas [3] have demonstrated progressive increment in tumor dimensions leading to neurological decline and death if left untreated, watchful waiting is usually not employed as the first line of treatment in most cases if the lesion is symptomatic. Middle-aged or elderly asymptomatic patients with multiple comorbidities who have been incidentally diagnosed with small PC lesions suggestive of a benign meningioma may be an appropriate exception. In such cases, first follow-up imaging is done at 3–4 months to rule out an aggressive variant of tumor, which may warrant surgical exploration. If there is no significant interval change in tumor dimensions at the first follow-up, serial scans can be safely deferred to once a year. Objective decision-making can also be aided by calculation of the tumor growth index. These patients are generally advised to avoid hormonal replacement therapy, which may potentially accelerate the growth rate of these tumors and cause early onset of neurological symptoms.

SRS has emerged as an invaluable alternative/adjunct to surgical resection for these tumors [17, 18]. Although long-term data supporting its efficacy and safety are limited, its short-term results are reassuring. Many neurosurgeons across the globe have switched from aggressive radical tumor resection to more tailored safe tumor decompression and use of SRS as adjuvant therapy for better functional outcome. SRS can be used as primary therapy for small, minimally symptomatic, PC lesions suggestive of meningioma with primary involvement of cavernous sinus, especially in elderly patients with multiple comorbidities and limited life expectancy [17, 18]. SRS is more often employed as adjunct/adjuvant therapy in the modern microneurosurgical era, particularly for residual tumors along the cavernous sinus for patients with any age group, tumors with higher histological grade, and remnant tumors showing progressive growth on serial imaging [17, 18]. Another school of thought believes that small, benign WHO grade I residual tumors can be safely monitored using serial imaging because many have already been devascularized during bone drilling and dural coagulation, thereby reducing their growth potential [12, 19]. This strategy is especially used in younger patients who have a higher risk of long-term radiation toxicity.

Surgical resection has been the standard of care for PC meningiomas in the present microneurosurgical era, although the aggressiveness of tumor resection has decreased over the past two decades in an effort to reduce iatrogenic neurological deficits. Surgery is primarily considered for young, symptomatic patients with rapidly growing tumors and no/minimal systemic comorbidities, patients with larger tumors causing brainstem compression and multiple cranial neuropathies, and cases where the diagnosis of benign lesion is in doubt [1, 3, 4]. The aim of the surgical intervention is maximal safe resection (complete if possible) of tumor without causing undue traction to surrounding neurovascular structures to minimize iatrogenic neurological deficits. The goals of surgery include establishing the histological diagnosis, achieving brainstem and cranial nerves decompression to facilitate improvement in functional outcome, and reducing tumor volume to smaller dimensions making it compatible to SRS adjuvant therapy (especially tumors extending into cavernous sinus). Intraoperative assessment of the tumor-brainstem interface is critical, as overzealous attempts at radically removing firm and adherent tumors stuck to brainstem may lead to catastrophic sequelae. Lastly, use of neuroendoscopy, neuronavigation, and electrophysiological monitoring intraoperatively can contribute toward a safe surgery and optimal patient outcome [11].

Surgical Approaches

The basic tenets of skull base surgery include optimal patient positioning to help gravity-assisted retraction; use of intraoperative lumbar drain to facilitate brain relaxation for easy access to the tumor, moving from one anatomical landmark to another to ensure precise surgical exposure and maximal use of the operative corridor; early devascularization of the tumor via drilling

of involved bone and coagulating tumor feeders along the involved dura mater; and maintaining the arachnoid plane between the tumor and the surrounding vital neurovascular structures. The rationale for choosing each skull base approach optimizes the balance between iatrogenic morbidity due to the approach and the need to limit brain retraction for good visualization of neurovascular structures involved. Broadly speaking, the surgical approaches to the PC region are divided into transfacial and transcranial approaches (Fig. 7.2) [11]. Transfacial approaches can utilize transoral, transsphenoidal, or transmaxillary surgical corridors for accessing the PC region. Advances in the realm of neuroendoscopy, the availability of precise neuronavigation systems, and development of better hemostatic agents have provided a much-needed boost to efforts to resect large PC meningiomas via minimally invasive transfacial approaches. At present, however, the data to support long-term safety and efficacy for this purpose are lacking.

On the contrary, transcranial approaches have stood the test of time for resecting PC meningiomas safely. They are further subdivided based on the surgical trajectory taken to reach the PC region: anterior/anterolateral and lateral/posterolateral approaches [1, 3, 4, 11]. The principal anterior approach is the transbasal transplanum transclival approach, which has traditionally been used for extensive and more midline tumors such as clival chordoma and craniopharyngioma, especially involving anterior and middle cranial fossa. Access to the petroclival region is limited for tumors involving the inferior half of the clivus and extending lateral to the internal acoustic meatus. Cavernous sinus and Meckel's cave involvement further limits surgical access via this approach. Anterolateral approaches include the pterional, orbitozygomatic, and transzygomatic subtemporal/pretemporal approaches [1, 3, 4, 11]. They are primarily utilized for tumors with their epicenters/tumor bulk in the supratentorial compartment, which are difficult to access via lateral/posterolateral approaches. The primary disadvantages to these approaches are limited access to tumor extending to the contralateral side across ventral brainstem, utilization of a

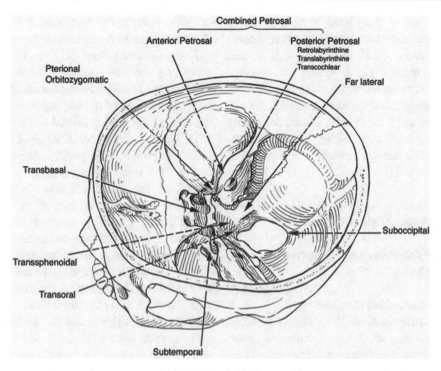

Fig. 7.2 Illustration demonstrating various transfacial and transcranial skull base approaches to the clivus and petroclival regions (Reproduced with permission from Liu and Couldwell [32])

long surgical access route to the tumor, and working in a narrow operative corridor between the optic apparatus, oculomotor nerves, and carotid vessels. Detailed description of these anterior/anterolateral approaches is beyond the scope of this chapter.

Lateral/posterolateral approaches include the transpetrosal and suboccipital approaches [1, 3, 4, 11]. Transpetrosal approaches are the workhorse for accessing PC tumors. They include anterior, posterior, and combined transpetrosal approaches, which are the primary focus of this chapter. The primary advantages of transpetrosal approaches over anterior/anterolateral approaches are wider, shorter, and direct access to the tumor and a much better surgical trajectory to access tumors extending across the midline along ventral brainstem. Limitations include the higher risk for retraction injury to the temporal lobe with consequent seizures and dysphasia, facial weakness, hearing loss, cerebrospinal fluid rhinorrhea, and iatrogenic injury to sigmoid sinus, transverse sinus, and vein of Labbé leading to venous

infarcts. The decision to use either of these approaches is governed by tumor size and extent, preoperative hearing status, and surgeon's preference [1, 3, 4, 11]. The retrosigmoid suboccipital approach (Fig. 7.1) is yet another option to resect lesions in PC region, although it is limited by the supratentorial extension of the tumor and contralateral extension across the ventral aspect of brainstem. The interposition of facial and cochlear cranial nerves between the tumor and the surgeon further limits the surgical freedom. The retrosigmoid suboccipital approach may also be used as a second-stage procedure after an anterior transpetrosal approach to resect the residual tumor lateral to the internal acoustic meatus and along the ventral brainstem. By choosing this surgical strategy, many neurosurgeons have been able to reduce the rate of iatrogenic complications arising from much more extensive combined (anterior and posterior) transpetrosal approaches (see below). Far/extreme lateral approaches can also be combined with retrosigmoid suboccipital approaches for tumors extending along lower third of the clivus and contralaterally along the ventral brainstem to optimize the surgical trajectory with limited brainstem traction [1, 3, 4, 11]. In addition, suprameatal extension of the conventional retrosigmoid suboccipital approach enhances the surgical access to Meckel's cave, an area commonly involved by these tumors (Fig. 7.1). The suboccipital approaches are described in depth elsewhere [1, 3, 4, 11].

Transpetrosal Approaches

Anterior Transpetrosal (Kawase's) Approach

Indications and Limitations
Small- to moderate-sized PC tumors centered on the petrous apex, which have a smaller supratentorial component and a larger infratentorial component, are good candidates for the anterior petrosal (Kawase) approach. It is an extremely handy approach that can be utilized for a large proportion of PC meningiomas. It has the advantage of providing direct access along the long axis of the tumor, offers the ability to devascularize the tumor first by drilling the involved bone extradurally and coagulating the dura mater feeders to the tumor, and carries lower risk of iatrogenic injury to vestibulocochlear apparatus and facial nerve. However, tumors extending lateral to internal acoustic canal (IAC) and inferior to the lower third of the clivus are difficult to access adequately using just this approach, which often needs to be combined with a posterior transpetrosal approach. There is also a risk of venous embarrassment of the temporal-parietal region with elevation of the middle fossa dura during dissection.

Surgical Technique and Nuances
Use of an intraoperative lumbar drain may be beneficial to prevent retraction injury to the temporal lobe. The patient is positioned supine in a comfortable beach chair position, with the head turned to contralateral side with slight extension so that the superior sagittal sinus is approximately parallel to the floor. This may be altered if a frontotemporal craniotomy is used, where the head is turned about 45° from midline. The pressure points are padded to prevent pressure sores and compression neuropathy. Intraoperative electrophysiological monitoring is useful in ruling out any positioning-related neurological deficits, which are reversible if identified early. Once the patient is positioned, the incision is marked in a small reverse question mark shape (based on the anterior division of superficial temporal artery and supratrochlear artery) or with a quadrangular flap (based on the posterior division of superficial temporal artery and posterior auricular artery) along the temporal area. The craniotomy is centered on the external auditory meatus and the root of the zygoma, flush with the skull base. Any opened air cells along the root of the zygoma and mastoid region are evaluated and filled with wax during bony exposure. Via an extradural approach, the two layers of the lateral cavernous sinus wall are separated so that the gasserian ganglion and inferior aspect of V3 are exposed adequately [20]. Next, the middle meningeal artery is identified ~2 cm inferior to the root of the zygoma, where it is coagulated and divided where it enters the foramen spinosum, just lateral and posterior to the foramen ovale. The greater superficial petrosal nerve (GSPN) is identified running posterior to the middle meningeal artery and is dissected free off the dura from a posterior-to-anterior trajectory to avoid traction and injury to the geniculate ganglion. The arcuate eminence is the next structure to be identified; it represents the upward projection of the superior semicircular canal (SCC). Once the boundaries of Kawase's triangle are identified—anteriorly the V3 nerve, laterally the GSPN, posteriorly the IAC, and medially Meckel's cave—the drilling can be safely performed to expose the posterior fossa dura mater. Dura is opened parallel to the base of the temporal lobe, followed by ligation of the superior petrosal sinus (SPS) proximal to the drainage of vein of Labbé. The tentorium is incised posterior to the entry of the trochlear nerve in its free margin to combine the supra- and infratentorial access [20].

Complications and Their Avoidance

Morbidity arising from this approach includes hearing loss, facial weakness, decreased tearing, CSF leak, and temporal lobe injury leading to seizures and dysphasia. The bony labyrinth surrounding the SCC and the cochlea can be identified by their distinct color and thickness of the bone, which facilitates avoiding these structures. The petrous segment of the ICA is also at risk of exposure and damage along the anterolateral aspect of Kawase's triangle. The GSPN is an accurate landmark for the underlying petrous ICA, and careful attention to its course can help prevent ICA injury. The use of neuronavigation can further reduce the risk of iatrogenic injury to bony and vascular structures. To prevent decreased tearing and to maintain the integrity of the GSPN, it is dissected off the periosteum invested over it in a posterior to anterior direction to prevent traction avulsion of the nerve from the geniculate ganglion and also indirect facial paresis that may ensue. CSF leaks can be avoided by meticulous waxing of exposed air cells. Use of appropriate autologous grafts (fat/pericranium/ muscle) or dural substitutes ensures optimal reconstruction of the dural defect along the skull base. SPS ligation distal to the drainage of the vein of Labbé can lead to disastrous sequelae, especially in the dominant lobes. To understand the venous drainage pattern, careful assessment of the preoperative CT/MR venogram is essential. The use of lumbar drainage and intermittent use of retraction can help prevent this complication.

Posterior Transpetrosal Approach

Indications and Limitations

The ideal candidates for posterior transpetrosal approach are patients with large PC tumors with their epicenter in the infratentorial compartment, extending across the midline as well as lateral to the IAC and inferiorly along the lower third of the clivus. Depending on the preoperative hearing status of the patient and the extent of the ventral brainstem exposure required, there is a choice of various modifications of the posterior transpetrosal

approach: retrolabyrinthine, transcrusal, translabyrinthine, and transcochlear approaches [21]. The advantages of these approaches include direct, short, and wide access to the PC region with adequate surgical freedom to access tumors extending across midline along ventral brainstem and lateral to IAC. These approaches demonstrate beautifully the principle of removing bone to avoid retracting the brain for visualization. Tumor vascularity is reduced by the approach, as all vascular supply emanating through the bone is removed with the approach. They are limited by the ability to visualize and resect the supratentorial component of the tumor, which may warrant a combined approach with anterior transpetrosal approach. Given the fact that these are essentially presigmoid approaches, dominance of the ipsilateral sigmoid sinus may limit the surgical view and easy maneuverability. Therefore, careful assessment of venous drainage patterns and anatomy is pivotal to ascertain the safety and feasibility of these approaches [13].

Surgical Technique and Nuances

The senior author prefers to perform these procedures with the patient in the lateral approach. This reduces neck rotation, and ventilation of the patient is unimpeded. Apart from the usual patient preparation, the abdomen is also prepared to harvest autologous fat graft. The incision is typically a C-shaped or curvilinear incision in the retroauricular region intended to expose the inferior aspect of the temporal bone, the mastoid process, and the suboccipital region. Next, the mastoidectomy is performed until the mastoid antrum—which lies posterior to the posterior ear canal and acts as an internal landmark for the vital middle ear structures—is opened. The mastoid antrum is also situated deep within the Macewen's triangle and posterior to the spine of Henle. Further drilling can be done using neuronavigation assistance or with the help of an otorhinolaryngologist to expose the sigmoid sinus and deeper otic capsule. The posterior semicircular canal can be identified deep to the mastoid antrum, and the fallopian bony canal of the facial nerve can be identified by a short process of incus and also by its location at the anterior and inferior border of the antrum [21]. Depending on the degree of removal of the vestibulocochlear structures to gain better access along ventral brainstem, the modifications of this approach can be retrolabyrinthine, transcrusal, translabyrinthine, and transcochlear, although at the cost of progressively greater hearing loss and facial weakness in the successive approaches [21]. The retrolabyrinthine approach preserves the hearing by leaving the otic capsule intact. The transcrusal approach has been modified from the classical translabyrinthine approach in that it only sacrifices the superior and posterior SCCs from their ampullae to the common crus. The translabyrinthine approach involves the removal of all three (superior, posterior, and lateral) SCCs including the common crus. With the openings of the SCCs and common crus occluded using bone dust and wax, the endolymph is contained within the otic capsule in the transcrusal approach, which helps preserve hearing in many instances; on the other hand, the translabyrinthine approach is almost inevitably associated with complete hearing loss [21]. The transcrusal approach also provides ~89% of the clival exposure afforded by the much more aggressive transcochlear approaches, which include removal of the complete vestibulocochlear apparatus and its otic capsule by drilling along the most anterior aspect of the petrous bone, ventral to the IAC [22, 23]. The transcochlear approaches also require facial nerve transposition from its bony canal, which leads to at least a transient grade III facial palsy. The posterior fossa dura is then opened to tackle the intradural pathology.

Complications and Their Avoidance

The morbidities most commonly associated with these approaches include hearing loss, vertigo, tinnitus, dizziness, facial palsy, CSF leak, and sigmoid sinus thrombosis. Hearing loss can be prevented by opting for hearing-preserving posterior transpetrosal approaches and using intraoperative brainstem auditory evoked response monitoring in select patients with preoperative serviceable hearing status. Careful application of bone dust and wax in occluding opened SCCs and common crus in the transcrusal approach helps prevent inadvertent hearing loss from the loss of endo-

lymph. Taking care to prevent fat graft filling the mastoidectomy defect from prolapsing in the middle ear cavity will reduce the incidence of conductive hearing loss after hearing preservation surgery [21]. Vertigo, tinnitus, and dizziness are often transient in nature, and the contralateral vestibular apparatus usually spontaneously compensates for the loss of ipsilateral vestibular function in a few days. Facial palsy is common with the transcochlear approaches but can also arise in translabyrinthine approaches while drilling in the vicinity of bony facial canal. Therefore, it is imperative that the facial nerve is not skeletonized if its transposition is not intended, and a thin layer of bone must remain to protect the nerve. Use of intraoperative facial nerve monitoring and neuronavigation may help reduce the risk of iatrogenic facial paresis. CSF leak is another common, preventable complication of transpetrosal approaches. Appropriate packing of the dural defect with autologous fat graft harvested from the abdomen helps to reduce the risk of postoperative CSF leak/paradoxical rhinorrhea. Use of a postoperative lumbar drain may further reduce the incidence of postoperative CSF leaks. Intraoperative injury to the sigmoid sinus predisposes for the risk of sinus thrombosis that can lead to catastrophic raised intracranial pressure symptoms and cerebellar venous infarct. Therefore, ensuring adequate hydration in such cases along with the use of antiplatelets/anticoagulants is mandatory, especially in cases of dominant sinus injury.

Combined Transpetrosal Approach

Indications and Limitations

The combined transpetrosal is the most versatile transpetrosal approach available for approaching PC meningiomas; it combines the advantages offered by both anterior and posterior transpetrosal approaches, although it is a much more aggressive skull base approach that carries a higher risk of iatrogenic complications and a greater propensity for longer operative duration, increased blood loss, and prolonged anesthesia [11]. Radical resection is afforded for almost the complete spectrum of PC meningiomas using this single approach, even tumors with significant supratentorial extension. This approach provides the widest exposure to PC tumors having multicompartmental spread and extensions across the midline, allowing their safe resection, along with good visualization of the tumor brainstem interface. In-depth evaluation of venous drainage patterns and anatomy is again pertinent to plan this approach to optimize the patient outcome.

Surgical Technique and Nuances

The senior surgeon prefers the lateral position for a combined petrosal approach. The incision is marked in a large quadrangular fashion with the anterior limb curving back from 1 cm in front of the tragus along superior temporal line and the posterior limb extending in the retroauricular region along the hairline, ending approximately 1 cm inferior to the mastoid tip [11, 24]. A combined supratentorial (temporal) and infratentorial (suboccipital) craniotomy is made across the transverse sinus (Fig. 7.3). The senior author performs a cosmetic mastoidectomy for the approach [25]. The outer table of the mastoid is undercut by an oscillating saw or drill to allow replacement as a bone flap at closure [24]. A complete mastoidectomy is performed next by drilling along the mastoid triangle, which is bounded anteriorly by the posterior ear canal, superiorly by the inferior temporal line, and posteriorly by the occipital bone. Next, the boundaries of Trautmann's triangle—the sigmoid sinus posteriorly, the superior petrosal sinus superiorly, and the posterior SCC anteriorly—are exposed. Once the appropriate bony exposure is completed to achieve the anterior petrosectomy and intended posterior petrosectomy, the dura is incised in a curvilinear fashion from the subtemporal region to the presigmoid region. The superior petrosal sinus is ligated and divided proximal to the drainage site of the vein of Labbé into the sigmoid transverse sinus junction to prevent venous infarct of the temporal lobe [11, 24]. The tentorium is then divided posterior to the entry point of the trochlear nerve to complete the exposure. The dural defect can be plugged using pericranial graft, myofascial flap, and autologous fat graft.

Complications and Their Avoidance

Apart from the typical set of complications and their prevention techniques for anterior and posterior transpetrosal approaches (see above), particular attention needs to be given to a few aspects including a risk of CSF leak and the risk of venous infarcts. If a cosmetic mastoidectomy is performed, there is no bony defect associated with the approach. A vascularized pedicled myofascial flap based on the sternocleidomastoid muscle and temporalis fascia is an invaluable option to plug the large dural defect created by combined petrosectomy approach to reduce the incidence of CSF leak [24]. The risk of venous infarct can be reduced by dividing the SPS as proximal as possible to maintain the petrosal vein drainage as well as that of vein of Labbé. Lastly, another important modification of the combined petrosectomy has been proposed to reduce the time of surgery and its associated anesthesia- and blood loss-related complications [26]. It includes anterior petrosectomy along with the petrous apicectomy in place of conventional posterior petrosectomy approaches, which helps reduce operative time and associated morbidity without sacrificing much of the operative exposure.

Treatment Outcomes in the Multimodality Management Era

The assessment of postoperative outcome has been done conventionally using tools such as Karnofsky Performance Status score, Glasgow Outcome Scale, and Modified Rankin Scale [24]. More recently, Morisako et al. [24] devised a petroclival meningioma impairment scale, which is specifically designed for more comprehensive assessment of patients with PC meningiomas. Gross total resection rates have improved over time, and they presently range from 20% to 79% [11]. Although new-onset iatrogenic cranial neuropathies or worsening of preexisting nerve deficits has been reported to occur in as many as 76% of patients, the majority are transient in nature, and long-term data suggest a return to preoperative status with no/minimal limitation of activi-

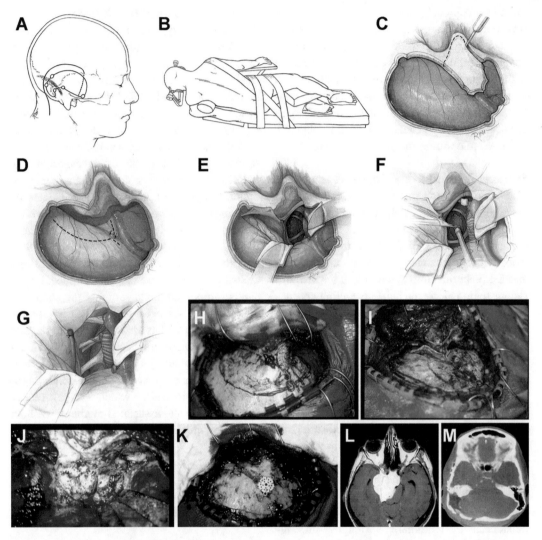

Fig. 7.3 The combined petrosal approach, which provides both infra- and supratentorial access (**a**). The patient is placed in the full lateral position (**b**), with extensive padding (**c**). After removal of the L-shaped bone flap extending in the temporal-occipital region to the suboccipital region, the outline of the cosmetic mastoidectomy is planned with cutting through the outer table of bone at the perimeter of the mastoid. After the outer table of the mastoid is removed, the mastoid resection is performed. The amount of bone removal is based on the status of hearing and need for basal exposure. The dural incision is then planned (**d**). Opening of the dura is done carefully in the region of the transverse-sigmoid junction, and the entrance of the vein of Labbé is preserved into this region. There is variability (and sometimes multiplicity) of venous drainage from the posterior temporal lobe in this region, and one must open the dura carefully to understand the individual drainage. The superior petrosal sinus is then ligated in a location to ensure the drainage of the temporal lobe is not embarrassed. After the superior petrosal sinus is ligated, the tentorium is then divided along the region of the petrous apex. The trochlear (fourth cranial) nerve is located, and the tentorium is cut posteriorly to where the nerve enters the tentorial edge. This maneuver then enables posterior retraction of the sigmoid sinus and cerebellum from the region of the petrous bone (**e**). (**f**) All cranial nerves are preserved during dissection and removal of the tumor. (**g**) Completion of tumor removal. (**h–j**) Case of large petroclival tumor that was removed with a combined petrosal approach. In this case, hearing was intact and the mastoidectomy was performed to preserve the labyrinth. The closure of the cosmetic mastoidectomy demonstrating replacement of the bone flap (**k**), preoperative MRI with gadolinium (**l**), and fat graft on placement on the postoperative CT scan (**m**) (**a–g** Reproduced with permission from Liu and Couldwell [32]; **k–m** Reproduced with permission from Couldwell and Fukushima [25])

ties of daily living [11]. The trochlear nerve is most commonly involved, followed by oculomotor and abducens nerve paresis [11]. Mortality in the perioperative period has reduced over the past few decades, and it varies from 0% to 7% in recently published series [11]. It is primarily due to poor neurological outcome secondary to a brainstem stroke, which reemphasizes the importance of preoperative and intraoperative assessment of the tumor-brainstem interface.

Tumor recurrence and progression rates up to 42% after surgical resection of PC meningiomas have been reported [11]. The primary factors contributing to higher risk of tumor recurrence include less extensive surgical resection, malignant histology, and cavernous sinus involvement. Use of adjuvant SRS for any residual tumor demonstrating progressive growth reduces the potential for tumor recurrence to approximately 4.5–22% with length of follow-up ranging from 6 to 8 years [12, 27, 28]. The studies assessing the role of SRS as a primary treatment modality for PC meningiomas have reported excellent tumor control rates (~100%), with an average follow-up of 3–4 years [28–30]. They also demonstrated favorable neurological outcome in 96–100% of patients [28, 30], along with improvement in cranial nerve function in ~50% of cases [29]. However, SRS has its own set of risks and side effects. Benign skull base meningiomas have been demonstrated to exhibit aggressive behavior following treatment failure with radiation treatment, especially with unpredictable growth pattern and growth rate. Primary radiosurgery treatment-resistant tumors are much more difficult to resect after receiving radiation therapy because of increased adhesiveness of the tumor, and surgery is often associated with higher complication rates if complete resection is attempted. Residual tumors >8 ml in volume are often associated with reduced efficacy of SRS treatment, highlighting the importance of adequate tumor resection as the primary modality for large tumors [17]. Because we lack sufficient data on long-term risks of SRS, the risk of radiation-induced malignancy must be considered. Finally, the limited long-term data available on the role of SRS in meningioma treatment have demonstrated less optimistic long-term survival. Rowe et al. [31] found a 53% 15-year survival, with 67% of patient mortality caused by meningioma after SRS treatment.

Direct comparison of radiation treatment and microsurgical resection cannot be aptly performed because of the lack of randomized controlled trials to assess the difference in treatment outcome and complications. In addition, the rarity of petroclival meningiomas, the heterogeneity in the clinical profile of patients, differential tumor characteristics among various studies, and institutional bias toward one modality over the other do not allow proper comparison of the two treatment modalities. These comparisons should be judiciously applied on a case-by-case basis. It is imperative to understand that the treatment modalities are not competitive but complementary to each other, and together they form an integral part of the armamentarium of the present-day neurosurgeon. The development of microneurosurgical skull base approaches, a better understanding of the surgical anatomy, the availability of newer imaging techniques, optimal electrophysiological monitoring and modern neuroanesthesia setups, and the introduction of radiosurgery have led to the modern multimodality management. In the current era of multimodality treatment aimed at preservation of the patient's functional status and quality of life, mortality rates have reduced to ~0% in the most recent reports, and a permanent morbidity rate of ~20% is observed, primarily in the form of cranial nerve deficits, which are often well compensated by patients in their day-to-day life [4].

Conclusions

During the inevitable evolution of modern-day neurosurgery, the aim for treatment of PC meningiomas has gradually shifted from primary aggressive resection and long-term survival to more selective resection and preservation of patient's quality of life using a multimodality approach comprising surgery, radiation treatment, and conservative management with close radiological surveillance. Therefore, appropriate decision-making is vital in choosing the best possible treatment strategy tailored to the individual patient's needs.

Acknowledgments We thank Kristin Kraus, MSc, our medical editor, for her contribution to manuscript editing and Vance Mortimer, our video editor, for his contribution to editing the operative videos.

References

1. Bambakidis NC, Kakarla UK, Kim LJ, et al. Evolution of surgical approaches in the treatment of petroclival meningiomas: a retrospective review. Neurosurgery. 2007;61(5 Suppl 2):202–9. discussion 9–11

2. Hunter JB, Weaver KD, Thompson RC, et al. Petroclival meningiomas. Otolaryngol Clin N Am. 2015;48(3):477–90.

3. Maurer AJ, Safavi-Abbasi S, Cheema AA, et al. Management of petroclival meningiomas: a review of the development of current therapy. J Neurol Surg B Skull Base. 2014;75(5):358–67.

4. Seifert V. Clinical management of petroclival meningiomas and the eternal quest for preservation of quality of life: personal experiences over a period of 20 years. Acta Neurochir (Wien). 2010;152(7):1099–116.

5. Olivecrona H. The surgical treatment of intracranial tumours. In: Olivecrona H, Tonnis W, editors. Handbuch der Neurochirurgie. Springer, Berlin Heidelberg New York; 1967. p 1–301.

6. Campbell E, Whitfield RD. Posterior fossa meningiomas. J Neurosurg. 1948;5(2):131–53.

7. Hakuba A, Nishimura S, Tanaka K, et al. Clivus meningioma: six cases of total removal. Neurol Med Chir (Tokyo). 1977;17(1 Pt 1):63–77.

8. Yasargil M, Mortara M, Curcic M. Meningioma of basal posterior cranial fossa. In: Krayenbuhl H, editor. Advances and technical standards in neurosurgery. Vienna: Springer-Verlag; 1980. p. 1–115.

9. Castellano F, Ruggiero G. Meningiomas of the posterior fossa. Acta Radiol Suppl. 1953;104:1–177.

10. Van Havenbergh T, Carvalho G, Tatagiba M, et al. Natural history of petroclival meningiomas. Neurosurgery. 2003;52(1):55–62. discussion – 4

11. Coppens J, Couldwell W. Clival and petroclival meningiomas. In: McDermott M, DeMonte F, editors. Al-Mefty's meningiomas. New York: Thieme; 2011.

12. Couldwell WT, Fukushima T, Giannotta SL, et al. Petroclival meningiomas: surgical experience in 109 cases. J Neurosurg. 1996;84(1):20–8.

13. Adachi K, Hayakawa M, Ishihara K, et al. Study of changing intracranial venous drainage patterns in Petroclival meningioma. World Neurosurg. 2016;92:339–48.

14. Liu JK, Couldwell WT. Interpositional carotid artery bypass strategies in the surgical management of aneurysms and tumors of the skull base. Neurosurg Focus. 2003;14(3):e2.

15. Yang T, Tariq F, Chabot J, et al. Cerebral revascularization for difficult skull base tumors: a contemporary series of 18 patients. World Neurosurg. 2014;82(5):660–71.

16. Kodama K, Javadi M, Seifert V, et al. Conjunct SEP and MEP monitoring in resection of infratentorial lesions: lessons learned in a cohort of 210 patients. J Neurosurg. 2014;121(6):1453–61.

17. Flannery TJ, Kano H, Lunsford LD, et al. Long-term control of petroclival meningiomas through radiosurgery. J Neurosurg. 2010;112(5):957–64.

18. Starke R, Kano H, Ding D, et al. Stereotactic radiosurgery of petroclival meningiomas: a multicenter study. J Neuro-Oncol. 2014;119(1):169–76.

19. Almefty R, Dunn IF, Pravdenkova S, et al. True petroclival meningiomas: results of surgical management. J Neurosurg. 2014;120(1):40–51.

20. Borghei-Razavi H, Tomio R, Fereshtehnejad SM, et al. Anterior petrosal approach: the safety of Kawase triangle as an anatomical landmark for anterior petrosectomy in petroclival meningiomas. Clin Neurol Neurosurg. 2015;139:282–7.

21. Sincoff EH, McMenomey SO, Delashaw JB Jr. Posterior transpetrosal approach: less is more. Neurosurgery. 2007;60(2 Suppl 1):ONS53–8. discussion ONS8–9

22. Horgan MA, Anderson GJ, Kellogg JX, et al. Classification and quantification of the petrosal approach to the petroclival region. J Neurosurg. 2000;93(1):108–12.

23. Horgan MA, Delashaw JB, Schwartz MS, et al. Transcrusal approach to the petroclival region with hearing preservation. Technical note and illustrative cases. J Neurosurg. 2001;94(4):660–6.

24. Morisako H, Goto T, Ohata K. Petroclival meningiomas resected via a combined transpetrosal approach: surgical outcomes in 60 cases and a new scoring system for clinical evaluation. J Neurosurg. 2015;122(2):373–80.

25. Couldwell WT, Fukushima T. Cosmetic mastoidectomy for the combined supra/infratentorial transtemporal approach. Technical note. J Neurosurg. 1993;79(3):460–1.

26. Shibao S, Borghei-Razavi H, Orii M, et al. Anterior transpetrosal approach combined with partial posterior petrosectomy for petroclival meningiomas with posterior extension. World Neurosurg. 2015;84(2):574–9.

27. Natarajan SK, Sekhar LN, Schessel D, et al. Petroclival meningiomas: multimodality treatment and outcomes at long-term follow-up. Neurosurgery. 2007;60(6):965–79. discussion 79–81

28. Park CK, Jung HW, Kim JE, et al. The selection of the optimal therapeutic strategy for petroclival meningiomas. Surg Neurol. 2006;66(2):160–5. discussion 5–6

29. Roche PH, Pellet W, Fuentes S, et al. Gamma knife radiosurgical management of petroclival meningiomas results and indications. Acta Neurochir (Wien). 2003;145(10):883–8. discussion 8

30. Subach BR, Lunsford LD, Kondziolka D, et al. Management of petroclival meningiomas by stereotactic radiosurgery. Neurosurgery. 1998;42(3):437–43. discussion 43–5

31. Rowe J, Grainger A, Walton L, et al. Risk of malignancy after gamma knife stereotactic radiosurgery. Neurosurgery. 2007;60(1):60–5. discussion 5–6

32. Liu J, Couldwell W. Petrosal approach for resection of petroclival meningiomas. In: Badie B, editor. Neurosurgical operative atlas 2E: neuro-oncology. New York: Thieme; 2006. p. 170–9.

Meningiomas of the Cerebellopontine Angle

8

Stephen T. Magill, Philip V. Theodosopoulos,
Aaron D. Tward, Steven W. Cheung,
and Michael W. McDermott

Anatomic Classification

The posterior face of the petrous temporal bone forms the lateral boundary of the CPA, while the pons and cerebellum form the medial boundary, the tentorium the superior boundary, and the jugular foramen the inferior boundary. Along the medial anterior aspect of the petrous bone runs the petro-occipital suture, which defines petroclival meningiomas when more than 25% of their attachment lies medial to this suture. Lateral to this and anterior to the internal auditory canal (IAC) is what can be referred to as the "anterior petrous face" meningiomas (APFM) (Fig. 8.1a, d). These tumors tend to present clinically with trigeminal symptoms such as numbness or pain (trigeminal neuralgia). Their arterial supply comes from non-internal carotid artery and non-tentorial artery dural feeders [10].

Tumors of the middle petrous face straddle the IAC and usually have a point of origin above the internal acoustic meatus and can be referred to as "middle petrous face" meningiomas (MPFM) (Fig. 8.1b, e). These are the tumors that Cushing referred to as "those simulating acoustic tumors," as they present with audiovestibular symptoms such as tinnitus, hearing loss, dizziness, and vertigo [9]. The hearing loss tends to manifest as decreased pure tone audiometry and impaired speech audiometry. Interestingly, high-frequency hearing is preserved, in contrast to the high-frequency sensorineural hearing loss that occurs with vestibular schwannoma [2].

Tumors arising from the region from the IAC posteriorly to the sigmoid sinus can be referred to as "posterior petrous face" meningiomas (PPFM) (Fig. 8.1c, f). In the lower 1/3 of the petrous face lies the vestibular aperture, an oblique opening in the bone for the vestibular aqueduct. The vestibular aqueduct terminates in a blind sac called the endolymphatic sac that lies partially embedded in folds of posterior petrous face dura. Even small tumors overlying the endolymphatic sac have been associated with audiovestibular symptoms resembling Meniere's syndrome. It is likely that compromise of the as yet poorly understood function of the endolymphatic sac gives rise to alterations in the fluid spaces of the inner ear, thus potentially giving rise to cochlear and vestibular dysfunction [8]. Large tumors of the posterior

S.T. Magill, MD, PhD (✉) • P.V. Theodosopoulos, MD
M.W. McDermott, MD
Department of Neurological Surgery, University of
California, San Francisco, CA, USA
e-mail: stephen.magill@ucsf.edu;
philip.theodosopoulos@ucsf.edu;
mike.mcdermott@ucsf.edu

A.D. Tward, MD, PhD • S.W. Cheung, MD
Department of Otolaryngology, University of
California, San Francisco, San Francisco, CA, USA
e-mail: aaron.tward@ucsf.edu; steven.cheung@ucsf.edu

© Springer International Publishing AG 2018
W.T. Couldwell (ed.), *Skull Base Surgery of the Posterior Fossa*,
https://doi.org/10.1007/978-3-319-67038-6_8

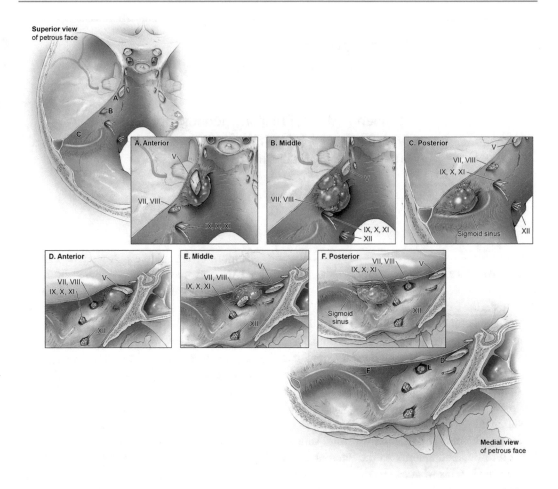

Fig. 8.1 Diagram of positions of meningiomas in axial and sagittal plane. APFM (**a, b**), MPFM (**b, e**). PPFM (**c, f**) (Published with permission)

petrous face are associated with symptoms of cerebellar dysfunction, ataxia, or elevated intracranial pressure. Figure 8.1 shows the proposed anatomic locations for each of the three petrous face locations and the approximate relationships to cranial nerves 5 and 7–12. Large tumors that span the entire petrous face can be referred to as AMPPF meningiomas.

Surgical Approaches

Most petrous face meningiomas can be exposed and resected via a standard retrosigmoid craniotomy. Preoperative preparation includes a volumetric magnetic resonance (MR) imaging study with

1.25 mm slices for image guidance during surgery. Since the approach is behind the mid-coronal plane of the skull, we use scalp-based fiducials for registering the image to physical space. An MR venogram can be included and is used to assess patency and dominance of the venous sinuses preoperatively.

The patient is positioned supine with a padded 1 Liter intravenous fluid bag under the ipsilateral shoulder, the head is secured with pins in the head holder, and the head is rotated 60° to the opposite side and then gently laterally extended down toward the floor. Kidney rests are placed along the side opposite of the exposure to secure the patient during rotation of the body away from the surgeon, which is used to obtain optimal lateral and superior views. Intraoperative neuromonitoring of cranial nerves 5, 7, 8 (Auditory Brain Responses (ABR)), and 11 is established. For larger tumors, somatosensory and motor-evoked potentials may also be monitored. Tumors with adjacent brainstem edema are usually not completely resectable due to the obscured pial-tumor interface. We have tried to move away from the routine use of a lumbar drain. A preoperative lumbar spinal tap for drainage of 30 mL of cerebrospinal fluid (CSF) is one option for decompression. The image guidance reference arc should be positioned anterior to the surgical field. After image registration, the position of the transverse-sigmoid sinus junction is marked on the scalp. A C-shaped incision is marked behind the ear using the top of the pinna and mastoid tip as the superior and inferior end points. The skin flap is dissected subcutaneously and rotated forward over the ear. Then the fascia over the mastoid process is incised with electrocautery from near the tip superiorly to the base of the mastoid process and then posteriorly along the superior nuchal line. The posterior aspect of the temporalis muscle is dissected subperiosteally forward and the suboccipital muscles posteriorly and inferiorly. Initially a self-retaining retractor is used but after the soft tissue dissection can be replaced by scalp hooks so as not to interfere with access to the operative field once under the microscope.

Once the soft tissue dissection is complete, image guidance is used to select burr hole positioning, and then a small craniotomy or craniectomy is completed exposing the inferior surface of the transverse sinus and the posterior surface of the sigmoid sinus. The mastoid emissary vein is a good landmark to follow toward the sigmoid sinus as it is posterior to the sinus. It can be isolated by removing the surrounding bone and can be coagulated and cut close to the sigmoid sinus, or it can be left in a bony canal up to the back edge of the sinus. Care must be taken to not use a volume of bone wax so as not to stuff in too much wax sufficient to encroach upon the lumen of the sigmoid sinus and thus cause thrombosis. In addition to bone wax, excessive use of any hemostatic agent, including liquid ones, can also lead to sinus thrombosis, so these should be avoided as well.

If bleeding is encountered, a simple Gelfoam placed over the sinus followed by a cotton patty should be sufficient to control bleeding without thrombosing the sinus. We typically avoid the "extended retrosigmoid approach" advocated by others [14] due to our experience with two cases of intraoperative sinus thrombosis and cerebellar swelling. During the standard retrosigmoid approach, opening the dura toward the foramen magnum and subsequently opening the cisterna magna arachnoid allow for drainage of CSF, cerebellar relaxation, and exposure of the tumor.

There are some nuances for each location, which will be covered below based on an experience of over 115 cases.

APFM

These tumors reside high and anteriorly in the CPA, and we perform suprameatal drilling in nearly every case to facilitate exposure of their base of attachment. It is our practice to do these cases with our neuro-otologists who perform the drilling. The removal of this bone is completed using a combination of round cutting and diamond burrs. The bone is removed over the midportion internal auditory canal until the dura is exposed to delimit the inferior portion of the dissection, and the bone is progressively removed superiorly. The subarcuate artery is drilled through and controlled with bone wax or drilling and can be taken without adverse sequelae. Posterolaterally, care must be taken to not enter the superior semicircular canal. Medially the dissection may be continued until the entry of the trigeminal nerve or tumor is clearly seen into Meckel's cave. Removal of this bone carries with it the advantage of removing a common site of the attachment of the meningioma to its dural base, which may devascularize the tumor and simplify further dissection. We typically preserve the superior petrosal vein when possible. The fifth nerve is usually displaced superiorly and medially to the tumor. Larger tumors have variable extension into Meckel's cave. While ultrasonic aspirators are efficient at tumor debulking, their size can pose a problem due to the depth of the tumor in the CPA. The CO_2 laser is small enough to fit easily into the angle and can be used to cut pieces of tumor out, debulk the central portion of the tumor, and vaporize the base of the tumor attachments.

MPFM

The main challenge in removing MPFMs is their relationship to the cranial nerve 7–8 complex and the risk of hearing loss or facial weakness. Similar to tumors around the optic apparatus, we have found it beneficial to debulk the tumor first before attempting to dissect the nerves from the surface of the tumor. Often there is a tongue of tumor or hypervascular tissue that extends into the internal auditory canal (IAC). Removal of the bone 270° surrounding the IAC with round diamond and cutting burrs permits the removal of these tumor extensions allowing more complete removal. If hearing preservation is a priority, then care should be taken to not enter the vestibule laterally. This limits the dissection of the lateral most few millimeters of the IAC. The preoperative scans should also be evaluated for evidence of a high-riding jugular bulb which may compromise the bony removal over the IAC. All of the drilling of the IAC should be completed prior to opening the dura of the IAC. If it appears that the meningioma extends into the IAC like a carpet, we accept near total removal while monitoring evoked potentials from the seventh and eighth nerve. It should be noted that there is often enhancement that extends into the IAC visible on preoperative MRI scans that may correspond to hypervascular dura rather than frank tumor involvement. Indeed, often residual enhancement seen on early post-op scans fades over the subsequent 12–18 months, suggesting in these cases that the enhancement was simply hypervascular tissue and not residual tumor.

PPFM

Small tumors in this location may be operated on when there is a consistent and disabling

audiovestibular syndrome presumably related to the function of the endolymphatic sac. Hyperostotic bone should be drilled down in this region when encountered. When the tumors are very large in this location, a modified far lateral approach can assist with CSF release in the upper cervical spine as reported previously by Sanai et al. [14].

Case Examples

Case 1: APFM

A 73-year-old woman presented after several years of left facial numbness and atypical facial pain, multiple dental procedures, and root canal surgery with no relief. She was evaluated by a neurologist who identified trigeminal sensory loss. MR imaging revealed a small/medium APFM impinging on the fifth nerve root entry zone (Fig. 8.2a). A retrosigmoid craniotomy was done with neuromonitoring, suprameatal drilling, and the use of the CO_2 laser to complete a Simpson Grade 2 removal (Fig. 8.2b). Her postoperative course was uncomplicated with relief of her facial pain syndrome and gradual improvement in facial numbness over the next 18 months.

Case 2: MPFM

A 43-year-old woman presented with reduced hearing, dizziness, and fullness in her right ear. She was unable to use the phone with her right ear due to reduced auditory perception. She was diagnosed with benign positional vertigo, but because of persistent symptoms, she requested an MR scan. The study showed a contrast-enhancing mass arising above the IAC, spanning the internal acoustic meatus with enhancement in the auditory canal (Fig. 8.3a). A right retrosigmoid craniotomy with superior and posterior meatal drilling with neuromonitoring was performed (Fig. 8.4). Gross total resection of the CPA mass and the extension into the first 5 mm of the IAC was achieved (Fig. 8.3b).

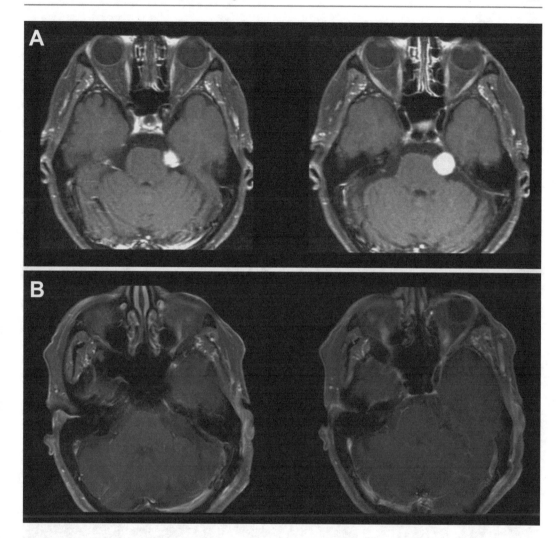

Fig. 8.2 Case example 1, APFM. Axial (**a**) preoperative and (**b**) postoperative T1 post-contrast MRI of APFM

Postoperative imaging showed residual enhancement of the IAC; however, at 118 months postoperative, there was no recurrence (Fig. 8.3d). Symptoms resolved and hearing improved so that she could again use her phone on the right side.

Case 3: PPFM: Small-Sized Tumor

A 35-year-old woman presented with a 3-year history of episodic dizziness and two episodes of true vertigo 2 years apart. There was no tinnitus and no change in hearing. MR imaging showed a meningioma attached to the dura near the vestibular aperture (Fig. 8.5). A left retrosigmoid crani-

otomy was performed and achieved a Simpson Grade 1 resection. The patient had marked improvement in audiovestibular symptoms.

Case 4: PPFM: Large-Sized Tumor

A 52-year-old woman presented with 6 months of right-sided suboccipital headache, worse with coughing, sneezing, and straining. She complained of dizziness and "walking like a drunk." She was seen by a neurologist who ordered a MR brain scan which revealed a 4.5 cm right PPFM with mass effect (Fig. 8.6). Surgery was recommended and a right-sided modified far lateral

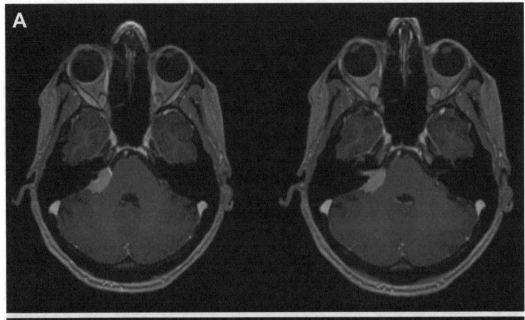

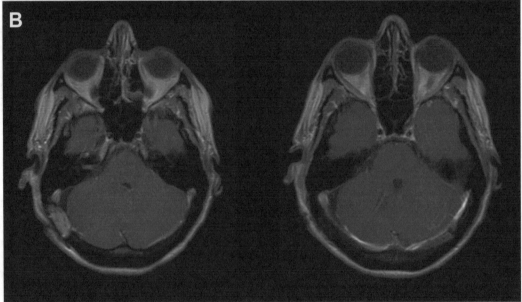

Fig. 8.3 Case example 2, MPFM. (**a**) Axial preoperative MPFM spanning IAC. The right-hand panel shows the tumor invading into the IAC. (**b**) Postoperative MR show-ing tumor removal with small residual enhancement deep in IAC (left panel)

suboccipital craniotomy was performed. A right C1 laminotomy allowed for opening of the cervical subarachnoid space below the circular sinus with release of CSF, which provided excellent relaxation for opening the convexity dura over the right cerebellum (Fig. 8.7).

Discussion

Meningiomas of the CPA are the second most common tumor in this location after vestibular schwannomas. While Cushing referred to them

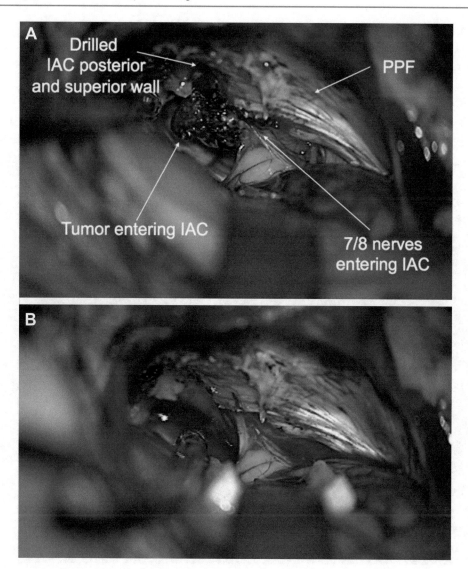

Fig. 8.4 Intraoperative photos from case example 2, small MPFM. (**a**) Intraoperative photo showing residual tumor superior and anterior to the IAC that extends into canal after drilling of superior and posterior wall of IAC. (**b**) Final result with gross tumor resection

collectively as "tumors of the cerebellar chamber," there are distinct clinical syndromes associated with location and size. Previously, we reported an early experience with 24 patients and now have accumulated over 50 such patients [9]. The senior author has divided these now into three distinct locations with four clinical syndromes, similar to the classification of Peyre et al. and the modified Desgeorges and Sterkers classification [6, 13]. The trends in presentation

size and symptomatology by location described in this chapter were also seen by Schaller et al. [16] Rather than dividing into three regions, they simply categorized the CPA meningiomas as pre- or retromeatal and found that smaller tumors were symptomatic anteriorly, while retromeatal tumors tended to grow much larger before causing symptoms. The importance of the tumor origin and dural attachment were emphasized in Robertson's series, where they demonstrated that

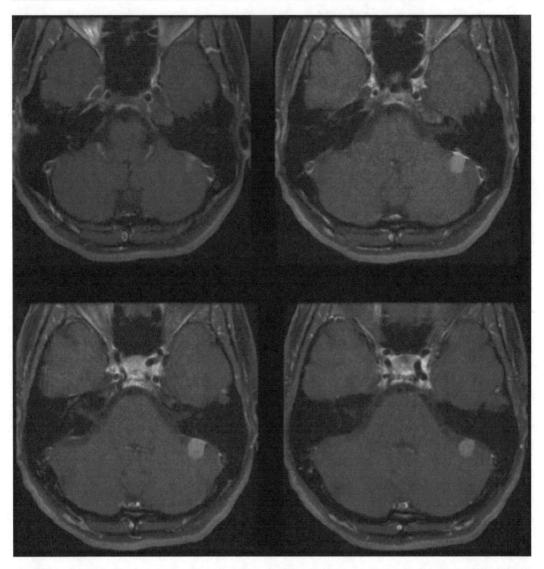

Fig. 8.5 Small PPFM. Preoperative axial T1 post-contrast MRI showing the tumor in the region of the vestibular aperture

tumor origin determined the direction of the seventh to eighth nerve displacement [18]. They used transpetrosal or translabyrinthine approaches to reach the tumors anterior to the 7–8 nerve complex, but we have been able to resect these using the retrosigmoid approach complemented by intradural drilling of the petrosal bone, which facilitates hearing preservation.

Over recent years, the surgical approach of choice has shifted from a transpetrosal or translabyrinthine approach to the retrosigmoid

approach. This has been driven by improved outcomes and hearing preservation with the retrosigmoid approach. When Thomas and King reported a series of CPA tumors and separated out the petrous face meningiomas from the petroclival tumors, they also observed the clinical syndromes described above [17]. They used a retrosigmoid approach for the posterior petrous tumors but required the more invasive translabyrinthine or transcochlear approach to the midpetrosal tumors. They used a middle fossa transtentorial approach

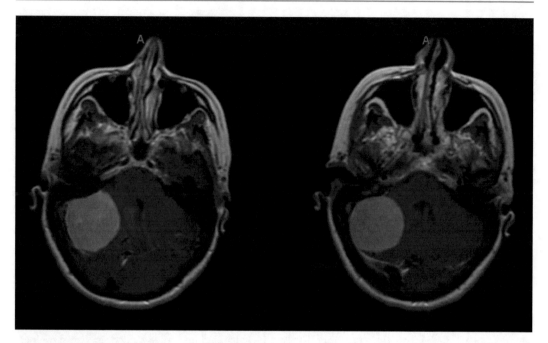

Fig. 8.6 Large PPFM. Preoperative axial T1 post-contrast MRI showing a large PPFM that required a modified far lateral approach

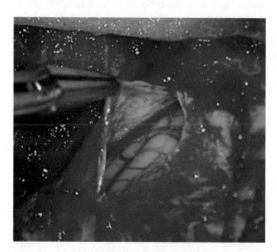

Fig. 8.7 Decompressed posterior fossa. Intraoperative photograph from Case 4, the large PPFM, demonstrating a relaxed cerebellum after CSF was released from the upper cervical subarachnoid space

to the anterior petrous/Meckel's cave tumors. We are able to use the retrosigmoid approach with additional petrous drilling to reach all these tumors. Overall, they had excellent results with most patients returning to full function and achieved gross total resection in all 13 cases.

Functional preservation is one of the keys to resection, with facial and hearing outcomes being the most important for petrous face tumors. The greatest experience reported in the literature belongs to Majid Samii, who presented his experience with more than 400 CPA meningiomas in two papers [12, 15]. He used a sitting suboccipital/retrosigmoid approach in 95% of cases and achieved Simpson Grade 1 or 2 resection in 86% of patients. The facial nerve was preserved in 89% of cases, and hearing was preserved in 91% of cases where the patient had functional hearing preoperatively. In tumors that invaded the IAC and required drilling of the petrosal bone around the internal auditory canal, facial nerve function was preserved in 80% of cases and hearing in 75% of cases. Deveze et al. evaluated outcomes in 43 patients with CPA meningiomas resected via a transpetrosal approach and found lower rates of gross total resection (79%), facial nerve preservation (73%), and hearing preservation (55%) [7]. Given these data, most modern surgeons use the retrosigmoid approach when resecting petrous face tumors. Baroncini et al. reported on 115

Table 8.1 Petrous face meningiomas: tumor size, clinical syndromes, and approaches

	APFM	MPFM	PPFM
Presentation size	Small or medium	Medium	Small, medium, or large
Symptom complex	Trigeminal neuropathy/neuralgia	Audiovestibular	Small – audiovestibular
			Large – ataxia, elevated ICP
Surgical approach	Retrosigmoid – suprameatal	Retrosigmoid	Small – retrosigmoid
			Large – modified far lateral

patients with CPA meningiomas that were resected with a retrosigmoid approach and achieved total removal in 91% of patients with facial nerve preservation in 91% of patients and hearing preservation in 83% [3]. A recent series advocated for subtotal resection followed by Gamma Knife radiosurgery for residual or small tumors with the goal of preserving facial nerve function, and they achieved similar functional results to Samii, with only 10% of patients having decreased facial function postoperatively but had a much lower rate of total resection (67%) [5]. Another recent smaller series that focused on functional preservation reported a low rate of facial deficits (5.9%) and no new hearing deficits in 34 patients [1]. Finally, a recent large Chinese series of 193 patients with CPA meningiomas found that gross total resection was markedly lower in tumors involving the IAC (30%) compared to no IAC involvement (71%) but did not report facial nerve or hearing outcomes.

The decision to treat with microsurgery or radiotherapy/radiosurgery depends on patient and tumor-specific factors. All patients with middle and posterior petrous face meningiomas should have preoperative audiometry to evaluate hearing. Observation with serial imaging is an option for asymptomatic small tumors. For tumors <2.5 cm in diameter, radiotherapy can be considered as an upfront treatment option and has excellent outcomes with regard to tumor growth arrest and preservation of cranial nerve function and avoids the morbidity of open surgery [5]. However, for larger tumors or symptomatic tumors, surgical resection is considered the standard of care and can lead to excellent outcomes, even in elderly patients [11]. Approach selection is determined by surgeon comfort and facility with the different

approaches; however, most tumors can be resected via a retrosigmoid or modified far lateral approach as discussed above. The presence of a neuro-otologist to assist with petrous drilling through the retrosigmoid approach has been very useful in our hands. Finally, patient preference must be taken into consideration, and a mutual decision on management should be made by the patient and surgeon.

In conclusion, petrous face meningiomas can be separated into three categories based on location, anterior, middle, and posterior. They present with distinct size and symptoms based on location. They can be resected via retrosigmoid or modified far lateral approaches, and surgical resection should be focused on maximal safe resection with preservation of facial and hearing function. Adjuvant postoperative radiotherapy or radiosurgery can be performed for small residuals with excellent tumor control (Table 8.1).

References

1. Agarwal V, Babu R, Grier J, Adogwa O, Back A, Friedman AH, et al. Cerebellopontine angle meningiomas: postoperative outcomes in a modern cohort. Neurosurg Focus. 2013;35:E10.
2. Baguley DM, Beynon GJ, Grey PL, Hardy DG, Moffat DA. Audio-vestibular findings in meningioma of the cerebello-pontine angle: a retrospective review. J Laryngol Otol. 1997;111:1022–6.
3. Baroncini M, Thines L, Reyns N, Schapira S, Vincent C, Lejeune J-P. Retrosigmoid approach for meningiomas of the cerebellopontine angle: results of surgery and place of additional treatments. Acta Neurochir (Wien). 2011;153:1931–1940.; discussion 1940.
4. Cushing H, Eisenhardt L. Meningiomas: their classification, regional behaviour, life history, and surgical ends results. Springfield: Charles C. Thomas; 1938.
5. D'Amico RS, Banu MA, Petridis P, Bercow AS, Malone H, Praver M, et al. Efficacy and outcomes

of facial nerve–sparing treatment approach to cerebellopontine angle meningiomas. J Neurosurg. 2017;10:1–11.

6. Desgeorges M, Sterkers O. Anatomo-radiological classification of meningioma of the posterior skull base. Neurochirurgie. 1994;40:273–95.

7. Devèze A, Franco-Vidal V, Liguoro D, Guérin J, Darrouzet V. Transpetrosal approaches for meningiomas of the posterior aspect of the petrous bone results in 43 consecutive patients. Clin Neurol Neurosurg. 2007;109:578–88.

8. Friedman RA, Nelson RA, Harris JP. Posterior fossa meningiomas intimately involved with the endolymphatic sac. Am J Otol. 1996;17:612–6.

9. Kane AJ, Sughrue ME, Rutkowski MJ, Berger MS, McDermott MW, Parsa AT. Clinical and surgical considerations for cerebellopontine angle meningiomas. J Clin Neurosci. 2011;18:755–9.

10. Kunii N, Ota T, Kin T, Kamada K, Morita A, Kawahara N, et al. Angiographic classification of tumor attachment of meningiomas at the cerebellopontine angle. World Neurosurg. 2011;75:114–21.

11. Nakamura M, Roser F, Dormiani M, Vorkapic P, Samii M. Surgical treatment of cerebellopontine angle meningiomas in elderly patients. Acta Neurochir (Wien). 2005;147:603–10.

12. Nakamura M, Roser F, Dormiani M, Matthies C, Vorkapic P, Samii M. Facial and cochlear nerve function after surgery of cerebellopontine angle meningiomas. Neurosurgery. 2005;57:77–90.–90.

13. Peyre M, Bozorg-Grayeli A, Rey A, Sterkers O, Kalamarides M. Posterior petrous bone meningiomas: surgical experience in 53 patients and literature review. Neurosurg Rev. 2012;35:53–66.

14. Sanai N1, McDermott MW. A modified far-lateral approach for large or giant meningiomas of the posterior fossa. J Neurosurg. 2010 May;112(5):907–12. https://www.ncbi.nlm.nih.gov/pubmed/19877805

15. Roser F, Nakamura M, Dormiani M, Matthies C, Vorkapic P, Samii M. Meningiomas of the cerebellopontine angle with extension into the internal auditory canal. J Neurosurg. 2005;102:17–23.

16. Schaller B, Merlo A, Gratzl O, Probst R. Premeatal and retromeatal cerebellopontine angle meningioma. Two distinct clinical entities. Acta Neurochir (Wien). 1999;141:465–71.

17. Thomas NW, King TT. Meningiomas of the cerebellopontine angle. A report of 41 cases. Br J Neurosurg. 1996;10:59–68.

18. Voss NF, Vrionis FD, Heilman CB, Robertson JH. Meningiomas of the cerebellopontine angle. Surg Neurol. 2000;53:439–67.

Tentorial Meningiomas

9

Hiroki Morisako, Takeo Goto, and Kenji Ohata

Introduction

The surgical treatment of tentorial meningiomas has been a challenge for most neurosurgeons over the years [1, 2]. Tentorial meningiomas are estimated to represent only 2–4% of all intracranial meningiomas [1]. Because of the intricate anatomical relationship of the tentorium to the surrounding neurovascular structures, their location and extension need to be precisely delineated before surgery [1].

The morphological features of the downward sloping of the tentorium from its apex anteriorly to the petrous bones laterally add a complicating factor when accessing these meningiomas. More recent advances in microsurgical techniques and skull base approaches have made access and resection of some of these larger and medially located tumors less difficult.

Tentorial meningiomas can be divided into incisural, falcotentorial, lateral, and posterior types according to their sites at the tentorium cerebelli (Fig. 9.1). In this chapter, the features of each type of tentorial meningioma are explained, with a focus on the surgical perspective.

H. Morisako, MD, PhD • T. Goto, MD, PhD
K. Ohata, MD, PhD (✉)
Department of Neurosurgery, Osaka City University
Graduate School of Medicine, 1-4-3 Asahi-machi,
Abeno-ku, Osaka 545-8585 Osaka, Japan
e-mail: hmorisako@med.osaka-cu.ac.jp;
gotot@med.osaka-cu.ac.jp; kohata@med.osaka-cu.ac.jp

Incisural Type

Surgical excision of meningiomas involving the tentorial incisura is a significant technical challenge, mainly due to access, especially for medially located lesions, as well as their relationship to the brain stem, cranial nerves, temporal lobe, blood vessels, and venous sinuses.

Meningiomas arising from the tentorial incisura grow up around the interpeduncular, crural, and ambient cisterns. Since they sometimes encase cranial nerves and blood vessels, such as the superior cerebellar artery or trochlear nerve, resection of the tumor requires great care to avoid any neurological dysfunction. If the tumor is huge, the tumor compresses the brain stem and adheres to it, thus making total resection relatively difficult.

Surgical Planning

Preoperative brain MRI scans and preoperative vascular studies (MRA, CTA, or angiogram) should be evaluated to identify the location of tumor extension, as well as the relationship to the brain stem, any encasement of vessels, and involvement of the cavernous sinus. In the case of incisura type, the venous system is crucial for planning surgery. Evaluation of the transverse and sigmoid sinuses and their connection at the torcular Herophili is important for lateral and posterior approaches. The venous drainage pattern of the

© Springer International Publishing AG 2018
W.T. Couldwell (ed.), *Skull Base Surgery of the Posterior Fossa*,
https://doi.org/10.1007/978-3-319-67038-6_9

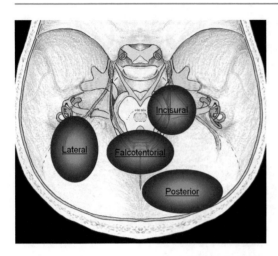

Fig. 9.1 Anatomical subclassification of tentorial meningiomas. Tentorial meningiomas are classified based on the tumor location. The four groups include the incisural type, falcotentorial type, lateral type, and posterior type

temporal lobe, including the vein of Labbe and basal temporal veins and the relationship between the superior petrosal sinus and petrosal vein, is also important to avoid any venous complications.

Different surgical approaches have been proposed for tentorial incisura meningiomas. A retrosigmoid approach and an anterior or combined transpetrosal approach are most frequently performed.

The retrosigmoid approach is appropriate for infratentorial tumor extension or older patients. This approach is simple and quickly performed, with no risk of temporal retraction. Its disadvantage is limited access to the prepontine region and clivus. If it is necessary to gain more access to the cerebellopontine angle, careful removal of the petrous apex with a high-speed drill is useful. The limits of this exposure are defined by the trigeminal nerve medially and the seventh and eighth cranial nerves laterally. If the petrosal vein is well developed, the surgical corridor is more obstructed.

The transpetrosal approach is reserved for relatively large meningiomas invading the cerebellopontine angle at the lateral incisura and the supratentorial region. By using the transpetrosal approach, the surgeon's operative distance to these regions is shorter than with the retrosigmoid approach, and a more multi-angled corridor leads to better control of the basilar artery and perforating vessels, with minimal retraction of the cerebellum and temporal lobe.

Illustrative Case

Case 1: Retrosigmoid Approach (Fig. 9.2)

A 43-year-old woman presented with a 1-year history of left facial pain. MR imaging demonstrated a mass lesion at the left tentorial incisura. The size of the tumor was 25 mm. The tumor compressed the brain stem slightly, and there was no edema into the brain stem. The tumor was excised via a retrosigmoid approach. The tumor had a well-defined plane of dissection from the brain stem and cranial nerves. The tumor could be totally removed with preservation of the petrosal veins, and there were no postoperative complications.

Case 2: Retrosigmoid Approach with Drilling of the Petrous Apex (Fig. 9.3)

A 52-year-old woman presented with a 2-year history of headache. Neurological examination showed instability of tandem gait. MR imaging demonstrated a mass lesion at the left tentorial incisura with extension into Meckel's cave. The tumor was removed via a retrosigmoid approach. After internal debulking of the tumor, the petrous apex was drilled out, and Meckel's cave was opened. Most of the tumor was resected except for around the porous part of the trochlear nerve. There were no postoperative complications.

Case 3: Anterior Transpetrosal Approach (Fig. 9.4)

A 67-year-old woman presented with a 1-year history of left facial pain. MR imaging demonstrated a mass lesion at the left tentorial incisura. Although the size of the tumor was not very large, the tumor compressed the brain stem slightly. The tumor was excised via a left anterior transpetrosal approach. The trigeminal nerve was compressed caudally, so that the tumor inside Meckel's cave was removed easily, and the tentorium was incised along the posterior edge of the tumor. The tumor was totally removed (Simpson G1), and there was no neurological worsening.

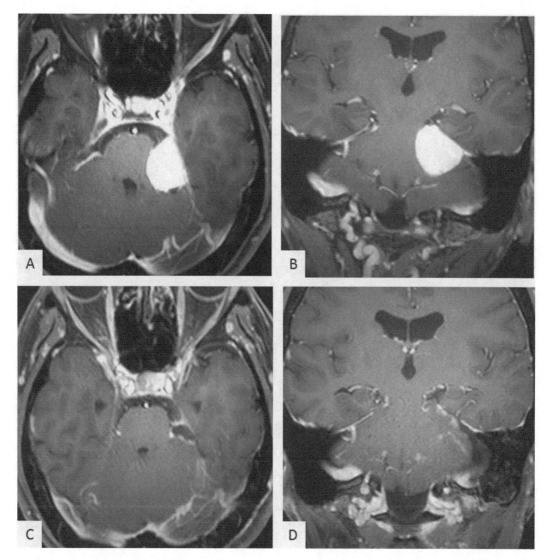

Fig. 9.2 Case 1. Preoperative axial (**a**) and coronal (**b**) T1-weighted magnetic resonance images with gadolinium showing the left incisural type of tentorial meningioma. Postoperative axial (**c**) and coronal (**d**) T1-weighted magnetic resonance images with gadolinium showing no tumor residual via a retrosigmoid approach

Case 4: Combined Transpetrosal Approach (Fig. 9.5)

A 39-year-old man presented with a 2-month history of gait disturbance. MR imaging showed a large mass lesion at the right tentorial incisura. The tumor severely compressed the brain stem and medial temporal lobe. Resection of the tumor was performed via a combined transpetrosal approach. The tumor adhered tightly to the midbrain at the interpeduncular cistern, leaving a small residual amount of tumor along the right oculomotor nerve. Subtotal resection of the tumor was performed with transient right oculomotor nerve palsy and left hemiparesis. These symptoms improved completely within 3 months.

Falcotentorial Type

Meningiomas arising from the falcotentorial junction are relatively rare, and only isolated case reports or small series related to surgical

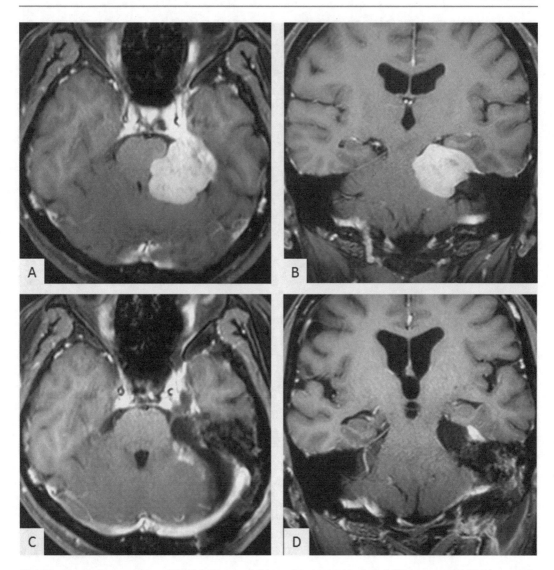

Fig. 9.3 Case 2. Preoperative axial (**a**) and coronal (**b**) T1-weighted magnetic resonance images with gadolinium showing the left incisural type of tentorial meningioma. Postoperative axial (**c**) and coronal (**d**) T1-weighted magnetic resonance images with gadolinium showing near-total resection of the tumor via a retrosigmoid approach with drilling of the petrous bone. After internal debulking of the tumor (**e**), the left SCA is exposed (**f**). The tumor is peeled from the brain stem (**g**), and the petrous apex is drilled out (**h**). The tumor in Meckel's cave is removed (**i**), and most of the tumor is resected, except for just around the porous part of the trochlear nerve (**j**). *SCA* superior cerebellar artery

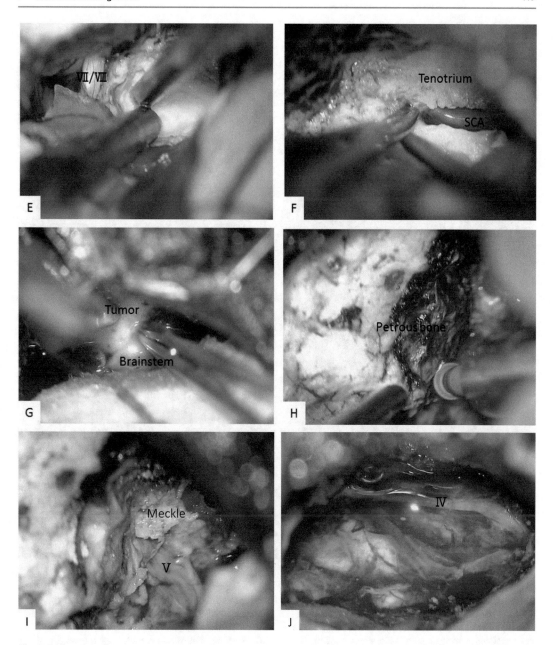

Fig. 9.3 (continued)

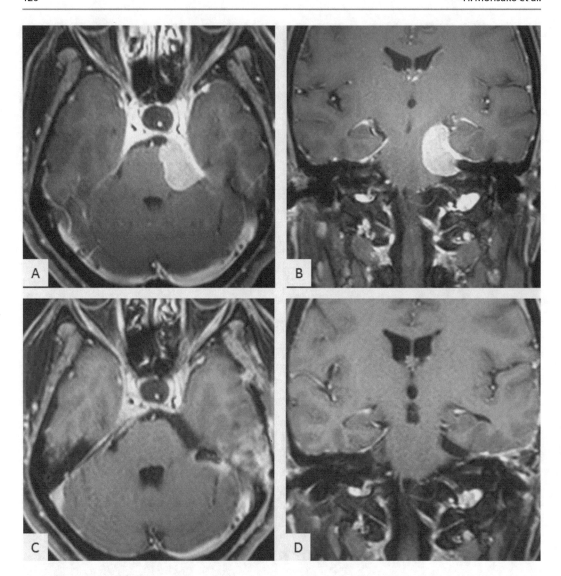

Fig. 9.4 Case 3. Preoperative axial (**a**) and coronal (**b**) T1-weighted magnetic resonance images with gadolinium showing the left incisural type of tentorial meningioma. Postoperative axial (**c**) and coronal (**d**) T1-weighted magnetic resonance images with gadolinium showing total removal of the tumor via an anterior transpetrosal approach. After opening of Meckel's cave (**e**), internal debulking of the tumor is performed. The tumor is carefully peeled from the trochlear nerve (**f**), and the tentorium is detached from the tumor (**g**). The tumor located around the trigeminal nerve and brain stem is removed (**h**). Residual tentorium, which was the origin of the tumor, is resected completely (**i**), and the tumor is totally removed (**j**)

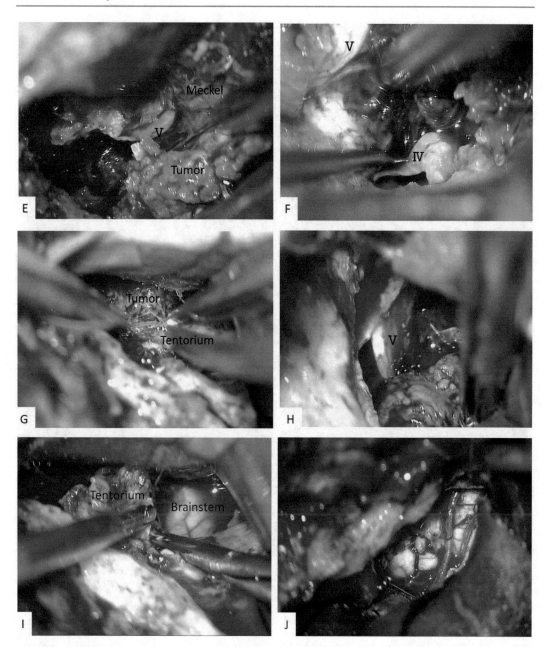

Fig. 9.4 (continued)

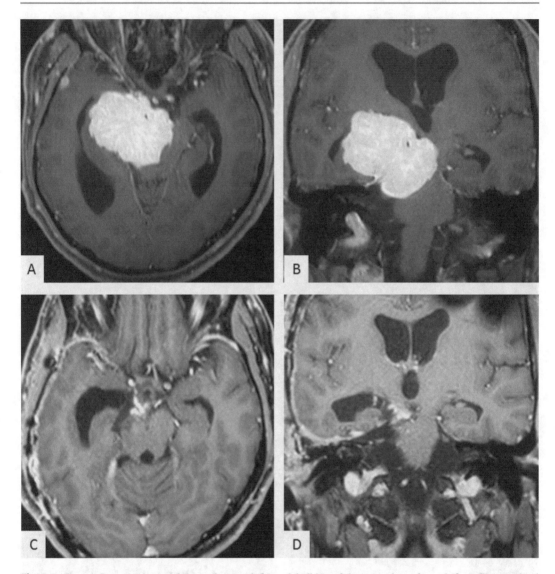

Fig. 9.5 Case 4. Preoperative axial (**a**) and coronal (**b**) T1-weighted magnetic resonance images with gadolinium showing the large right incisural type of tentorial meningioma. Postoperative axial (**c**) and coronal (**d**) T1-weighted magnetic resonance images with gadolinium showing near-total resection of the tumor via a right combined transpetrosal approach. After cutting of the superior petrosal sinus (**e**) and opening of Meckel's cave, internal debulking of the tumor is performed (**f**, **g**). The proximal portion of the right SCA is exposed (**h**). The distal portion of the right SCA and brain stem are peeled from the tumor (**i**). Near-total resection of the tumor is achieved with a small residual tumor along the right oculomotor nerve (**j**). *SPS* superior petrosal sinus, *SCA* superior cerebellar artery, * residual tumor

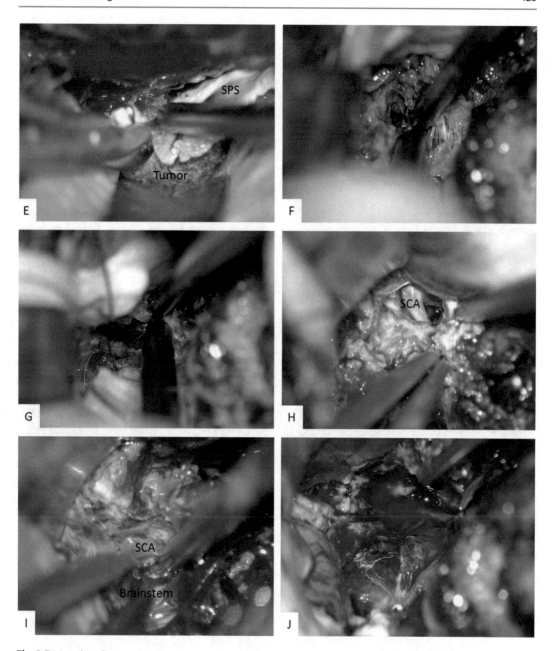

Fig. 9.5 (continued)

technique are available in the literature [1, 3]. Because of the lesion's depth from the surface and its anatomical proximity to critical neural and vascular structures, surgical access and technique are complex issues. A variety of factors, including the tumor location and the patency of the vein of Galen and the straight sinus, influence surgery and the outcomes. Falcotentorial meningiomas are difficult to treat, but they can be well controlled by meticulous strategy.

Surgical Planning

Preoperative neuroimaging investigations include MR imaging, MR venography, CT venography, and angiography. Apart from evaluating the physical characteristics of the tumor, the relationship of the tumor to the great vein of Galen, the patency of the vein of Galen and the straight sinus are evaluated, and pre-existing occlusion of the Galenic system and the subsequent development of collateral venous circulation are important factors when considering surgery on pineal region tumors, including falcotentorial junction meningiomas [3].

Depending on the relationship of the tumor to the great vein of Galen, tumors are classified into two types: tumors located superior to the vein and compressing it downward are labeled the superior type, whereas those displacing it superiorly are labeled the inferior type (Fig. 9.6).

The superior type of falcotentorial meningioma growing inside the posterior pericallosal cistern might compress deep veins over the arachnoid membrane. In this situation, a thick arachnoid membrane septum between the posterior pericallosal cistern and the quadrigeminal cistern protects the deep veins from direct tumor invasion, which enables the surgeon to dissect the lesion from the deep veins. Therefore, in the case of superior type tumor, even when the vein of Galen is patent, careful surgical technique enables the surgeon to separate the tumor from the vein of Galen. Thus, complete surgical removal can be relatively safely performed in the case of superior type tumors.

The inferior type of falcotentorial meningioma growing in the quadrigeminal cistern might compress the deep veins and dorsal midbrain in direct contact with it. Accordingly, in many cases of inferior type, the tumor adheres tightly to the vein of Galen, basal vein, collateral veins, and midbrain. In cases of inferior type tumor with an occluded Galenic system, dissecting the

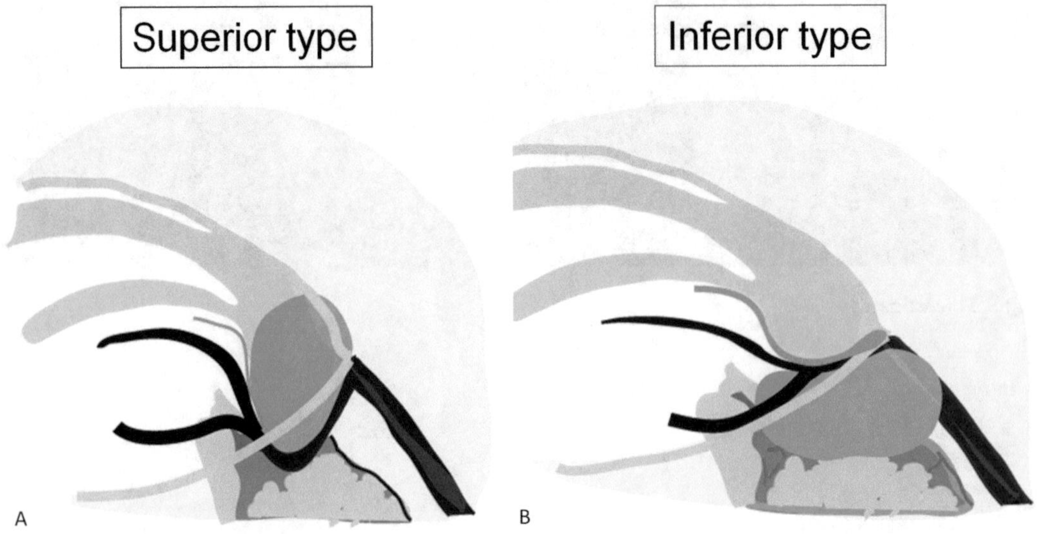

Fig. 9.6 Illustration demonstrating the type of tumor by location. A tumor located over the vein of Galen and compressing it downward is classified as the superior type (**a**), and one situated under the vein of Galen and dislocating it upward is the inferior type (**b**)

tumor from surrounding collateral veins and brain stem is relatively difficult technically. Resection of the tumor in such cases leads to damage of the surrounding structures with additional neurological deficits. In cases in which the Galenic venous system is patent, the surgical procedure is more difficult because the tumor adheres tightly to the venous system. To prevent injury to the deep veins, a small amount of the tumor can be left behind around the deep veins to avoid their injury in the context of an inferior type tumor. Considering the surgical risk involved in excising the inferior type of meningioma, a combination of subtotal tumor resection and stereotactic radiotherapy might be recommended.

As a surgical strategy, the superior type tumor is accessed using a posterior interhemispheric transtentorial approach, and there may be some who prefer a posterior interhemispheric transtentorial approach for inferior type tumors. With inferior tumors located below the vein of Galen, a supracerebellar approach might be advantageous because the vein of Galen would not be directly in harm's way. Surgeons would not have to work through the vein and its tributaries. Therefore, a supracerebellar infratentorial approach to inferior type tumors should be considered [3].

Illustrative Case

Case 5: Posterior Interhemispheric Transtentorial Approach (Fig. 9.7)

A 36-year-old woman presented with a headache. MR imaging demonstrated a mass lesion at the falcotentorial junction. The size of the tumor was 42 mm, and the main part of the tumor was located below the vein of Galen. CT venography showed stenosis of the vein of Galen due to tumor compression. The tumor was excised via a posterior interhemispheric transtentorial approach. Subtotal resection of the tumor was performed with some residual tumor just around the vein of Galen to preserve the deep venous system. There were no neurological deficits after the operation.

Lateral Type

Surgical resection of meningiomas located at the lateral tentorium is relatively simple.

Surgical Planning

Preoperative neuroimaging including MR imaging and MR venography or CT venography is complementary.

Meningiomas located at the lateral tentorial region and extending mainly into the cerebellopontine angle are very well managed through a retrosigmoid approach. This allows the early identification of the cranial nerves, especially the seventh to eighth complex. During tumor dissection, care should be taken to respect the arachnoidal layer to preserve the cranial nerves that are usually compressed dorsally.

Meningiomas located at the lateral tentorial region and extending mainly into the supratentorial region are resected via a subtemporal approach. The ventral or lateral aspect of the midbrain and pons can be accessed by a simple temporal craniotomy. Additional zygomatic osteotomy enhances extensive superior exposure, and anterior petrosectomy enlarges the surgical corridor to the infratentorial region.

Large tentorial leaf meningiomas with superior extension into the occipital lobe and inferior extension into the cerebellum can be approached using a supra-infratentorial approach. In this approach, wide exposure of the transverse sinus is achieved above and below without sinus sacrifice.

Illustrative Case

Case 6: Retrosigmoid Approach (Fig. 9.8)

A 53-year-old man presented with a 2-month history of headache, floating sensation, and gait disturbance. MR imaging demonstrated a large mass lesion at the left lateral tentorium with no invasion of the venous sinuses. The tumor was removed via a left retrosigmoid approach. Simpson G2 removal of the tumor was performed. Postoperatively, the patient's symptoms recovered completely.

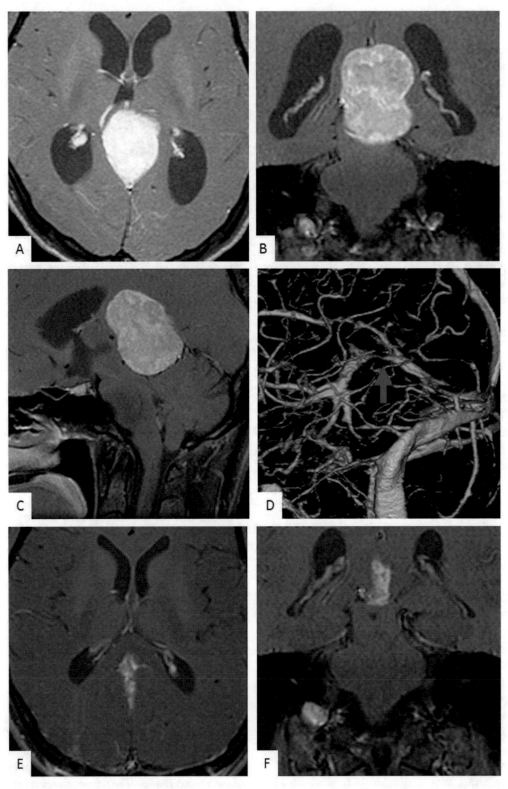

Fig. 9.7 Case 5. Preoperative axial (**a**), coronal (**b**), and sagittal (**c**) T1-weighted magnetic resonance images with gadolinium showing the large falcotentorial type of meningioma. Preoperative CT venography shows stenosis of the vein of Galen (**d**). Postoperative axial (**e**), coronal (**f**), and sagittal **g**) T1-weighted magnetic resonance images with gadolinium showing subtotal resection of the tumor via a posterior interhemispheric transtentorial approach.

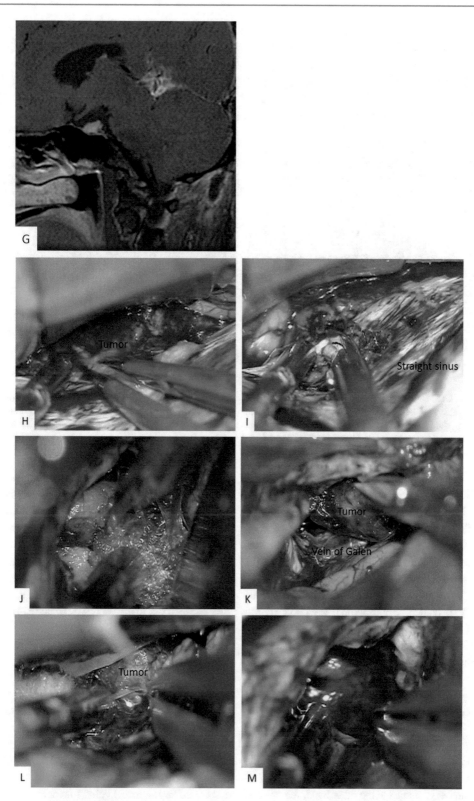

Fig. 9.7 (continued) The tumor is exposed via a left posterior interhemi spheric approach (**h**), and the tentorium is cut (**i**). After internal debulking of the tumor (**j**), the vein of Galen is exposed (**k**). The tumor is peeled from the deep venous system (**l**), and subtotal resection of the tumor is performed

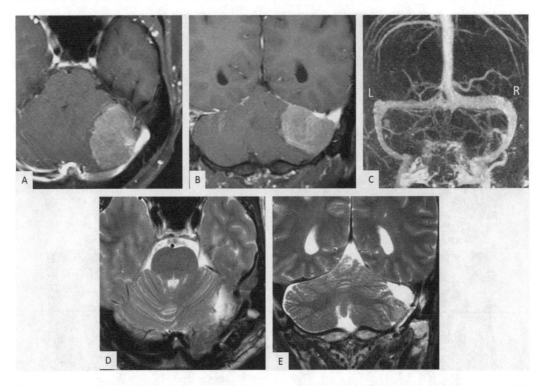

Fig. 9.8 Case 6. Preoperative axial (**a**) and coronal (**b**) T1-weighted magnetic resonance images with gadolinium showing the lateral type of tentorial meningioma. Preoperative MR venography shows no invasion of the venous sinuses (**c**). Postoperative axial (**d**) and coronal (**e**) T2-weighted magnetic resonance images show total resection of the tumor via a retrosigmoid approach

Case 7: Combined Presigmoid and Retrosigmoid Approach with Resection of Tumor Invading the Sigmoid Sinus (Fig. 9.9)

A 35-year-old woman was found to have an intracranial lesion incidentally. MR imaging demonstrated a large mass lesion at the right lateral tentorium. CT venography showed the right sigmoid sinus that was already occluded. Simpson G1 resection of the tumor was performed via a left combined presigmoid and retrosigmoid approach. There were no neurological deficits postoperatively.

Posterior Type

The surgical management of meningiomas located in the posterior tentorium is relatively simple if the tumor has no relationship to the torcular Herophili and transverse sinus. On the other hand, the optimal surgical management of meningiomas involving the major venous sinuses represents a therapeutic dilemma. The operative approach should be planned according to the MRI results, and the venous sinuses should be preserved. Stereotactic radiation therapy might be a beneficial auxiliary treatment of meningiomas in the torcular Herophili region. The decision is whether to leave a fragment of the lesion and have a higher recurrence rate, especially for higher grade meningiomas, or to attempt total removal, which may increase risk to the venous circulation [4].

Surgical Planning

Preoperative MR imaging to determine the extent of the tumor and the degree of brain and venous sinus invasion and vascular imaging in the form of digital subtraction angiography, MR venography, or CT venography are essential. The degree of occlusion of the sinus, anatomy of the sinus and associated large cortical veins, and development of venous collaterals are evaluated preoperatively in cases with invasion into the venous sinuses.

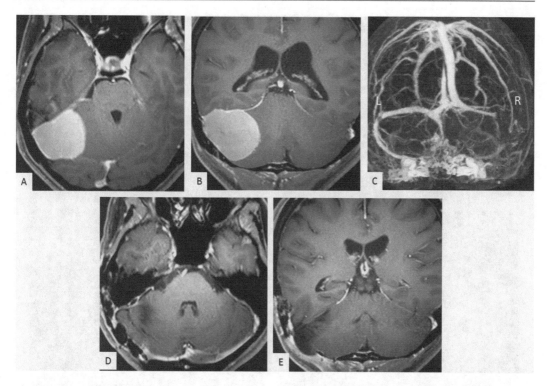

Fig. 9.9 Case 7. Preoperative axial (**a**) and coronal (**b**) T1-weighted magnetic resonance images with gadolinium showing the lateral type of tentorial meningioma. Preoperative CT venography shows occlusion of the right sigmoid sinus (**c**). Postoperative axial (**d**) and coronal (**e**) T1-weighted magnetic resonance images with gadolinium show total resection of the tumor via a combined presigmoid and retrosigmoid approach. Right temporal craniotomy and suboccipital craniotomy with partial petrosectomy is performed (**f**). After internal debulking of the tumor though a retrosigmoid approach (**g**), the right sigmoid sinus is cut at the distal side (**h**). Additional resection of the tumor into the right sigmoid sinus is performed via a presigmoid approach (**i**). The right transverse sinus is cut on the margin of the tumor (**j**), and the tentorium is resected through a presigmoid approach (**k**). The tumor is totally removed (**l**)

Aggressive resection is contraindicated for meningiomas located at the posterior tentorial region invading the sinus partially with sinus patency [5]. After a conservative approach, the residual tumor may be observed or stereotactically irradiated either initially or at the time of recurrence [6].

In the case of total sinus occlusion, particularly if collateral venous channels have developed, complete removal of the tumor, including the segment of the invaded sinus, can be performed safely without venous flow restoration [7].

An aggressive removal may be needed for a higher-grade meningioma with reconstruction of the sinus, especially in younger patients [4].

Illustrative Case

Case 8: Suboccipital Approach with Resection of Invasion into the Transverse Sinus (Fig. 9.10)

A 67-year-old woman presented with headache. MR imaging demonstrated a mass lesion at the right posterior tentorium, invading the right transverse sinus. MR venography showed the already occluded right transverse sinus. The tumor was removed, including the part invading the right transverse sinus, via a suboccipital approach. Postoperatively, there were no complications.

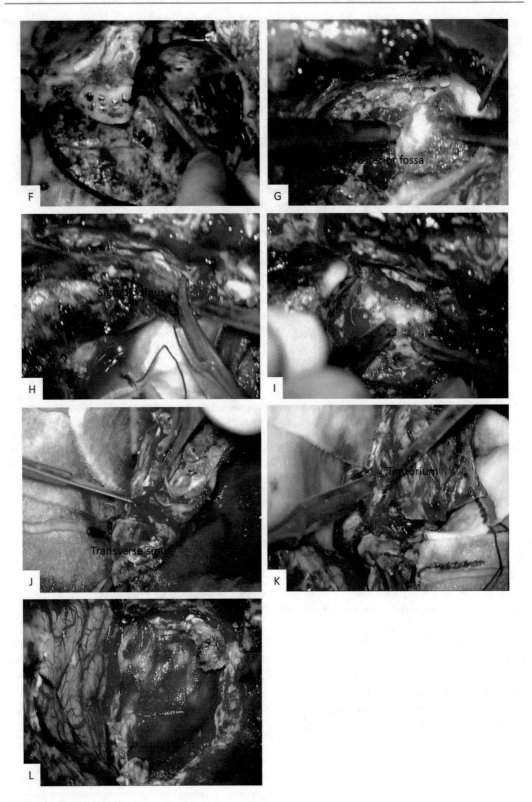

Fig. 9.9 (continued)

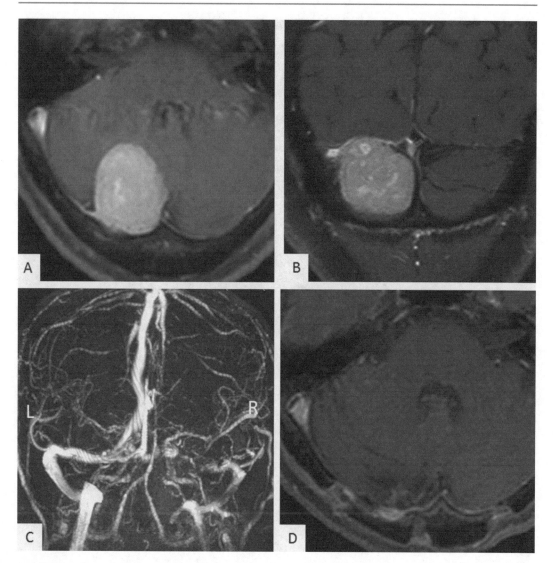

Fig. 9.10 Case 8. Preoperative axial (**a**) and coronal (**b**) T1-weighted magnetic resonance images with gadolinium showing the posterior type of tentorial meningioma. Preoperative MR venography shows invasion of the right transverse sinus (**c**). Postoperative axial (**d**) T1-weighted magnetic resonance images with gadolinium showing total resection of the tumor, including the part invading the sinus, via a suboccipital approach

Case 9: Aggressive Resection with Reconstruction of the Superior Sagittal Sinus (Fig. 9.11)

A 47-year-old woman who had twice undergone tumor resection and γ-knife treatment at a previous hospital showed recurrent tumor at the torcular Herophili. Preoperative CT venography demonstrated occlusion of the straight sinus and left transverse sinus, but venous flow from the superior sagittal sinus to the right transverse sinus was preserved. Thus, an aggressive resection with reconstruction of the sinus using a saphenous vein graft was performed. Simpson G1 removal of the tumor was performed without any complications.

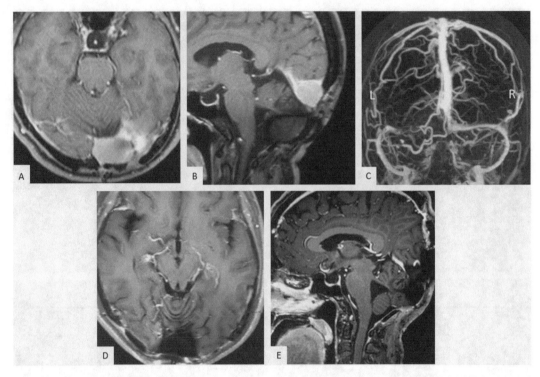

Fig. 9.11 Case 9. Preoperative axial (**a**) and sagittal (**b**) T1-weighted magnetic resonance images with gadolinium showing the posterior type of tentorial meningioma. Preoperative CT venography shows occlusion of the straight sinus and left transverse sinus, although venous flow from the superior sagittal sinus to the right transvers sinus is preserved (**c**). Postoperative axial (**d**) and sagittal (**e**) T1-weighted magnetic resonance images with gadolinium show total resection of the tumor. After craniotomy, the tumor, superior sagittal sinus, and right transverse sinus are exposed (**f**). The left transverse sinus and tentorial edge are cut at the lateral and anterior margins of the tumor (**g, h**). The cerebellar surface is peeled from the torcular Herophili (**i**). Most of the tumor is resected with no residual tumor around the torcular Herophili (**j**). After anastomosis between the right transverse sinus and superior sagittal sinus using a saphenous vein graft is performed (**k, l**), the tumor is totally removed (**m**)

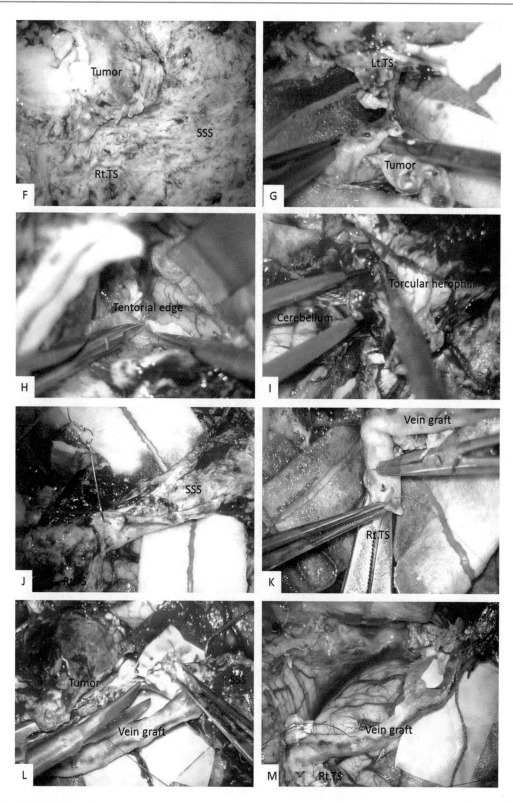

Fig. 9.11 (continued)

Conclusions

- Surgical difficulty is related to tumor location.
- Incisural lesions require a skull base approach.
- Falcotentorial lesions are difficult but can be well controlled by meticulous strategy.
- Lateral lesions and posterior lesions that do not involve the major venous sinuses are relatively simple to treat.
- Surgical management of posterior lesions invading the sinus remains controversial.
- The normal deep venous system should be preserved to avoid any complications.

References

1. Samii M, Carvalho GA, Tatagiba M, Matthies C, Vorkapic P. Meningiomas of the tentorial notch: surgical anatomy and management. J Neurosurg. 1996;84(3):375–81.
2. Sekhar LN, Jannetta PJ, Maroon JC. Tentorial meningiomas: surgical management and results. Neurosurgery. 1984;14(3):268–75.
3. Goto T, Ohata K, Morino M, et al. Falcotentorial meningioma: surgical outcome in 14 patients. J Neurosurg. 2006;104(1):47–53.
4. Mantovani A, Di Malio S, Ferreira MJ, Sekhar LN. Management of meningiomas invading the major dural venous sinuses: operative technique, results, and potential benefit for higher grade tumors. World Neurosurg. 2014;82(3–4):455–67.
5. Raza SM, Gallia GL, Berm H, Weingart JD, Long DM, Olivi A. Perioperative and long-term outcomes from the management of parasagittal meningiomas invading the superior sagittal sinus. Neurosurgery. 2010;67(4):885–93.
6. Stafford SL, Pollock BE, Foote RL, et al. Meningioma radiosurgery: tumor control, outcomes, and complications among 190 consecutive patients. Neurosurgery. 2001;49(5):1029–37.
7. DiMeco F, Li KW, Casali C, et al. Meningiomas invading the superior sagittal sinus: surgical experience in 108 cases. Neurosurgery. 2004;55(6):1263–72.

Foramen Magnum Meningiomas

10

Angela M. Richardson, Karolyn Au,
and Jacques Morcos

Introduction

Foramen magnum meningiomas (FMMs) are a rare entity; they account for 2.5% of all intracranial meningiomas and 4% of posterior fossa meningiomas [22]. The pathologic entity of FMM was first described in 1872; the first publication describing surgical removal was in 1922 [10]. That same year Cushing described a nomenclature for these lesions and published his series. The location of these lesions at the craniocervical junction in proximity to, and possibly encasing, the lower cranial nerves or vertebral arteries makes successful removal particularly challenging [14, 20]. A meningioma is considered to arise from the foramen magnum if the insertion of the tumor is in the region bounded anteriorly by the lower third of the clivus and the upper edge of the body of C2, laterally by the jugular tubercles and the upper aspect of the C1 laminas, and posteriorly by the anterior edge of the squamous occipital bone and C2 spinous process [8]. The large majority (90%) of these tumors are located ventrally or ventrolaterally requiring a lateral or anterior trajectory for successful surgical removal [8, 21, 23].

A.M. Richardson, MD, PhD • K. Au, MD, MSc
J. Morcos, MD, FRCS(Eng), FRCS(Ed), FAANS (✉)
Department of Neurological Surgery, University of
Miami/Jackson Memorial Hospital, Miami, FL, USA
e-mail: jmorcos@med.miami.edu

Clinical Presentation

FMMs are typically slow growing with an indolent course, but when they become symptomatic, they most commonly present with quadriparesis, sensory abnormalities, ataxia, and dysfunction of cranial nerves (CN) IX and X [22]. Patients often describe suboccipital headache or upper cervical pain, exacerbated by coughing or straining [10]. The vague nature of symptoms often prevents early diagnosis with a mean of 31 months to diagnosis from symptom onset [7]. The classic presentation of weakness associated with a FMM is initial weakness in the ipsilateral arm. Progression then occurs to the ipsilateral leg, then the contralateral leg, and finally the contralateral arm [7]. With compression at the craniocervical junction, patients may also have downbeat nystagmus on physical exam. Other signs that may be present include wasting of the sternocleidomastoid, trapezius, or intrinsic muscles of the hands [10].

Evolution of Surgical Approach to FMM

A suboccipital craniotomy with drilling of the condyle/jugular tubercle was initially described for resection of craniospinal lesions in 1978 [22]. Heros then described the far-lateral approach

© Springer International Publishing AG 2018
W.T. Couldwell (ed.), *Skull Base Surgery of the Posterior Fossa*,
https://doi.org/10.1007/978-3-319-67038-6_10

in 1986 for the treatment of lesions of the verte-brobasilar system [13]. A similar technique was then described in 1988 for the resection of anterior foramen magnum pathology [12]. Since those early descriptions, many variations on the far-lateral approach have been described with differing degrees of mastoidectomy, condylectomy, the extent of the cervical laminectomy, and mobilization of the vertebral artery depending on the specifics of the case [5, 21]. In 1991, six variations of the dorsolateral approach for meningioma resection were reported: transfacetal, retrocondylar, partial transcondylar, complete transcondylar, extreme-lateral transjugular, and transtubercular [17].

Classification

Foramen magnum meningiomas may be classified based on their compartment of development (intradural or extradural), their relation to the vertebral artery (below, above, or on both sides), and the location of their dural attachments (posterior, lateral, or anterior) [8]. FMMs are considered anterior if the origin is bilateral with respect to the anterior midline (Fig. 10.1), lateral if the origin is between midline and the dentate ligament, and posterior if the origin is posterior to the dentate ligament. Extradural meningiomas at the foramen magnum are less common than intradural tumors, but complete resection is more challenging due to their invasive nature [8, 15]. In tumors that originate beneath the vertebral artery, the cranial nerves are displaced cranially and posteriorly. However, in tumors that originate above the vertebral artery, the location of the cranial nerves is variable, and great care must be taken to avoid injury during tumor resection [15].

Preoperative Assessment

Preoperative workup is aimed at determining the best surgical approach and proximity to nearby structures in order to accurately assess surgical risks. CT is the best tool for assessing bony anatomy in regard to hyperostosis and calcifications, as well as allowing for preoperative determination of the surgical corridor and the degree of bony removal required. In the event of significant bony erosion by the tumor, the patient may require surgical fusion to prevent instability at the craniocervical junction. MRI remains the imaging modality of choice for assessing soft tissues, including the origin of the tumor and the involvement of the critical neurovascular structures located nearby [19].

Many advocate vascular imaging (CTA, MRA, or conventional angiography) preoperatively to evaluate arterial feeders, venous drainage, and the extent of vascular involvement. In particular, defining the V3 and V4 segments of the vertebral artery along with the origin of the PICA will aid in operative planning and the avoidance of complications [8]. Identification and analysis of vessels that are encased in tumor are particularly important. The presence of significant stenosis is suggestive of tumor invasion of the adventitia. In these cases, conventional angiography allows the surgeon to determine if vessel sacrifice is a feasible option based on the results of balloon occlusion test and the presence or absence of collaterals [4].

Surgical Considerations

Patients presenting with FMMs are usually considered for surgery if the lesion is symptomatic, has experienced growth, or is causing mass effect on the brainstem. In these patients, radiosurgery is considered difficult due to the absence of a plane between the tumor and the brainstem and the likelihood of ongoing compression of the brainstem.

As most foramen magnum meningiomas are located ventrally, surgical resection via a far-lateral or extreme-lateral approach may be utilized (see chapter on the far-lateral approach). For midline posterior tumors that do not cross the

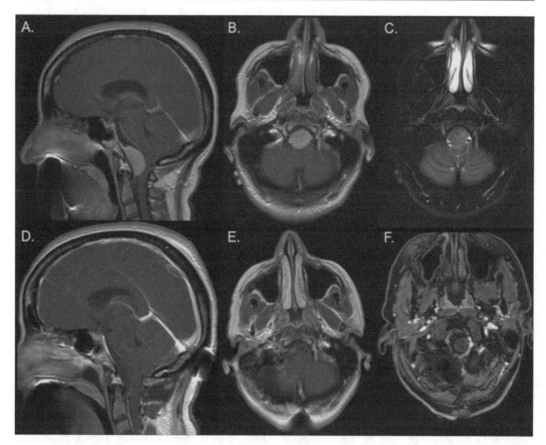

Fig. 10.1 MRI of a 38-year-old female presenting with headaches and dysphagia. (**a–c**) Preoperative imaging. (**a, b**) T1-weighted image with gadolinium demonstrating an anteriorly located FMM eccentric to the right. (**c**) T2-weighted image. (**d–f**) Postoperative imaging T1 weighted with gadolinium demonstrating successful resection of the tumor

plane of the dentate ligament, a midline posterior approach is indicated. Midline anterior tumors without significant spinal extension may appear at first glance to be best approached via an endoscopic endonasal route (EEA), if the tumor is located on the anterior rim of the foramen magnum, the origin is medial to the hypoglossal canal and jugular foramen with posterior and lateral displacement of the lower cranial nerves. However, significant inferior extension would necessitate removal of the anterior arch of C1, the C2 odontoid process, and the ligamentous complex that provides stability at the craniocervical junction. Therefore these tumors are usually managed via a posterolateral approach [4]. The

proponents of the EEA would state that it allows for tumor resection without retraction of brain tissue and does not necessitate crossing the plane of the cranial nerves. In anteriorly based tumors, this approach allows for early access to the dural blood supply with improved visualization during tumor resection and decreased intraoperative blood loss. Also, involved bone and dura may be resected more easily as compared to a more lateral trajectory. Our objection to utilizing the EEA to intradural meningiomas is based on five categories of pitfalls. First, the bony removal in this approach necessitates reconstruction of the skull base and is accompanied by a significant risk of CSF leak [11]. Second, lower rates of complete resection are achieved. Similar to the case with tuberculum sella meningiomas, the dural tails, not well appreciated on preoperative MRIs, often extend lateral to the "presumed" margins of the tumor and are missed or not seen properly during an endoscopic approach. Third, the current, even state-of-the-art instrumentation available for endoscopic skull base surgery lags behind the more mature microscopic arsenal available to microsurgeons. Fourth, the nasal/nasopharyngeal mucosa postoperative morbidity is not trivial and often mischaracterized. Lastly, if a transoral approach is combined with a transnasal route, there is the risk of velo-palatine insufficiency [9]. Additionally, this approach requires a multidisciplinary team and not all surgeons are familiar or adept with it.

The vertebral artery is identified early in lateral surgical approaches, and the decision must be made to work around the artery or mobilize it. We agree with those surgeons who argue against mobilization of the vertebral artery in most cases [6, 14, 15, 23], although, others routinely employ this tactic [16, 20]. Encasement of the vertebral artery by tumor can be seen, and if identified preoperatively, the consequences of vessel sacrifice can be anticipated with balloon occlusion testing. Both extradural encasement and repeat surgery are associated with increased risk of vessel rupture as well as incomplete removal (41% and 51%, respectively) [20, 23].

Monitoring

Many surgeons recommend the use of somatosensory evoked potentials, brainstem auditory evoked potentials, and electromyographic monitoring of the lower cranial nerves (CN X, XI, XII), and this is good practice for this type of surgery [8]. Approaching via a transnasal route mandates monitoring CN VI motor and sensory evoked potentials as this cranial nerve will be encountered early during the approach to the tumor [4]. The senior author has experienced cases where the radicular artery traveling with the C1 nerve root would have been sacrificed (with devastating consequences) to improve exposure for a foramen

magnum meningioma during a far-lateral approach, had it not been for a change in evoked potentials when a temporary clip was placed on the artery to test its contribution to the vascular supply of the upper cervical cord.

Specific Microsurgical Considerations

A detailed discussion of the far-lateral approach is described in the chapter dedicated to that subject. Patient positioning, location of the incision, and drilling of the foramen magnum are addressed there. Once the approach to a foramen magnum meningioma has been completed, be it a far lateral or unilateral suboccipital, there are some general principles to be respected.

The dura is opened in a linear or C-shaped manner based laterally. The dentate ligament should be divided, with particular attention to not confuse it with a portion of the spinal accessory nerve (located posterior to the dentate). The other relational anatomy of relevance is that the V4 segment of the vertebral artery is anterior to the 12th nerve rootlets, which in turn are anterior to the 9/10/11th nerve complex, while the PICA originates at variable heights along the V4 and also courses in a variable direction between the nerves (Fig. 10.2). Once the dentate ligament is divided, the rostrocaudal extent of the tumor needs to be defined. A good practice is to lyse all arachnoidal fibers above and below the tumor, then posterior and medial to the tumor, to allow the cerebellum and other structures to "fall away" from the tumor with gravity. This helps define the "boundaries" of the resection and focuses the surgery. Self-retaining retractors are almost never used. We favor the use of nonstick Telfa strips to create the surgical boundaries.

Ideally, the next step should then be an exposure to the dural base of the tumor for early bipolar devascularization (Fig. 10.3). This step is always straightforward in the case of a lateral origin of the tumor, but may be more problematic in the case of a large midline base covered by a large bulk of tumor, particularly when the vertebral artery and its perforators may be

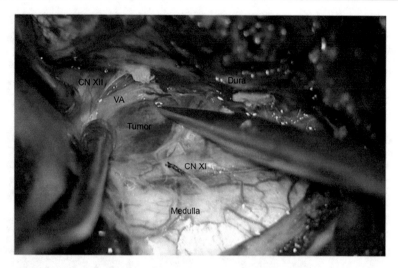

Fig. 10.2 Intraoperative photograph during resection of a FMM (patient shown in Fig. 10.1) from the right side. At the superior aspect of the field, the dura can be appreciated lying flat due to complete drilling of the foramen magnum. This allows optimal visualization of the surgical field. The tumor can be seen displacing the medulla and CN XI posteriorly, creating a working corridor. Distortions of the normal anatomy are common with these tumors, and care must be taken to identify the key neural and vascular structures

Fig. 10.3 The inferior aspect of the tumor has been identified, and early coagulation of the base using the bipolar devascularizes the mass, simplifying piecemeal removal as resection progresses

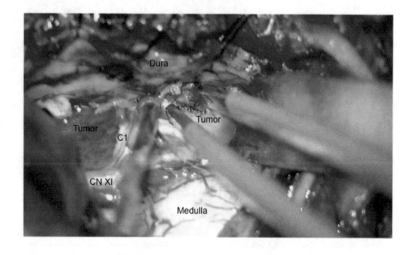

engulfed in the tumor. Here, a "test" resection of an accessible piece of tumor is done first to see how vascular it might be. Piecemeal resection can continue if the tumor is not too bloody, without further consideration given to reaching the base first (Figs. 10.4, 10.5). If on the other hand the vascularity is significant, then a tailored corridor to the dural base should be created through a careful and systematic partial debulking of the most accessible part of the tumor. Once part of the base is reached, the tumor can be devascularized, leading to incremental exposure of more of the base, more debulking, and so on with sequential steps of increasing returns. The tumor shell most adherent to neurovascular structures is naturally left for the end of the resection, when more space is available to tease it out safely. It has been our observation that no matter how large or fibrous or invasive a foramen magnum meningioma is, it never transgresses the pia of the medulla, which, for unclear reasons, is not the case for large petroclival meningiomas that unfortunately often invade the pons subpially.

Fig. 10.4 With this same exposure, the jugular foramen can be seen. Inspection of the superior portion of the tumor allows visualization of the CN IX, X complex with an appreciation for the distortion of normal anatomic relationships caused by the tumor. CN XII can be seen displaced posteriorly (in comparison to the CN IX and X) as it is draped over the tumor surface

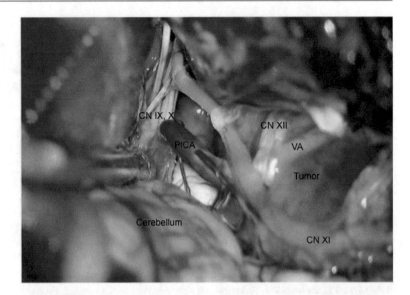

Fig. 10.5 Depending on the particular anatomy of the tumor and locations of the neural and vascular structures, the surgeon may work through one or more surgical corridors that are offered. Debulking continues through these various approaches

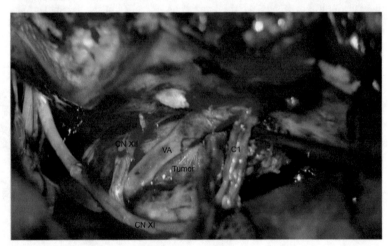

As in most meningioma surgeries, the principles of using sharp dissection and measured countertraction cannot be overemphasized. Ultrasonic aspirators must be used with caution, as they will not respect perforators or buried arteries and nerves (Fig. 10.6).

Once the bulk of visible tumor is removed, one can then address the dural base (Figs. 10.7, 10.8). It is not at all uncommon for a segment of meningioma to extend in the interdural space, which is why the dural base has to be resected as completely as possible. The depth of the resection rarely needs to go through and through to the bone, as FMM rarely invades that deeply.

Outcomes and Complications

Over the past 20 years, the overall reported mortality for FMM resection is 6.2% with a lower rate of permanent morbidity in the far-lateral approach as compared to the extreme-lateral approach (0–17% vs. 21–56%) [8]. In Yasargil's review of 114 FMMs, a good outcome was achieved in 69% of patients, fair in 8%, and poor in 10% [24]. In larger series (>10 patients), neurological improvement was seen in 70–100% of patients [8]. Cerebellar and long tract signs tend to improve postoperatively; however, only a minority of patients experience recovery of pre-

Fig. 10.6 Debulking of the tumor can be performed using sharp dissection. An ultrasonic aspirator may also be used, but this must be done with caution to avoid damage to the surrounding structures

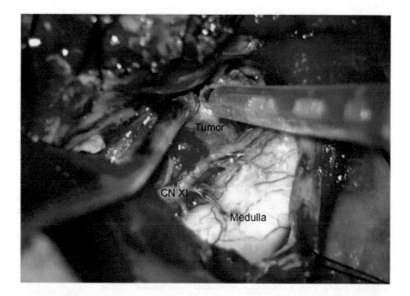

Fig. 10.7 With progressive debulking, portions of the tumor can be pushed away from the surrounding structures and removed

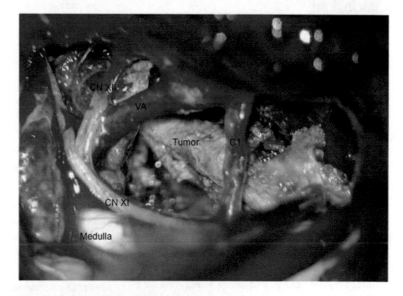

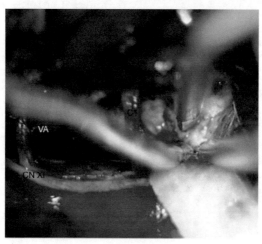

Fig. 10.8 Adequate visualization provided by the exposure allows bipolaring of the dural base following tumor resection, yielding a Simpson Grade 2

existing cranial nerve deficits [22]. Lower cranial nerve palsies are the most commonly observed postoperative deficit, although these deficits (unlike those present preoperatively) have a tendency to recover with time [1–3]. Dysphagia with an attendant risk of aspiration pneumonia may be seen in up to 10% of patients. Multiple regression analysis identified tumor recurrence, arachnoid scarring, prevalent cranial extension, and absence of preoperative lower CN dysfunction as significantly associated with aspiration pneumonia [18]. Vigilance is required postoperatively to minimize these risks.

Conclusions

Foramen magnum meningiomas are a rare entity with the potential for significant symptoms preoperatively and significant complications postoperatively. Thorough preoperative imaging and evaluation aids in determining the extent of neurovascular involvement and in detailing the bony anatomy in the region of the tumor. With adequate surgeon experience and selection of the optimal surgical approach, successful extirpation of the tumor may be achieved.

References

1. Arnautovic KI, Al-Mefty O, Husain M. Ventral foramen magnum meningiomas. J Neurosurg. 2000;92(1 Suppl):71–80.
2. Babu RP, Sekhar LN, Wright DC. Extreme lateral transcondylar approach: technical improvements and lessons learned. J Neurosurg. 1994;81(1):49–59. https://doi.org/10.3171/jns.1994.81.1.0049.
3. Bassiouni H, Ntoukas V, Asgari S, Sandalcioglu EI, Stolke D, Seifert V. Foramen magnum meningiomas: clinical outcome after microsurgical resection via a posterolateral suboccipital retrocondylar approach. Neurosurgery. 2006;59(6):1177–1185.; discussion 1185-1177. https://doi.org/10.1227/01.NEU.0000245629.77968.37.
4. Beer-Furlan A, Vellutini EA, Balsalobre L, Stamm AC. Endoscopic endonasal approach to ventral posterior fossa meningiomas: from case selection to surgical management. Neurosurg Clin N Am. 2015;26(3):413–26. https://doi.org/10.1016/j.nec.2015.03.006.
5. Bertalanffy H, Gilsbach JM, Mayfrank L, Klein HM, Kawase T, Seeger W. Microsurgical management of ventral and ventrolateral foramen magnum meningiomas. Acta Neurochir Suppl. 1996;65:82–5.
6. Borba LA, de Oliveira JG, Giudicissi-Filho M, Colli BO. Surgical management of foramen magnum meningiomas. Neurosurg Rev. 2009;32(1):49–58.; discussion 59–60. https://doi.org/10.1007/s10143-008-0161-5.
7. Boulton MR, Cusimano MD. Foramen magnum meningiomas: concepts, classifications, and nuances. Neurosurg Focus. 2003;14(6):e10.
8. Bruneau M, George B. Foramen magnum meningiomas: detailed surgical approaches and technical aspects at Lariboisiere Hospital and review of the literature. Neurosurg Rev. 2008;31(1):19–32.; discussion 32–13. https://doi.org/10.1007/s10143-007-0097-1.
9. Crockard HA, Sen CN. The transoral approach for the management of intradural lesions at the craniovertebral junction: review of 7 cases. Neurosurgery. 1991;28(1):88–97. discussion 97–88
10. Flores BC, Boudreaux BP, Klinger DR, Mickey BE, Barnett SL. The far-lateral approach for foramen magnum meningiomas. Neurosurg Focus. 2013;35(6):E12. https://doi.org/10.3171/2013.10.FOCUS13332.
11. Fraser JF, Nyquist GG, Moore N, Anand VK, Schwartz TH. Endoscopic endonasal minimal access approach to the clivus: case series and technical nuances. Neurosurgery. 2010;67(3 Suppl Operative):ons150–ons158.; discussion ons158. https://doi.org/10.1227/01.NEU.0000383130.80179.41.
12. George B, Dematons C, Cophignon J. Lateral approach to the anterior portion of the foramen magnum. Application to surgical removal of 14 benign tumors: technical note. Surg Neurol. 1988;29(6):484–90.
13. Heros RC. Lateral suboccipital approach for vertebral and vertebrobasilar artery lesions. J Neurosurg. 1986;64(4):559–62. https://doi.org/10.3171/jns.1986.64.4.0559.
14. Kano T, Kawase T, Horiguchi T, Yoshida K. Meningiomas of the ventral foramen magnum and lower clivus: factors influencing surgical morbidity, the extent of tumour resection, and tumour recurrence. Acta Neurochir. 2010;152(1):79–86.; discussion 86. https://doi.org/10.1007/s00701-009-0511-2.
15. Margalit NS, Lesser JB, Singer M, Sen C. Lateral approach to anterolateral tumors at the foramen magnum: factors determining surgical procedure. Neurosurgery. 2005;56(2 Suppl):324–36. discussion 324–336
16. Park HH, Lee KS, Hong CK. Vertebral artery transposition via an extreme-lateral approach for anterior foramen magnum meningioma or Craniocervical junction tumors. World Neurosurg. 2016;88:154–65. https://doi.org/10.1016/j.wneu.2015.12.073.
17. Salas E, Sekhar LN, Ziyal IM, Caputy AJ, Wright DC. Variations of the extreme-lateral craniocervical approach: anatomical study and clinical analysis of 69 patients. J Neurosurg. 1999;90 (2 Suppl):206–19.

18. Samii M, Klekamp J, Carvalho G. Surgical results for meningiomas of the craniocervical junction. Neurosurgery. 1996;39(6):1086–94. discussion 1094–1085

19. Sekhar LN, Jannetta PJ, Burkhart LE, Janosky JE. Meningiomas involving the clivus: a six-year experience with 41 patients. Neurosurgery. 1990;27(5):764–81. discussion 781

20. Sekhar LN, Javed T. Meningiomas with vertebrobasilar artery encasement: review of 17 cases. Skull Base Surg. 1993;3(2):91–106.

21. Sen CN, Sekhar LN. An extreme lateral approach to intradural lesions of the cervical spine and foramen magnum. Neurosurgery. 1990;27(2):197–204.

22. Talacchi A, Biroli A, Soda C, Masotto B, Bricolo A. Surgical management of ventral and ventrolateral foramen magnum meningiomas: report on a 64-case series and review of the literature. Neurosurg Rev. 2012;35(3):359–367.; discussion 367–358. https://doi.org/10.1007/s10143-012-0381-6.

23. Wu Z, Hao S, Zhang J, Zhang L, Jia G, Tang J, et al. Foramen magnum meningiomas: experiences in 114 patients at a single institute over 15 years. Surg Neurol. 2009;72(4):376–382.; discussion 382. https://doi.org/10.1016/j.surneu.2009.05.006.

24. Yaşargil MG, Mortara RW, Curcic M. Meningiomas of basal posterior cranial fossa. In: Krayenbühl H, Brihaye J, Loew F, Logue V, Mingrino S, Pertuiset B, Symon L, Troupp H, Yasargil MG, editors. Advances and technical standards in neurosurgery. Vienna: Springer Vienna; 1980. p. 3–115.

Vestibular Schwannomas

Gmaan Alzhrani, Clough Shelton,
and William T. Couldwell

Introduction

Vestibular schwannomas (VSs) are benign nerve sheath tumors originating along the vestibulocochlear nerve course that account for 6–8% of all intracranial tumors. VS is the most common pathology found in the cerebellopontine angle (CPA), accounting for up to 80% of tumors there [19]. The management options of these tumors are observation, radiation therapy, and surgical removal, depending on imaging findings and clinical presentation. The surgical removal of VSs is accomplished through three main surgical routes: the middle fossa approach (MFA), the translabyrinthine approach, and the retrosigmoid approach.

The choice of microsurgical approach for VS tumors is multifactorial and depends on the tumor size, patient age, tumor site and extent of internal auditory canal (IAC) involvement, anatomy of the vestibule, amount of tumor extension in the CPA, brainstem involvement, preoperative hearing status, and surgeon's preference [1, 16, 26, 34].

The availability of superior microscopes, safer high-speed drills, better hemostatic agents, and intraoperative neuromonitoring has led to an evolution in the goals of microsurgery for VS, which have progressed from preserving life to preserving facial nerve function and now to hearing preservation [8, 11, 20]. Whereas the translabyrinthine approach sacrifices hearing to achieve greater exposure, the MFA and retrosigmoid approaches to resection of VS tumors offer the possibility of hearing preservation. In this chapter, we describe these three most commonly used approaches for the removal of VSs and their technical nuances.

Retrosigmoid Approach

Indications

The retrosigmoid approach is indicated in patients undergoing removal of VS of any size or when an attempt at hearing preservation is to be made with smaller tumors, either intercanalicular or extracanalicular. From a practical standpoint, the retrosigmoid approach is used by the senior authors for large tumors, as it offers expansive view of the posterior fossa for rapid verification of neurovascular anatomy, and for medial acoustic tumors in which hearing preservation is the goal of surgery.

G. Alzhrani, MD • W.T. Couldwell, MD, PhD (✉)
Department of Neurosurgery, Clinical Neurosciences Center, University of Utah, 175 N. Medical Drive East, Salt Lake City, UT 84132, USA
e-mail: neuropub@hsc.utah.edu

C. Shelton, MD
Division of Otolaryngology – Head and Neck Surgery, University of Utah School of Medicine, Salt Lake City, UT, USA

© Springer International Publishing AG 2018
W.T. Couldwell (ed.), *Skull Base Surgery of the Posterior Fossa*,
https://doi.org/10.1007/978-3-319-67038-6_11

Surgical Technique

The steps of the retrosigmoid technique for hearing preservation are illustrated in Fig. 11.1, and those for the non-hearing preservation procedure are illustrated in Fig. 11.2. At our institution, we use the lateral position with the head held in a Mayfield three-point pin headrest. We try to minimize the rotation of the head and flex the neck in a lateral direction to offer increased working distance between the suboccipital region and the upper shoulder of the nondependent arm. The arm is placed on an airplane rest and retracted gently inferiorly. An axillary roll and a Foley

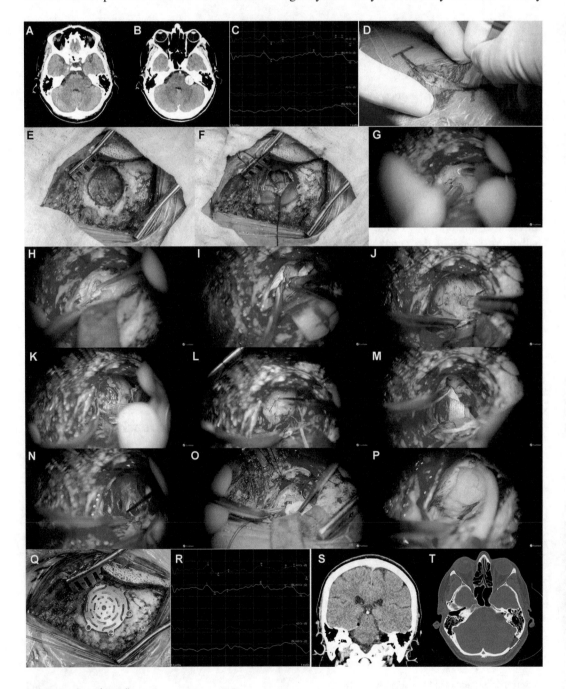

Fig. 11.1 (continued)

catheter are placed, and pillows are positioned between the legs. For all surgeries in the posterior fossa, we use a total intravenous anesthesia technique. The benefits of this have been described elsewhere [5]. The patient is given corticosteroids, antibiotics, and mannitol for brain relaxation.

The incision used is a gently curved incision of one to two fingerbreadths behind the mastoid. The course of the transverse and sigmoid junction and transverse and sigmoid sinuses can be anticipated based on the bony anatomy. A straight line is drawn between the roots of the zygoma to the inion, and the transverse sinus lies along this line. It curves inferiorly into the sigmoid sinus at the region of the asterion. The incision is infiltrated with lidocaine and opened with a sharp blade. After self-retaining retractors are placed, we attempt to identify the region of the mastoid emissary vein, which is a guide to the location of the sigmoid sinus. Bleeding from the mastoid emissary is controlled with bone wax. We perform either a craniectomy or a craniotomy, located just below the transverse sigmoid junction at its most superior extent. We look to identify the inferior aspect of the transverse sinus and the posterior aspect of the sigmoid sinus along the course after the bone flap is removed. This ensures an adequate trajectory and maximal visualization of the CPA. A roughly 2- to 3-cm oval opening is made extending from the transverse sinus down along the posterior aspect of the sigmoid sinus. The dura is usually opened in a cruci-ate fashion that allows the flap to be reflected superiorly or laterally along the transverse and sigmoid sinuses, respectively. Alternatively, a cuff of dura may be left adjacent, and the opening may follow the sinuses. This allows the cuff to be reflected with sutures for added retraction. After the dura is opened, we bring the operating microscope in the field and identify the superior and lateral aspects of the cerebellum. We then continue our dissection down along the petrous ridge at its junction with the tentorium and identify the petrosal vein. The arachnoid is opened in this location to allow egress of cerebrospinal fluid (CSF). Immediately inferior to the petrosal sinus, we look for evidence of the VS.

Upon visualization of the tumor, the outer layer of arachnoid is reflected down to expose the posterior aspect of the tumor. We use soft cottonoids to reflect the arachnoid and the vasculature from the tumor and expose the tumor to develop the window for resection. We immediately stimulate the back of the tumor to see if there is an aberrant location of the facial nerve. At this time, we use a dissector and identify the IAC. The cuff of dura over the IAC is opened approximately 1–2 cm, and the lateral aspect of the IAC is drilled to enable visualization of the limits of tumor within the canal. This then enables identification of the location of the facial nerve early in the dissection. If the facial nerve is running along the anterior aspect of the tumor as in the vast majority of cases, a window is opened in the posterior aspect of the tumor, and a specimen is removed for pathological analysis. We

---

Fig. 11.1 (continued) Images showing steps of a retrosigmoid approach for resection of a *left* small VS. Axial CT brain cuts without contrast (**a**) and with contrast (**b**) demonstrating medially located VS. (**c**) Preoperative BAEP responses demonstrate symmetric hearing. (**d**) Skin incision. (**e**) A 2.5-cm-diameter craniectomy is performed exposing the transverse and sigmoid sinuses. (**f**) Dural opening along the margins of the transverse and sigmoid junction. (**g**) IAC drilling intradural. (**h**) Sealing of the opened air cells using bone wax after IAC exposure is completed. (**i**) Dura is opened over the medial aspect of the tumor. (**j**) The posterior aspect of the tumor exposure and a window is cut after verifying the facial nerve is not located on the posterior aspect of the tumor. (**k**) The ultrasonic aspirator is used to debulk the center of the tumor. (**l**) The tumor capsule is gently elevated from the cerebellum and brainstem, and the facial and vestibulocochlear nerves are located at their brainstem exit and entry, respectively. (**m**) Continued dissection of the capsule from the facial and vestibulocochlear nerves. We carefully use soft cottonoids to protect the nerves during the dissection. (**n**) The tumor has been removed and the facial nerve is stimulated at the brainstem to verify continuity. (**o**) The region of the IAC that was drilled is coated with bone wax to prevent any possibility for CSF leak. (**p**) Fat graft is placed over the drilled IAC and fibrin glue is applied. (**q**) Large bur hole cover is used to cover craniectomy defect. (**r**) Postoperative BAER demonstrates preserved hearing. (**s, t**) Postoperative CT in the coronal and axial planes demonstrating region of bone drilling and tumor removal

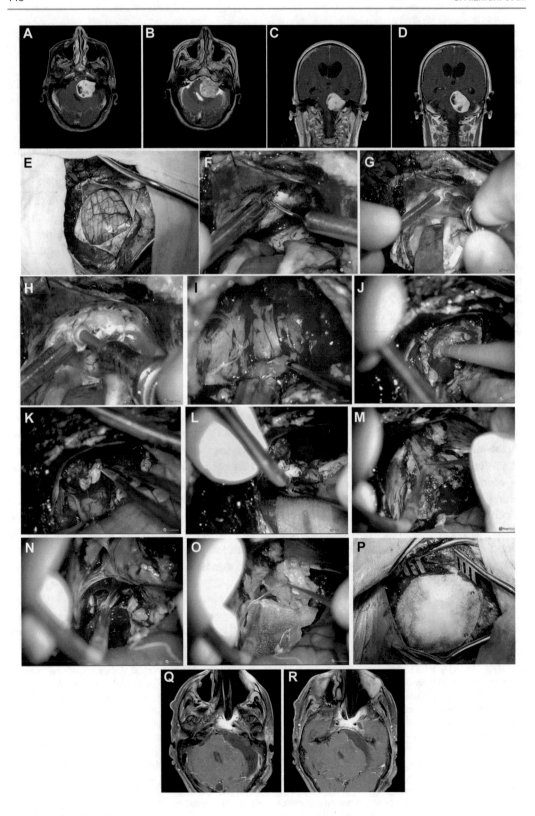

Fig. 11.2 (continued)

then debulk the center of the tumor. The amount of removal of the interior aspect of the tumor is determined by the size of the tumor on the scan, with the objective of leaving a margin of the tumor along the tumor capsule to enable the capsule to be dissected from the surrounding cerebellum, brainstem, and nerves.

Attention is then paid to activity of the facial and vestibulocochlear nerves as measured by the electromyographic activity of the facial nerve and the brainstem auditory evoked responses (BAERs) of the cochlear nerve. If the tumor is large and the hearing is nonserviceable, vestibulocochlear nerve monitoring is not performed. We then start a dissection around the capsule of the tumor to identify the CPA and the location of the vestibulocochlear and facial nerves at the brainstem. The vestibulocochlear nerve is more posteriorly located in the brainstem and is usually found without difficulty on the medial aspect of the tumor. If hearing preservation is not a goal, the vestibulocochlear nerve is stimulated to ensure there is no aberrant course of the facial nerve and then is divided sharply. We then continue to rotate the capsule of the tumor laterally and identify the facial nerve, which is located anterior to the root entry zone of the vestibulocochlear nerve. The root exit zone of the facial nerve is identified visually and verified electrophysiologically with stimulation from the Prass electrode. Once the facial nerve is identified at the brainstem, dissection is then continued with debulking of the tumor, removal of the capsule, and slow dissection of the capsule in a medial-to-

lateral direction from the facial and possibly vestibulocochlear nerves if hearing preservation is a goal (Fig. 11.1). The most adherent aspect of the tumor to the facial nerve is usually at the region of the lip of the porus acusticus. The nerve often flares in dimension at this location, but in most cases, judicious dissection from medial to lateral can be performed and the nerve dissected free of the tumor. The remaining tumor is removed from the IAC, and careful dissection is performed to sharply divide the vestibular nerve lateral to the attachment to the nerve. At this point, we verify functional continuity of the facial nerve by stimulating the nerve at the brainstem to assess its function. The BAER is recorded carefully after resection of the tumor.

The drilled posterior aspect of the IAC is inspected carefully to see if any air cells have been entered. If air cells have been entered, bone wax is used to obliterate them, and a small piece of abdominal fat is placed over the drilled area and held in place with fibrin glue. Hemostasis is obtained, and a small piece of Surgicel is placed over the region of the brainstem where the tumor has been dissected free. The dura is closed in a watertight fashion using dural substitute if necessary. AlloDerm is our preferred material. The bone is carefully waxed over the region of the mastoid where any air cells have been entered. We either replace the bone flap at this point or place a small titanium or MEDPOR (Stryker, Kalamazoo, MI) cranioplasty over the defect. The muscle is closed in separate layers, and the skin is closed with a 3-0 nylon suture.

Fig. 11.2 (continued) Images showing steps of a retrosigmoid approach for resection of a left large VS. (**a**) Axial T1-weighted MRI with gadolinium demonstrating large tumor. (**b**) Axial T2-weighted MRI demonstrating CSF cleft between tumor, brainstem, and cerebellar peduncle. (**c, d**) Coronal T1-weighted MRI with gadolinium demonstrating large tumor. (**e**) Dural opening with flaps of dura adjacent to transverse and sigmoid sinuses. (**f**) Tumor exposure in the CPA and the petrous surface dural opening is made in a semilunar fashion behind Fig. 11.2 (continued) the posterior lip of the IAC. (**g, h**) Posterior lip of IAC is drilled. (**i**) IAC is opened and the tumor is identified and the facial nerve is located. (**j**) The ultrasonic aspirator is used to debulk the tumor. (**k**) The vestibular nerve is identified entering the tumor. It is then divided sharply at the brainstem. (**l**) The facial nerve is identified at its root exit zone from the brainstem. It is verified with the stimulator. (**m**) Continued dissection of the tumor from the facial nerve at the IAC. (**n**) The capsule of the tumor is dissected from the facial nerve from the brainstem in a medial-to-lateral direction. (**o**) The remaining portion of tumor is dissected off the facial nerve near the lip of the porus acusticus. (**p**) A small MEDPOR cranioplasty is used to cover the craniectomy defect. (**q, r**) Postoperative axial MRI with gadolinium demonstrating complete resection of the tumor

Surgical Risks and Complications

The reported mortality rate for retrosigmoid approach for VS is 0.3% [1]. Morbidities including CSF leak in 10.3%, postoperative headache in 17.5%, postoperative symptomatic hemorrhage in 2.2%, major neurological complications in 1.8%, postoperative hydrocephalus in 2.3%, and meningitis in 3% have been reported [1, 27]. Inspection for air cells while opening and drilling the IAC, careful tumor dissection, and meticulous dural closure may help reduce the risk of these morbidities. A systematic review for this approach found residual tumor on imaging postoperatively in 5.6% of the patients planned for gross-total resection and tumor recurred in 6.2% [1].

Surgical Outcome

The hearing preservation rates after retrosigmoid approach are 55.7%, 35.7%, and 28.4% for intracanalicular, <1.5 cm, and 1.5–3-cm tumors, respectively [1]. The facial nerve function preservation rate is >90% for intercanalicular tumors ≤3 cm in diameter and 69.8% for tumors >3 cm [1].

Middle Fossa Approach

The MFA was used by otolaryngologists to treat pathologies involving the inner and middle ear long before it was adapted by neurosurgeons for resection of intracanalicular VSs. This approach and its modifications provide an excellent corridor for middle and posterior fossa pathologies. The MFA was first performed in Glasgow by R. H. Parry, a Scotch otolaryngologist, in 1904 to treat a 30-year-old patient with left ear pain, tinnitus, and vertigo. The surgery was carried out to divide the vestibular nerve, but unfortunately, the facial nerve was injured when additional bone was removed over the most proximal portion of the fallopian canal during the approach [23]. For this reason, the MFA did not gain popularity until William House and Theodore Kurze described their microsurgical technique in 1961; they used the MFA in 14 patients for treatment of Ménière's disease and otosclerosis of the middle ear and later treated 106 patients with intracanalicular VS via the MFA without permanent facial nerve paralysis [12–14]. This approach has undergone few modifications over the years, most of which are related to the methods for localization of the IAC.

Indications

Ménière's disease, dehiscence of the posterior semicircular canal, and VS are the most common indications for MFA. Other indications include facial nerve decompression and repair in trauma and Bell's palsy, facial nerve neuroma, cholesteatoma drainage, middle fossa encephalocele, CSF leak through the middle ear, petrous carotid exposure for high-flow intracranial bypass for complex aneurysms, skull base tumors, and fungal infections. For patients with VS, we use the MFA for hearing preservation in relatively young patients with purely intracanalicular tumor, for VS located in the IAC with cisternal extension of less than 1–1.5 cm (Fig. 11.3), and for tumor extending to the fundus of the IAC (lateral VS).

Relevant Surgical Anatomy

The middle fossa is bordered by the sphenoid ridge anteriorly, squamosal bone laterally, mastoid bone posterolaterally, petrous ridge posteromedially, and cavernous sinus and sella medially. The floor of the middle fossa hosts a number of important structures. Rhoton et al. [33] divided the floor of the middle fossa using a vertical plane through the anterior border of the cochlea into anterior and posterior parts. The anterior part contains, from lateral to medial, respectively, the eustachian tube, tensor tympani, and petrous carotid artery, parallel and deep to the greater superficial petrosal nerve (GSPN) in the space between the V3 divisions of the trigeminal nerve anteriorly and the cochlea posteriorly. The eustachian tube and tensor tympani are almost always covered by the bone, but in 63% of cadaveric specimens, the horizontal segment of the petrous

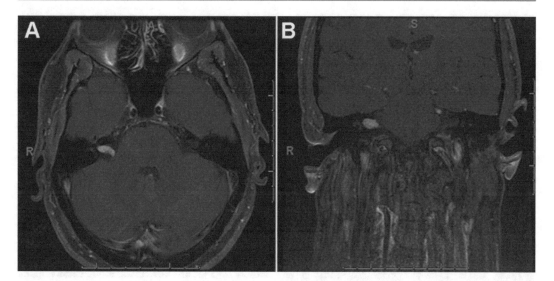

Fig. 11.3 Axial (**a**) and coronal (**b**) T1-weighted MRI with gadolinium showing patient who presented with progressive vestibular symptoms and preserved hearing. The cuts demonstrate a small VS located at the right IAC extending from the fundus of the IAC to the prepontine cistern

carotid artery is apparent with only a very thin or no bony covering [21, 33]. The posterior part of the middle fossa floor contains the bony labyrinth with its three components: the cochlea, vestibule, and semicircular canals. The posterior part of the middle fossa is more vulnerable to injury during surgery given its intimate relationship with the lateral part of the IAC. The cochlea is located at the cochlear angle between the GSPN and the labyrinthine part of the facial nerve just anterior to the IAC fundus. The semicircular canals open inferomedially into the vestibule, which is a small cavity located in the posterolateral margin of the IAC fundus.

Along the petrous ridge on the floor of the middle fossa, a few bony landmarks can be identified: the petrous apex, trigeminal impression, trigeminal prominence, meatal depression, arcuate eminence (AE), and tegmen from medial to lateral, respectively. The superior semicircular canal (SSC) projects toward the middle fossa floor and makes a bony elevation known as the AE. In the anterior part of the middle fossa, the foramen spinosum and foramen ovale are very important landmarks that must be identified. The foramen spinosum, with the middle meningeal artery (MMA) passing through it, is located just posterior and lateral to the foramen ovale. The

GSPN carries the preganglionic parasympathetic fiber of the facial nerve to the lacrimal gland, and some taste fibers from the soft palate originate at the geniculate ganglion. It passes anteriorly in the sphenopetrosal groove, where it runs beneath the V3 division of the trigeminal nerve toward the foramen lacerum, and then joins the lesser petrosal nerve to form the vidian nerve in the vidian canal (Fig. 11.4). The lateral extent of the IAC is divided into four quadrants: Bill's bar (vertical crest) separates the facial nerve in the superior-anterior quadrant from the superior vestibular nerve in the superior-posterior quadrant; the transverse crest separates the superior vestibular nerve in the superior-posterior quadrant from the inferior vestibular nerve in the inferior-posterior quadrant. The cochlear nerve is located in the inferior-posterior quadrant of the IAC.

IAC Localization Techniques in the Petrous Bone

Four techniques are commonly reported in the literature to localize the IAC during MFA. The House technique follows the GSPN posteriorly to the area of the Gasserian ganglion (GG) and the labyrinthine segment of the facial nerve medially toward porus

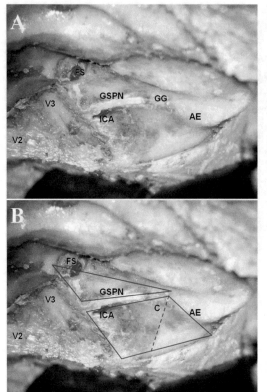

Fig. 11.4 (**a**) Cadaveric dissection (*right-sided approach*) photograph demonstrating the anatomy of the middle fossa. The temporal lobe is elevated extradurally to expose the floor of the middle fossa. This is performed in a posterior-to-anterior direction to avoid traction injury to the facial nerve by putting stretch on the greater superficial petrosal nerve (GSPN). The horizontal segment of the petrous internal carotid artery (ICA) is visible through a bony dehiscence. The arcuate eminence (AE) initially is identified along the petrous ridge. Extradural elevation then is continued anteromedially to expose the geniculate ganglion (GG) and the GSPN. The middle meningeal artery at the foramen spinosum (FS) is divided to allow further release of the temporal dura from the middle fossa cranial base to expose the posterior cavernous sinus and the V2 and V3 branches of the trigeminal nerve. (**b**) Cadaveric dissection photograph showing the middle fossa rhomboid (*red*) is bordered by the V3 anteriorly, the GSPN laterally, the AE posteriorly, and the petrous edge medially. The horizontal segment of the petrous ICA courses parallel to and beneath the GSPN. The internal auditory canal (IAC, *blue dotted line*) lies approximately in the plane that bisects the angle between the GSPN and AE. The cochlea (C) is situated anteromedial and inferior to the geniculate ganglion. Glasscock's triangle (*blue*) is bordered by the posterior rim of the foramen ovale, the foramen spinosum, the posterior border of V3, and the cochlear apex. (Liu et al. [18], by permission of Congress of Neurological Surgeons [18])

acusticus in a lateral-to-medial direction [12]. The Fisch technique exposes the blue line of the SSC, and the IAC plane is approximated by drawing an imaginary line angled 60° to the SSC plane directed toward the posterior fossa dura [9]. Both techniques expose the IAC in a lateral-to-medial direction where the facial nerve is most superficial in the petrous bone, increasing the risk for facial nerve, SSC, and cochlear injury. The Garcia-Ibanez technique uses the GSPN and AE to locate the IAC [10]. The IAC is localized using a line bisecting the angle between GSPN and AE, and then the drilling is directed toward the porus acusticus to expose the IAC in a medial-to-lateral direction, decreasing the risk for facial nerve injury; this technique does not require exposure of the SSC. Another less popular technique involves drilling a point away from the tip of the GG about 9.9 mm on a line angled with the GSPN about 96° [17].

Given the variation in the middle fossa anatomy, there is no one technique fit for all patients. We generally prefer the Garcia-Ibanez technique (Fig. 11.4) because of the lower risk for injuring the facial nerve and inner ear structures.

Surgical Technique

Bony Exposure

After general anesthesia and intubation, the patient is positioned in either a completely lateral position with the side of the surgery up and the head fixed in a Mayfield head clamp or a supine position with small shoulder post under the ipsilateral side with head turned 60° to the contralateral side (Fig. 11.5). We tilt the head toward the contralateral shoulder until the ipsilateral sigmoid sinus becomes parallel to the floor. Facial nerve monitoring and auditory BAER are used routinely for all VS cases. A lazy "S" skin incision is marked starting at the zygomatic root just anterior to the tragus and then extending superiorly, curving posteriorly and then anteriorly just above the superior temporal line and behind the coronal suture. Preoperative antibiotics, dexamethasone, and mannitol are administered. The incision line is injected with local anesthetic and a vasoconstrictor, after which the skin incision is

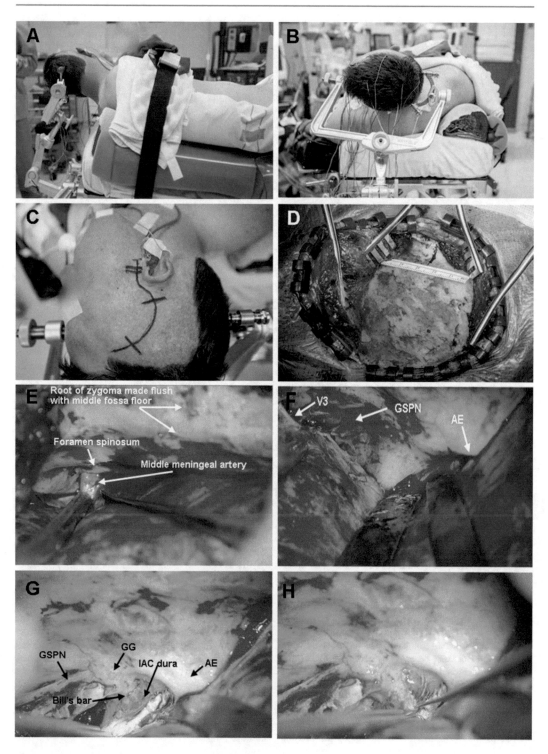

Fig. 11.5 (continued)

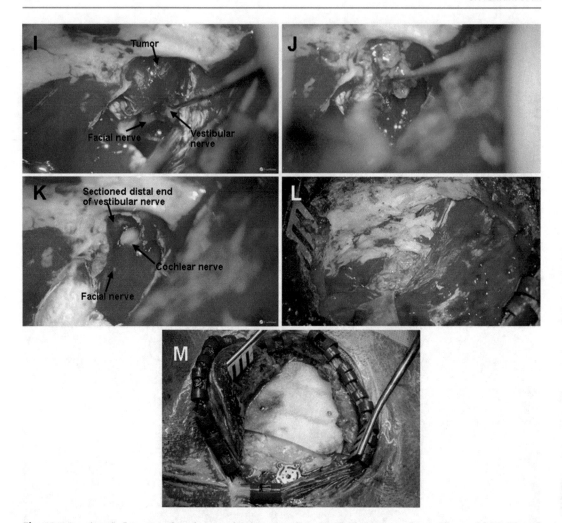

Fig. 11.5 (continued) Intraoperative photographs showing a right middle fossa approach for an intracanalicular tumor with small cisternal extension. (**a, b**) Surgical positioning. (**c**) Planned surgical incision extending from the superior temporal line to the front of the tragus. (**d**) Exposure of the zygomatic process, which is centered at the inferior end of the planned craniotomy (measuring 2.5 cm anterior and 2.5 cm posterior to the zygomatic root). (**e**) Exposure of the middle meningeal artery (MMA) at the foramen spinosum, which then coagulated and divided. Note that the zygomatic root is made flush with the middle fossa floor. (**f**) Completed temporal dural elevation in the posterior-to-anterior direction with exposed arcuate eminence (AE), greater superficial petrosal nerve (GSPN), and V3 division of the trigeminal nerve at foramen ovale. Note the placement of the retractor blades' tips just underneath the lip of the petrous ridge. (**g**) Drilled petrous bone ridge and IAC lip and exposure of the IAC dura as far laterally as Bill's bar. Note the relation between the AE, GG, GSPN, and IAC. (**h**) Dural opening along the superior and posterior margin of the IAC long axis to avoid injuring the facial nerve anteriorly. (**i, j**) Complete exposure of the IAC with identification of the facial nerve and the tumor attachment to the vestibular nerve. The tumor may need to be debulked internally to be able to manipulate and dissect away from the nerves. Note the elevation of the tumor from a medial-to-lateral direction. (**k**) Complete resection of the tumor with intact cochlear nerve and sectioned distal end of the vestibular nerve posterior to the facial nerve. (**l**) Placement of a fat graft over the IAC and fibrin glue to prevent CSF leak. (**m**) Bone flap placement with placement of MEDPOR to cover the drilled part of the temporal bone inferiorly

made down to the galea. This is followed by opening the temporalis fascia and muscle using a monopolar cautery down to the bone. The skin incision is often extended inferiorly over the zygomatic root to allow for a wider exposure when the retractors are placed. Care must be taken not to injure the frontal branch of the facial nerve below the zygomatic arch. A periosteal elevator is used to dissect the temporalis along with the periosteum from the bone anteriorly and posteriorly, making sure the root of the zygoma is completely exposed and centered at the lower margin of the bony exposure. A self-retaining retractor is placed, and two bur holes are made. One bur hole is placed just above the root of the zygoma and the other one just above the squamosal suture in the same plan. A craniotome is used to make the bony cuts; and a bone flap (~5 × 5 cm) is elevated while maintaining the integrity of the dura, which is then tacked up to the edge of the craniotomy superiorly. The lower edge of the craniotomy is made flush with the middle fossa floor using a cutting drill. Air cells of the temporal bone may be encountered in some cases and must be closed using bone wax to prevent the risk of CSF leak. Under microscopic visualization, the dural elevation is commenced. A small suction and a dural dissector are used to elevate the dural from the middle fossa floor. This process is started by identifying the foramen spinosum and the MMA in the middle fossa floor, which is considered a very important landmark. The foramen spinosum is always located posterolateral to the foramen ovale and V3, so injury of the GSPN at this stage of the operation is unlikely. We then identify the foramen ovale and the V3 anteriorly and medially. The foramen spinosum and ovale with the MMA and V3 mark the anterior limit of the surgical exposure. The MMA is coagulated and divided sharply, which will release the dural tethering and ease the dural elevation to identify the foramen ovale and V3. Bipolar cautery is avoided in this area to prevent thermal injury to the GSPN or GG. Bleeding from small emissary veins from both foramina is not uncommon and is easily controlled by using a hemostatic agent. Once that is done, attention is turned toward the petrous ridge posteriorly, where the dura is ele-

vated from lateral to medial along the ridge, identifying the tegmen, AE, meatal depression, and trigeminal prominence. The trigeminal impression and petrous apex do not need to be exposed. Dissection then is continued in a posterior-to-anterior direction along the floor of the middle fossa toward the foramen ovale to identify the GSPN, which is dissected from the dura and followed to where it enters under V3. A malleable self-retaining retractor is placed as far deep as the superior petrosal sinus to expose the petrous ridge and retract the temporal dura superiorly. The IAC location is now approximated using a line bisecting the angle between the GSPN anteriorly and the AE (SSC) posteriorly. A 3-mm diamond drill is used with a continuous suction-irrigation system to expose the IAC. The drilling starts medially close to the petrous ridge and deepens inferiorly until the medial portion of the IAC dura is identified. The drilling is continued laterally until we identify Bill's bar, which can serve as an important landmark for the facial nerve at the lateral canal. Drilling continues ~270° around the IAC dura to provide a room for maneuverability after dural opening. Care must be taken not to open the cochlear angle just anteromedial to the junction of the labyrinthine facial segment and the GG or the vestibule, which is located posterolateral to this lateral end of the IAC (Fig. 11.5).

Dural Opening and Tumor Dissection Techniques

Once the IAC dura is exposed, it is incised along its posterior length parallel to the superior vestibular nerve to avoid injury to the facial nerve, which lies in the anterosuperior portion of the IAC. A facial nerve stimulation probe is used to identify the location of the facial nerve in the lateral portion of the IAC. A sharp hook is used to transect the superior vestibular nerve just in the posterior margin of Bill's bar using very gentle movement to protect the labyrinthine segment of the facial nerve. The transverse crest at this lateral aspect of the canal may prevent adequate visualization of the cochlear nerve anteroinferiorly; however, when the dura of the IAC is removed along the axis of the IAC posteriorly to the area of the porus acusticus and the CSF is allowed to egress, more brain relaxation and better middle fossa retraction can be accomplished. This will allow for better surgical trajectory to the lateral aspect of the IAC and cochlear nerve.

The facial nerve is identified first in the medial portion of the IAC proximal to the tumor using the facial nerve stimulator, and then the proximal vestibular nerve is divided sharply. The tumor is now elevated slowly and gently from the facial nerve and the cochlear nerve in a medial-to-lateral direction to minimize the risk of tearing the cochlear nerve fibers entering the lamina cribrosa from the hair cell. In some cases, tumor debulking is completed using a microscissor or ultrasonic aspirator to facilitate tumor manipulation and dissection from the facial and cochlear nerve. A sharp hook is used to create the plan between the tumor and the facial and cochlear nerves and to divide the facial-vestibular communication fibers. Bipolar cautery is avoided during this surgery to prevent thermal injury to the delicate facial and cochlear nerve. Bleeding in these small tumors in the IAC is minimal and usually controlled easily with hemostatic agents and continuous irrigation; however, when bleeding obscures the dissection plan and the surgical cavity, the operative table can be placed in reverse Trendelenburg position to decrease the venous congestion and allow the blood and the irrigation to egress out of the surgical field until the tumor is completely removed. Care must be taken not to injure the labyrinthine artery or its branches during tumor dissection. Any exposed air cells are sealed off using bone wax. After hemostasis is achieved, a small piece of fat is harvested from the abdomen or thigh and placed over the IAC. The lower margin of the craniotomy is inspected for any open air cells, and bone wax is used to seal them. The bone flap is placed back, and the lower end of the drilled bone is covered using a small piece of MEDPOR cranioplasty (Fig. 11.5). Temporalis muscle is closed as a separate layer followed by closure of the fascia, galea, and skin. A routine postoperative CT scan of the brain is obtained showing the surgical corridor and the amount of bony drilling (Fig. 11.6).

Limitations of the MFA

Although it offers a short operative time and easy approach with minimal morbidity and mortality for carefully selected patients with VSs, there are several limitations to the MFA. The surgical cor-

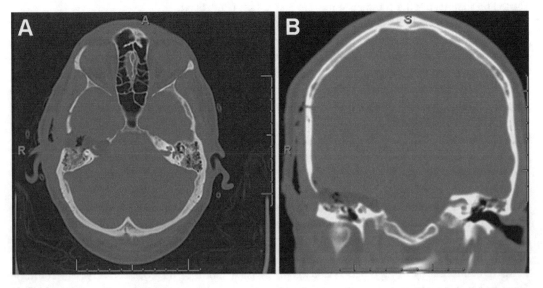

Fig. 11.6 Axial (**a**) and coronal (**b**) CT scan brain bone window demonstrating the extent of the bone removed during middle fossa approach to reach the right IAC postoperatively

ridor is narrow. Tumors with significant burden in the cisternal space of the CPA are difficult to remove. Furthermore, the infrequent use of this approach and limited familiarity with the petrous bone anatomy can be disadvantageous for the inexperienced neurosurgeon, but with experience the approach is desirable for well-selected tumors.

Surgical Risk and Complications

All middle fossa structures are at risk during the MFA including the temporal lobe, vein of Labbé in the dominant side, trigeminal nerve (V3), GSPN, GG, petrous carotid artery, cochlea, vestibule, facial nerve, cochlear nerve, and labyrinthine artery. Air cell openings in either the inferior or lateral aspect of the temporal bone or in the middle ear should be recognized and sealed adequately on the way in and out during this approach. Although the reported rate of CSF leak following MFA is 5.3–8% because of unsealed air cells (early, within 3 days) or hydrocephalus (late, more than 3 days) [1, 6], in our series, there was 0% incidence of postoperative CSF leak, which has been attributed to meticulous closure technique and continuous bone dust irrigation and clearance during bony drilling [25]. Increasing body mass index and prolonged operative time have been suggested as independent risk factors for CSF leak [6]. A systematic review of VS resections done using MFA reported 8% incidence of postoperative headache, 2.6% incidence of residual tumor, 1.1% rate for tumor recurrence, and 0.4% mortality rate [1]. In our series, there was no residual tumor, no recurrence, and no deaths at 15 months of follow-up [25]. Postoperative temporal lobe venous infarction, intracranial hemorrhage, epidural hematoma, subdural hematoma, seizure, and aphasia are also potential risks during the MFA.

Surgical Outcome for MFA

The reported hearing preservation rate with the MFA has ranged from 37% to 82% in the most recently published series [3, 7, 15, 24, 29, 30, 32, 34, 35]. In a systematic review of 35 studies for VS resection, the hearing preservation rate was 56.4% for tumors <1.5 cm and 59.4% for purely intracanalicular tumors. The facial nerve function preservation rate was found to be 96.7% for tumors <1.5 cm and 83.3% for purely intracanalicular tumors [1]. The authors demonstrated that the MFA is superior to the retrosigmoid approach for hearing preservation and superior to the translabyrinthine approach for facial nerve function preservation for tumors <1.5 cm [1]. In our experience, the hearing preservation rate is 75.5%, and the facial function preservation rate is 90% at 15 months postoperatively with MFA for VS [25].

Translabyrinthine Approach for Vestibular Schwannoma

Indications

The translabyrinthine approach is indicated for VS resection in patients with nonserviceable hearing or complete hearing loss preoperatively. This approach provides the most direct access to the CPA. Generally, all VSs that can be approached through a retrosigmoid route can be removed through a translabyrinthine route; however, this approach is particularly useful for tumors that extend to the fundus of the IAC laterally and into the CPA angle medially (Fig. 11.7). The entire length of the facial verve is exposed routinely from the origin of the brainstem to the fundus of IAC. This approach allows surgeons to identify the facial nerve early during surgery, minimal or no cerebellar retraction is required as opposed to the retrosigmoid approach, and the approach allows for early CSF drainage and relaxation to the cerebellum [2, 4, 22]. The surgical positioning and bony exposure have been described elsewhere in this book.

Tumor Removal Techniques

After the presigmoid dura and IAC dura are exposed, under microscopic vision, the dura is opened first superoposteriorly along the axis of the IAC away from the presumed position of the

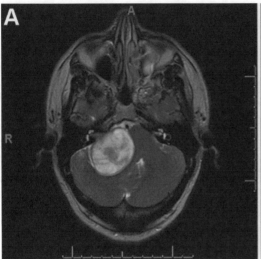
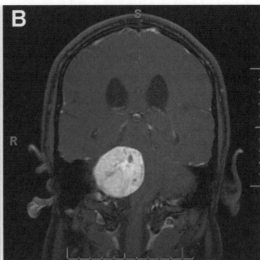

Fig. 11.7 (a) Axial T2-weighted and (b) coronal T1-weighted MRI of the brain with gadolinium demonstrate a large *right* CPA VS extending into the *right* IAC fundus. Note the significant brainstem and fourth ventricle compression causing hydrocephalus

facial nerve under the dura. The tumor is followed laterally, and the vestibular nerve is identified posterior to Bill's bar and transected by using a sharp hook. The facial nerve is identified first distal in the canal just anterior to Bill's bar and is confirmed using a facial nerve stimulator. Because the translabyrinthine approach is a non-hearing preservation procedure, the tumor can be partially dissected off the facial nerve in this position in a medial-to-lateral direction. Next, a linear incision is made anterior to the sigmoid sinus and inferior to the sinodural angle. Care must be taken not to injure the underlying cerebellar tissue, veins, or arteries. This dural opening is widened superiorly and inferiorly in a funnel shape toward the upper and lower extent of the IAC. The dural flap between the IAC and presigmoid region is transected and removed to expose the tumor. The arachnoid of the CPA is divided sharply, and the tumor should be apparent. Every effort is made to preserve the arachnoid plan and preserve all neurovascular structures of the CPA. In most cases, the facial nerve is located in the anterior surface of the tumor, running anterior-superior or anterior-inferior; however, the facial nerve stimulator is used to stimulate the posterior surface of the tumor to ensure absence of stimulation where the tumor is opened. Bipolar cautery at a low setting

can be used to coagulate the posterior surface of the tumor, and a small window is made in the back side of the tumor using a microscissors. A piece of tumor is removed and sent for pathological analysis. An ultrasonic aspirator is used next to debulk the tumor from the center. During this step, it is important to stay inside the tumor capsule and avoid aggressive debulking so that the tumor capsule can be manipulated during tumor dissection off the brainstem and facial nerve. A small hook is used to visualize the thickness of the remaining capsule after debulking to ensure enough debulking and maneuverability of the tumor. The goal of this maneuver is to make the tumor smaller and easier to manipulate without too much traction on the facial nerve or brainstem.

Once enough debulking is achieved, the facial nerve should be identified at the root exit zone at the brainstem level. The origin of the facial nerve is located ventral and caudal to the vestibulocochlear nerve origin. A hook is used to gently lift the tumor capsule away from the brainstem, and the space between the tumor capsule and brainstem is inspected. The facial nerve stimulator is used to confirm the position of the facial nerve, and the vestibulocochlear nerve is divided sharply. Tumor capsule is peeled away gently from the facial nerve in a medial-to-lateral direction. As the tumor is dissected, the redundant capsule can be debulked more with microscissors or an ultrasonic aspirator. This is continued until just before the porus acusticus, where the maximum adhesion between the tumor and the facial nerve usually exists. The dissection now is directed toward the lateral extent of the tumor in the IAC. The tumor is debulked similarly at the lateral end of the IAC and then dissected sharply off the facial nerve in a lateral-to-medial fashion. A back-and-forth dissection–debulking technique is used to remove this last piece of tumor from the facial nerve until both dissection plans are met at the porus acusticus. All opened air cells must be checked and sealed with bone wax. Similar to the MFA, the closure is done using just enough pieces of fat to fill the surgical corridor in the mastoid. It is important to ensure that these fat grafts do not fall into the intradural space in the CPA angle. On the other hand, too much fat packing may compress the sigmoid sinus and should be avoided. The first fat piece may be made just big enough to plug the dural opening, and the other small fat pieces are placed over it. A small absorbable plate is placed over the mastoid to buttress the fat. The muscle and galea are closed in layers; the skin is closed using a simple running or locking nylon stitches (Fig. 11.8). The extent of the bone removal and tumor removal using the translabyrinthine approach can be seen in Fig. 11.9.

Surgical Risks and Complications

The operative-related mortality rate for the translabyrinthine approach for VS resection ranges from 1% to 1.3% [1, 31], mainly in elderly patients with tumors larger than 3 cm [31]. CSF leak postoperatively has been reported to occur in 1.8–14% of patients [28, 31]. Major neurological deficits such as stroke, seizure disorder, and persistent cerebellar dysfunction have been reported in 2.6% of patients [1]. In a large series of 1244 patients with VS who underwent translabyrinthine approach, the risk of the following complications was <1%: subdural hemorrhage, CPA hematoma, cerebellar edema, brainstem hematoma, transient aphasia, and lower cranial nerve

dysfunction [31]. In cases where gross-total resection was planned, residual tumor was reported in 5.6% of patients [1].

Facial Nerve Preservation with the Translabyrinthine Approach

The overall facial nerve preservation rate reported with the translabyrinthine approach was 89.5% in a large systematic review [1]. The reported rates of facial nerve preservation are 100%, 84.2%, and 57.7% for intracanalicular tumors, tumors measuring 1.5–3 cm, and tumors larger than 3 cm, respectively [1].

Limitations of Translabyrinthine Approach

The translabyrinthine approach is usually indicated for resection of VS in patients with unserviceable hearing or with poor hearing preservation prognosis preoperatively. The size of the tumor is not a limiting factor for this approach; however, in some cases, the jugular bulb is located very close to the IAC, and careful studying of the jugular bulb height in the preoperative MRI and CT scans is important to ensure adequate distance between the IAC and jugular bulb, especially in large VSs.

Specific Perioperative Considerations

Thin-cut axial, sagittal, and coronal MRIs of the skull base should be studied preoperatively. The dominant temporal lobe and vein of Labbé must be kept in mind for complication avoidance. Neuronavigation systems that use stereotactic CT scan or MRI may be useful surgical adjuncts to localize the IAC and define the limits of bony drilling. Facial nerve monitoring and BAER are used routinely for all VS cases. Muscle paralysis agents should be avoided during anesthesia. Dexamethasone and mannitol can be used to relax the brain and prevent dural tear during bone elevation. Early mobilization and physiotherapy postoperatively are important parts of the treat-

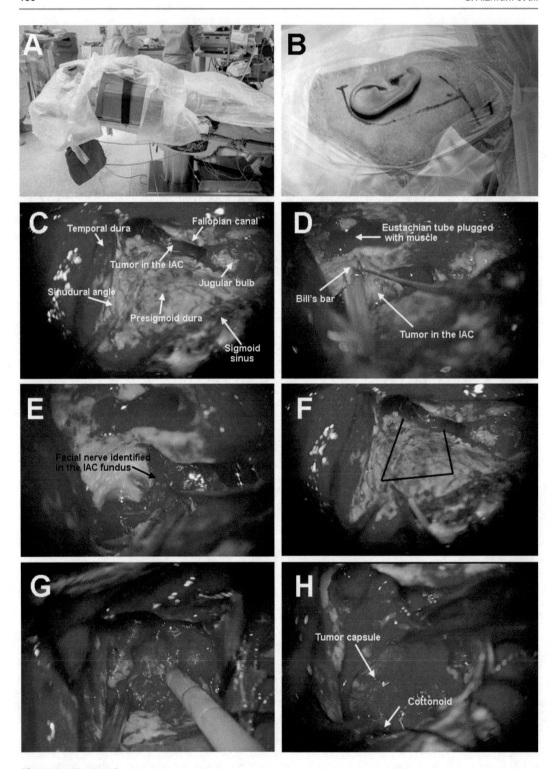

Fig. 11.8 (Continued)

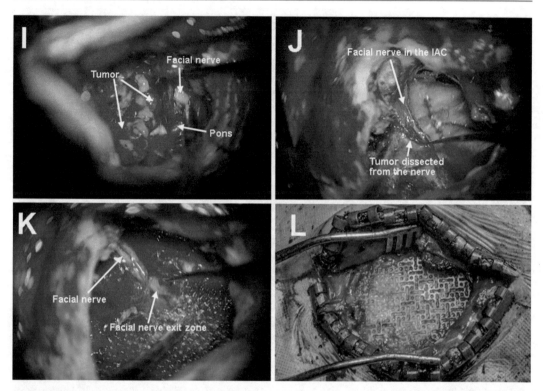

Fig. 11.8 Translabyrinthine approach for a large VS. (**a, b**) Surgical position and skin incision marking. (**c**) Completed bone removal of the mastoid air cells and exposure of the presigmoid dura and the tumor in the right IAC. Note the complete skeletonization of the sigmoid sinus with only a thin shell of the bone left over the jugular bulb. (**d**) Identification of the Bell's bar and opening the IAC dura just posterior to it. Note the eustachian tube plugged with muscle. (**e**) Further dissection of the tumor off the facial nerve in the IAC. (**f**) Opening of the presigmoid dura parallel and inferior to the sinodural angle. The *black lines* denote the dural opening Fig. 11.8 (continued) around the IAC. (**g**) Debulking of the tumor after opening a window in the backside of the tumor (facial nerve stimulator is used to confirm the absence of aberrant facial nerve course along the incision line of the tumor capsule). (**h**) Lifting the tumor capsule off the cerebellum and brainstem after adequate tumor debulking is achieved. Note the use of cottonoids to gently dissect the tumor capsule from the brainstem using traction-countertraction technique in medial-to-lateral direction. (**i**) Identifying the facial nerve at the inferior and anterior part of the tumor. (**j**) Tumor remnant dissected from lateral-to-medial direction off the facial nerve after more tumor debulking. (**k**) Complete tumor removal with intact facial nerve. Note the view provided by translabyrinthine approach at the end of the dissection (ability to see the whole length of the facial nerve from the root exit zone to the IAC fundus). (**l**) The use of an absorbable plate for mastoidectomy repair after placement of fat graft over the presigmoid dura

ment plan for postoperative complication avoidance and vestibular function rehabilitation.

Conclusion

Detailed anatomical understanding of the middle fossa, inner ear, and IAC anatomy is the key to achieving the desired outcome with very low morbidity and mortalities in the retrosigmoid, MFA, and translabyrinthine approaches for VS resection. Unlike otolaryngologists, many neurosurgeons are not familiar with these approaches because of the rarity of VSs compared with the other pathological processes that may involve the inner or middle ear. Nevertheless, learning the technical nuances of these approaches is advantageous. Having dedicated skull base and ear, nose, and throat surgical teams during the preoperative, operative, and postoperative care for patients with VSs treated using these approaches is an important aspect for management of this pathology.

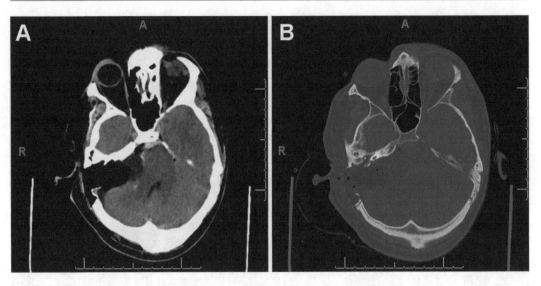

Fig. 11.9 Postoperative CT scan brain. (**a**) Axial brain and (**b**) axial bone window demonstrate complete resection of right VS. Note the extent of the bone exposure for the translabyrinthine approach

References

1. Ansari SF, Terry C, Cohen-Gadol AA. Surgery for vestibular schwannomas: a systematic review of complications by approach. Neurosurg Focus. 2012;33(3):E14.
2. Arriaga MA, Lin J. Translabyrinthine approach: indications, techniques, and results. Otolaryngol Clin N Am. 2012;45:399–415.
3. Brackmann DE, Owens RM, Friedman RA, Hitselberger WE, De la Cruz A, House JW, et al. Prognostic factors for hearing preservation in vestibular schwannoma surgery. Am J Otolaryngol. 2000;21:417–24.
4. Chamoun R, MacDonald J, Shelton C, Couldwell WT. Surgical approaches for resection of vestibular schwannomas: translabyrinthine, retrosigmoid, and middle fossa approaches. Neurosurg Focus. 2012;33(3):E9.
5. Cole CD, Gottfried ON, Gupta DK, Couldwell WT. Total intravenous anesthesia: advantages for intracranial surgery. Neurosurgery. 2007;61:369–377; discussion 377–378.
6. Copeland W, Mallory G, Neff B, Driscoll C, Link M. Are there modifiable risk factors to prevent a cerebrospinal fluid leak following vestibular schwannoma surgery? J Neurosurg. 2015;122:312–6.
7. DeMonte F, Gidley PW. Hearing preservation surgery for vestibular schwannoma: experience with the middle fossa approach. Neurosurg Focus. 2012;33(3):E10.
8. Dutton JE, Ramsden RT, Lye RH, Morris K, Keith AO, Page R, et al. Acoustic neuroma (schwannoma) surgery 1978-1990. J Laryngol Otol. 1991;105:165–73.
9. Fisch U. Transtemporal surgery of the internal auditory canal. Report of 92 cases, technique, indications and results. Adv Otorhinolaryngol. 1970;17:203–40.
10. Garcia-Ibanez E, Garcia-Ibanez JL. Middle fossa vestibular neurectomy: a report of 373 cases. Otolaryngol Head Neck Surg. 1980;88:486–90.
11. Gormley WB, Sekhar LN, Wright DC, Kamerer D, Schessel D. Acoustic neuromas: results of current surgical management. Neurosurgery. 1997;41:50–58; discussion 58–60.
12. House WF. Surgical exposure of the internal auditory canal and its contents through the middle, cranial fossa. Laryngoscope. 1961;71:1363–85.
13. House WF, Gardner G, Hughes RL. Middle cranial fossa approach to acoustic tumor surgery. Arch Otolaryngol. 1968;88:631–41.
14. House WF, Shelton C. Middle fossa approach for acoustic tumor removal. Otolaryngol Clin N Am. 1992;25:347–59.
15. Jacob A, Robinson LL, Bortman JS, Yu L, Dodson EE, Welling DB. Nerve of origin, tumor size, hearing preservation, and facial nerve outcomes in 359 vestibular schwannoma resections at a tertiary care academic center. Laryngoscope. 2007;117:2087–92.
16. Kutz JW Jr, Scoresby T, Isaacson B, Mickey BE, Madden CJ, Barnett SL, et al. Hearing preservation using the middle fossa approach for the treatment of vestibular schwannoma. Neurosurgery. 2012;70:334–340; discussion 340–341.
17. Lan M-Y, Shiao J-Y. Using greater superficial petrosal nerve and geniculate ganglion as the only two landmarks for identifying internal auditory canal in middle fossa approach. Eur Arch Otorhinolaryngol. 2010;267:1867–71.

18. Liu JK, Fukushima T, Sameshima T, Al-Mefty O, Couldwell WT. Increasing exposure of the petrous internal carotid artery for revascularization using the transzygomatic extended middle fossa approach: a cadaveric morphometric study. Neurosurgery. 2006;59:ONS309–18.

19. Mahaley MS Jr, Mettlin C, Natarajan N, Laws ER Jr, Peace BB. Analysis of patterns of care of brain tumor patients in the United States: a study of the brain tumor section of the AANS and the CNS and the commission on cancer of the ACS. Clin Neurosurg. 1990;36:347–52.

20. Misra BK, Purandare HR, Ved RS, Bagdia AA, Mare PB. Current treatment strategy in the management of vestibular schwannoma. Neurol India. 2009;57:257–63.

21. Mortini P, Mandelli C, Gerevini S, Giovanelli M. Exposure of the petrous segment of the internal carotid artery through the extradural subtemporal middle cranial fossa approach: a systematic anatomical study. Skull Base. 2001;11:177–87.

22. Nickele CM, Akture E, Gubbels SP, Baskaya MK. A stepwise illustration of the translabyrinthine approach to a large cystic vestibular schwannoma. Neurosurg Focus. 2012;33(3):E11.

23. Parry RH. A case of tinnitus and vertigo treated by division of the auditory nerve. 1904. J Laryngol Otol. 1991;105:1099–100.

24. Quist TS, Givens DJ, Gurgel RK, Chamoun R, Shelton C. Hearing preservation after middle fossa vestibular schwannoma removal: are the results durable? Otolaryngol Head Neck Surg. 2015;152:706–11.

25. Raheja A, Bowers CA, MacDonald JD, Shelton C, Gurgel RK, Brimley C, et al. Middle fossa approach for vestibular schwannoma: good hearing and facial nerve outcomes with low morbidity. World Neurosurg. 2016;92:37–46.

26. Sameshima T, Fukushima T, McElveen JT Jr, Friedman AH. Critical assessment of operative approaches for hearing preservation in small acoustic neuroma surgery: retrosigmoid vs middle fossa approach. Neurosurgery. 2010;67:640–644; discussion 644–645.

27. Samii M, Matthies C. Management of 1000 vestibular schwannomas (acoustic neuromas): surgical management and results with an emphasis on complications and how to avoid them. Neurosurgery. 1997;40:11–21; discussion 21–23.

28. Sanna M, Taibah A, Russo A, Falcioni M, Agarwal M. Perioperative complications in acoustic neuroma (vestibular schwannoma) surgery. Otol Neurotol. 2004;25:379–86.

29. Satar B, Jackler RK, Oghalai J, Pitts LH, Yates PD. Risk-benefit analysis of using the middle fossa approach for acoustic neuromas with >10 mm cerebellopontine angle component. Laryngoscope. 2002;112:1500–6.

30. Shelton C, Hitselberger WE, House WF, Brackmann DE. Hearing preservation after acoustic tumor removal: long-term results. Laryngoscope. 1990;100:115–9.

31. Springborg JB, Fugleholm K, Poulsgaard L, Caye-Thomasen P, Thomsen J, Stangerup SE. Outcome after translabyrinthine surgery for vestibular schwannomas: report on 1244 patients. J Neurol Surg B Skull Base. 2012;73:168–74.

32. Sughrue ME, Yang I, Aranda D, Kane AJ, Parsa AT. Hearing preservation rates after microsurgical resection of vestibular schwannoma. J Clin Neurosci. 2010;17:1126–9.

33. Tanriover N, Sanus GZ, Ulu MO, Tanriverdi T, Akar Z, Rubino PA, et al. Middle fossa approach: microsurgical anatomy and surgical technique from the neurosurgical perspective. Surg Neurol. 2009;71:586–596.; discussion 596.

34. Wang AC, Chinn SB, Than KD, Arts HA, Telian SA, El-Kashlan HK, et al. Durability of hearing preservation after microsurgical treatment of vestibular schwannoma using the middle cranial fossa approach. J Neurosurg. 2013;119:131–8.

35. Wilkinson EP, Roberts DS, Cassis A, Schwartz MS. Hearing outcomes after middle fossa or retrosigmoid craniotomy for vestibular schwannoma tumors. J Neurol Surg B Skull Base. 2016;77:333–40.

Epidermoid Cyst

12

Gmaan Alzhrani and William T. Couldwell

Introduction

Epithelial inclusion cysts generally form congenitally between the third and fifth weeks of gestation secondary to an early dysjunction and entrapment of the ectoderm before neural tube closure [11, 27, 29]. Iatrogenic implantation of the skin after lumbar puncture and traumatic implantation after gunshot wound have been proposed as rare mechanisms underlying the development of these lesions [12, 32]. Epidermoid cyst walls are lined with stratified squamous epithelium overlying a connective tissue lamina that closely adheres to the pia mater and is grossly anatomically indistinguishable from the latter. Tumor growth results from continuous desquamation and degradation of epithelial cells inside the cyst, forming pearly and shiny debris composed of cholesterol crystals and keratin [7, 9, 23]. These cysts constitute 0.2–1.8% of all intracranial tumors [11, 17, 18, 25]. The most common location for epidermoid tumors is the cerebellopontine angle (CPA). In the posterior fossa, these represent 5–7% of all CPA lesions [11, 31], and 40–50% of all intra-

cranial epidermoid cysts are located in the CPA [11, 31]. The paramedian location of this lesion is thought to be related to the otic vesicles displacing the epithelia rest more peripherally toward the CPA [3, 4, 19]. The second most common location in the posterior fossa is the fourth ventricle, accounting for 5–18.5% of all intracranial epidermoid tumors [9, 20, 35].

Clinical Presentation

Epidermoid cysts can remain asymptomatic clinically for a long time because they have a slow and linear growth pattern similar to the normal epidermis but are insinuated into the surrounding subarachnoid spaces [2, 11, 14]. Patients usually become symptomatic between the third and fifth decades of life, and a latency period of clinical presentation of CPA epidermoids of 2–4.6 years has been reported [1]. This latency period may be shorter for fourth ventricular epidermoids, which have a reported average of 1.6 years from the onset of symptoms to diagnosis [11, 34]. The pathophysiological mechanism for symptoms and signs of onset of posterior fossa epidermoid cysts may be related to compression of neurovascular structures, encasement and strangulation of the cranial nerves and blood vessels, or irritation of the neurovascular structures secondary to the cyst rupture and spillage of its content into the subarachnoid space (Mollaret's meningitis) [14].

G. Alzhrani, MD • W.T. Couldwell, MD, PhD (✉)
Department of Neurosurgery, Clinical Neurosciences Center, University of Utah, 175 N. Medical Drive East, Salt Lake City, UT 84132, USA
e-mail: neuropub@hsc.utah.edu

Trigeminal neuralgia, hearing impairment, dizziness, headaches, diplopia, and facial paralysis are common presenting symptoms of CPA epidermoid cysts [7, 8, 17], whereas gait disturbance, abducens and facial nerve palsy, and hydrocephalus are common presentations for fourth ventricular epidermoids [33]. Seizures and diplopia can also be a presenting symptom for epidermoids of the CPA extending to the middle fossa secondary of mesial temporal structure compression [33].

Imaging and Differential Diagnosis

The signal characteristics of epidermoid tumor on CT (Fig. 12.1) and standard MRI (Fig. 12.2) are similar to those of cerebrospinal fluid (CSF). Typically, these cysts appear as an extra-axial hypodense lesion on CT scan, are hypointense on T1-weighted MRI and hyperintense on T2-weighted MRI, and display no contrast enhancement on MRI. However, a rare CT scan characteristic of some epidermoid cysts has been referred to as "dense epidermoid cysts" or "white epidermoids" [5, 26]. These lesions have atypical CT scan hyperdensity that has been variously described as being a result of liquefaction of the cyst content, representing high protein content or prior hemorrhage into the cyst, indicating the presence of ferro-calcium or iron-containing pigment or denoting the presence of polymorphonuclear leukocytes based on intraoperative observation and pathological correlation [22, 26, 31, 36]. Other radiological features including cal-

cifications have been reported in 10–25% of cases, and capsular enhancement related to perilesional inflammation in the MRI has been described [7, 31]. Fluid-attenuated inversion recover (FLAIR) sequence may show heterogeneous signal with central hyperintensity in epidermoid cysts and can be used to differentiate epidermoids from other cystic lesion of the CPA [16, 31]. True restricted diffusion on diffusion-weighted MRI (hyperintense signal) and apparent diffusion coefficient MRI (hypointense signal) is the most characteristic MRI finding for typical epidermoid cysts [6]. The main differential diagnosis for epidermoid cysts in the CPA is arachnoid cysts. Uncomplicated arachnoid cysts are usually isointense in FLAIR with no restricted diffusion. The differential diagnosis for atypical epidermoid cysts should include atypical appearance of meningioma, cystic schwannoma, endolymphatic sac tumors, teratoma, pilocytic astrocytoma, hemangioblastoma, and ganglioglioma [15, 31].

Management

Epidermoid cysts are slow growing and benign and do not respond to chemotherapy or radiotherapy, and asymptomatic small epidermoid cysts of the CPA can be monitored with serial imaging. However, for symptomatic or large asymptomatic cysts with significant mass effect on the brainstem, surgical removal is indicated. Complete surgical resection of the epidermoid tumor along with its

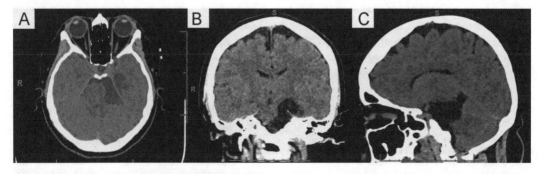

Fig. 12.1 Axial (**a**), coronal (**b**), and sagittal (**c**) CT scans of the brain demonstrating a hypodense lesion located at the left CPA angle. Note the supratentorial extension of the lesion and the mass effect on the brainstem and mesiotemporal structures

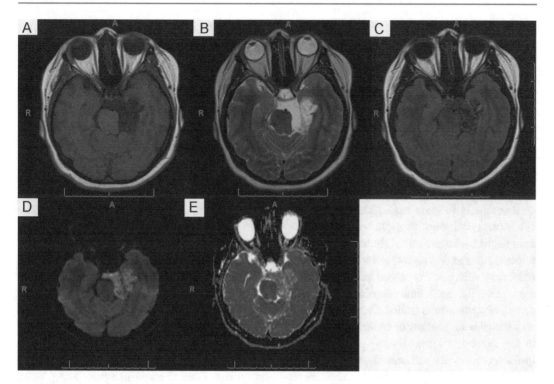

Fig. 12.2 Brain MRI demonstrating a right CPA epidermoid cyst with characteristic T1-weighted hypointense signal (**a**), T2-weighted hyperintense signal (**b**), heterogeneous signal intensity in FLAIR (**c**), and restricted diffusion signal in DWI (**d**) and ADC (**e**) sequences. Note the supratentorial extension and the mass effect on the brainstem and mesiotemporal structures

capsule is ideal to reduce the risk of recurrence, but it is almost impossible to predict preoperatively how adherent the cyst capsule is to the brainstem and the traversing CPA neurovascular structures. Hence, the goal of surgical resection for these lesions should be maximum safe resection. Some studies have demonstrated that recurrence risk for CPA epidermoid cysts is the same with complete removal and incomplete removal [17, 30]. However, these studies are limited by short follow-up periods. Epidermoid cysts are composed of soft white material and are often amenable to suctioning. In some cases, however, the lesion grows around the cranial nerves and blood vessels in the CPA, making it difficult to distinguish between the cyst contents and the cranial nerves, especially the sixth and fourth cranial nerves, which are small and fragile and can be easily injured during surgery. Identifying the cranial nerves where they enter the skull base foramina

during surgery may be a helpful trick during surgery for safe resection.

Surgery is the mainstay of treatment for epidermoid cysts. Epidermoid cysts of the fourth ventricle are removed using a standard midline suboccipital craniotomy. Most of the epidermoid cysts confined to the CPA are removed using a standard retrosigmoid approach [17, 30, 33], but epidermoids that extend into the middle fossa can be removed using a combined retrosigmoid and subtemporal transtentorial approach simultaneously or in separate stages [28, 30] or an extended retrosigmoid transtentorial approach. More recently, the endoscopic-assisted retrosigmoid approach [28] or pure endoscopic retrosigmoid approach has been described [24]. In the following section, we describe the keyhole retrosigmoid transtentorial approach for epidermoid cyst of the CPA extending into the supratentorial (middle fossa) compartment.

Surgical Approach

After general anesthesia induction and patient intubation, the patient is positioned in a lateral decubitus position with the head held in a three-point fixation head clamp. Muscle paralytic agents are avoided, and neuromonitoring—including motor evoked and somatosensory evoked potentials, facial nerve and auditory brainstem evoked responses, and 9th, 10th, 11th, and 12th cranial nerve monitoring—is used routinely in these cases. The head is kept in a neutral position with slight lateral neck flexion toward the contralateral shoulder so that the mastoid tip is at the highest point in the surgical field. An axillary roll is placed under the dependent side; the ipsilateral shoulder is slightly flexed, and the arm is pulled down and secured with a tape over a bellow or an arm support fixed in the operating table. Undue traction of the ipsilateral shoulder and arm should be avoided to prevent brachial plexus injury. The operating table is reflexed, and the patient is secured onto the operating table using an adhesive tape for airplane positioning during the surgery. The pressure points are checked and padded appropriately. Neurophysiological baseline studies are obtained after positioning is complete so that undue traction of the brachial plexus or neck lateral flexion is detected and readjusted before starting the procedure. A neuronavigation system can be used to help localize the position of the skin incision and the bony removal in relation to the sigmoid and transverse sinuses.

Anatomically, a straight line connecting the ipsilateral root of the zygoma and the inion along the superior nuchal line is a landmark for the ipsilateral transverse sinus. The asterion is located 4 cm posterior to the ipsilateral external auditory meatus and can usually be felt as a bony depression just superior and posterior to the mastoid notch. This point marks the inferior margin of the sigmoid-transverse sinus junction. A line extending from the asterion inferiorly just posterior to the mastoid tip marks the posterior margin of the sigmoid sinus. A curved skin incision is planned 0.5–1 cm posterior to the mastoid notch so that one third is above and two thirds are below the asterion. The hair above the ipsilateral pinna is clipped and draped in case a subtemporal bony window is necessary for resection of the supratentorial part of the lesion.

Once the skin incision and the bony exposure are complete, a small craniotomy or craniectomy is performed. It is very important to expose the posterior third of the sigmoid sinus and the inferior third of the transverse sinus to be able to reflect the dural edges or leaflet and to see along the posterior petrous and the inferior tentorial surface without difficulties. In cases where hydrocephalus is present on preoperative imaging, a preoperative or intraoperative frontal or occipitoparietal external ventricular drain may be inserted and used to relax the brain during the surgery and to prevent postoperative CSF leak. The dura is opened in a cruciate fashion or curved along the inferior sinus border leaving a small cuff of dura for watertight closure at the end. The dural margins are tacked up superiorly and anteriorly over the sinuses margins using dural stitches. Under microscopic vision, the prepontine and/or the pontomedullary cistern arachnoid membrane is opened sharply, and CSF is allowed to egress to aid cerebellar relaxation. The cyst should be visible at this stage, and the arachnoid membrane covering the cyst is dissected sharply A small, self-retaining retractor with a brain spatula may be used with minimal retraction over the lateral part of the cerebellum to allow better visualization. Care must be taken not to cause traction injury of the seventh and eighth cranial nerves or petrosal veins during this stage. The seventh and eighth nerve complex should be identified early. Attempts should be made to preserve all petrosal veins, but in certain cases, some petrosal veins may have to be sacrificed to prevent accidental tears or to provide better visualization for the deeper portion of the CPA cistern. At this stage, the cyst contents are debulked using careful microdissection techniques. It is important to remember that the cranial nerves and posterior circulation blood vessels and the perforators may be embedded within or displaced by the cyst and should be preserved at all costs. Careful attention to the abducens and trochlear nerves is important because these two nerves are small and can be difficult to visualize during the debulking of epidermoids. The abducens nerve can be identified below the seventh and eighth cranial nerve complex from its brainstem origin before going back up to its clival intradural fold before it enters Dorello's canal. The trochlear nerve should be sought just medial to the dural free margin at the incisura. Enough debulking is achieved once the 4th, 5th, 6th, 7th, and 8th complexes; the 9th, 10th, 11th, and 12th cranial nerves; the basilar artery; and the anterior inferior cerebellar artery are identified and decompressed. At this stage, the arachnoid-epidermoid cyst wall adhesions are identified and divided sharply, and the cyst wall is removed. In cases where the cyst wall is very adherent to the brainstem, cranial nerves, or blood vessels, the adherent part of the cyst is left behind to prevent neurological or vascular injury.

Attention now is turned toward the supratentorial middle fossa portion of the cyst. The tentorial surface posterior to the superior petrosal sinus and medial to the petrosal vein is divided sharply using a sharp blade and extended toward the tentorial free margin using a microscissor. The trochlear nerve is at risk during this step and must be visualized and protected before completing the tentorial cut, which is performed posterior to where the trochlear nerve enters the tentorial edge. Bleeding from the tentorium can be controlled with hemostatic agent and bipolar cautery. The supratentorial portion of the cyst can now be debulked, and the third cranial nerve, posterior cerebellar artery, and posterior communicating artery can be identified and freed using microsurgical techniques. The endoscope can be brought at this stage and 30-, 45-, and 70-degree angled scopes can be introduced into the surgical field so the remaining pieces of the lesion can be visualized and removed using curved suction and microinstruments.

In cases where the supratentorial portion of the cyst proves difficult to resect microscopically or endoscopically from the retrosigmoid window, the skin incision can be extended superiorly by curving forward and then inferiorly to the level of the root of the zygoma just anterior to the tragus, and a separate subtemporal bone window is made. Once the bone window is elevated, the inferior margin of the temporal bone is drilled away until the root of the zygoma is flush with the middle fossa floor. The dura is opened in an inverted U shape and reflected inferiorly. The temporal lobe is elevated, and the tentorium is followed medially to the free margin. The arachnoid over the ambient cistern is divided sharply, and the lesion should be evident at this stage. In a similar fashion, the epidermoid is debulked, and the oculomotor and trochlear nerves, the posterior cerebellar artery, and the posterior communicating artery should be identified and freed (Fig. 12.3).

The dura is closed in a watertight fashion either primarily or using a dural substitute. Bone wax is used to seal the middle fossa and mastoid bone to ensure obliteration of any opened air cells. Muscle and fascia, galea, and skin are closed in a multilayered fashion.

Complication Avoidance

Surgical position-related neuropathy is not uncommon, especially in an obese patient with a short neck when lateral positioning is used. In our experience, somatosensory and motor evoked potentials may provide invaluable information after final positioning and may be used to adjust the extremity position of neck position before starting the procedure.

To avoid sigmoid or transverse injury during surgical exposure and to ensure adequate bony removal before opening the dura, a neuronavigation system is a useful surgical adjunct when available. Careful attention to the sigmoid and transverse dominance in the preoperative imaging is important in all posterior fossa approaches. When sinus injury occurs during surgery, every effort is made to repair the injured sinus primarily using a vascular stitch; depending on the extent of the injury, postoperative antiplatelet treatment using aspirin may be considered. When a subtemporal window is planned, the superficial sylvian vein drainage patterns and vein of Labbé, especially in the dominant temporal lobe, should be identified in the preoperative imaging and protected during surgery.

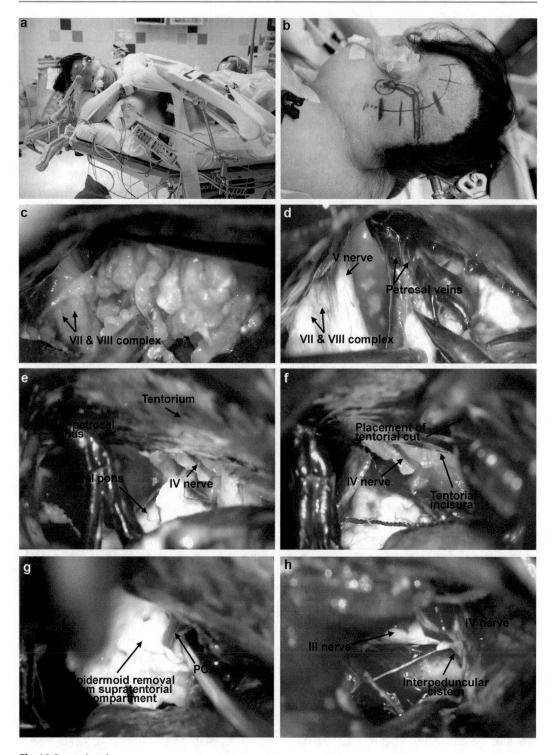

Fig. 12.3 continued

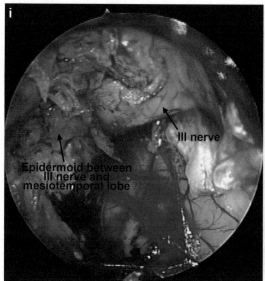
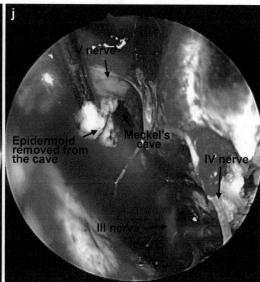

Fig. 12.3 (continued) Patient positioning (**a**, **b**) and microscopic (**c–h**) and endoscopic (**i**, **j**) views of left retrosigmoid transtentorial approach for resection of a left CPA epidermoid cyst with supratentorial extension into the left middle fossa. (**a**) The patient is positioned in a right lateral position with slight operative table reflex to help with decreasing the venous congestion and bleeding. (**b**) The location of the surgical incision in relation to the sigmoid and transverse sinus. Note the extension of the incision toward the left temporal bone in cases were a middle fossa window for the supratentorial portion is required. (**c**) Microscopic view of the left seventh and eighth cranial nerve complex entering the internal auditory canal after freeing the complex from the epidermoid cyst. (**d**) Microscopic view of the fifth cranial nerve pushed toward the seventh and eighth cranial nerve complex as well as preservation of the petrosal veins. (**e**) Microscopic view of the tentorial surface, tentorial free margin, and the fourth cranial nerve. (**f**) Microscopic view of the opening of the tentorium toward the incisura with direct visualization of the fourth cranial nerve. (**g**) Microscopic view of the removal of the supratentorial part of the epidermoid cyst with identification of the left posterior cerebral artery. (**h**) Microscopic view of the fourth cranial nerve, the interpeduncular cistern, and the third cranial nerve after partial removal of the supratentorial part of the epidermoid cyst. (**i**) Endoscopic view of the supratentorial compartment demonstrating a residual epidermoid cyst located between the third cranial nerve and the mesiotemporal lobe. (**j**) Endoscopic view shows the removal of the a small piece of epidermoid cyst from the Meckel's cave around the fifth cranial nerve

When preoperative hydrocephalus or significant perilesional edema is evident preoperatively, insertion of an external ventricular drain before starting the procedure can be of clinical benefit to avoid intraoperative intracranial hypertension and postoperative acute deterioration. The drain is inserted preoperatively and opened at high pressure or kept closed until the bone is removed. Once this is done, the drain is opened, and CSF is drained to allow for cerebellar relaxation just before dural opening. The drain can be kept in place to prevent postoperative CSF leak for few days, and then a weaning trial is attempted. If the trial fails, then a shunt should be inserted.

Most of these surgical cases can be done with dynamic brain retraction using the suction instrument in the nondominant hand; however, when a fixed brain retractor is used, care must be taken not to apply too much retraction on the cerebellum to prevent cranial nerve (especially seventh and eighth nerve complex) traction injury or petrosal vein tears. During cyst wall dissection off of the cranial nerve, manipulation of the seventh and eighth nerve complex should be avoided to prevent postoperative facial nerve weakness or hearing loss. On the other hand, the trigeminal nerve is more resilient to manipulation and can be maneuvered with impunity.

Approaching the supratentorial portion of the cyst from the posterior fossa can be challenging. Care must be taken not to injure the trochlear nerve when performing the tentorial cut by identifying the nerve before completing the cut. When dissecting the middle fossa portion, care must be taken not to injure the oculomotor nerve, posterior cerebral artery, or posterior communicating artery. The adherent portion of the cyst wall should be kept in place, with no attempt to pull or dissect it, because these lesions are benign and slow growing. Any residual tumor can be monitored with serial imaging postoperatively.

In cases where the epidermoid cyst wall is liquefied or ruptured, and the cyst contents are spilled in the arachnoid space, the risk of aseptic meningitis is high. The reported incidence of this complication is as high as 18.2% [7]. Preoperative steroid administration, intraoperative surgical field irrigation with normal saline and hydrocortisone solution [30, 33], and long-term postoperative steroid administration have been advocated in these patients [7, 8, 17].

Surgical Outcome

The rate of gross total resection for posterior fossa epidermoid cysts varies widely in the literature. It is evident in the contemporary series for posterior fossa epidermoid cysts that complete resection is achievable in no more than 75% of the cases (Table 12.1). In one study, the reported recurrence-free survival rates for gross total resection and subtotal resection after 13 years of follow-up were 95% and 65%, respectively [33]. In another study, the recurrence-free survival for gross total resection and subtotal resection after 15 years of follow-up were 91% and 7%, respectively [11]. Fourth ventricle epidermoid has a higher rate for gross total removal when compared with CPA epidermoid cysts.

A perioperative mortality rate related to neurovascular structure injuries for posterior fossa epidermoid cysts of 2–12% was reported in the literature published before 2002; however, advancement in microsurgical techniques and

Table 12.1 A summary for the major publications of the CPA and PF epidermoid cyst

Author	Location	No. of cases	Total removal (%)	Mortality	Recurrence (%)	Follow-up (years)
Sabin et al. (1987)	CPA	20	5	5	10	6
Salazar et al. (1987)	CPA	17	0	6	24	6.8
Yamakawa et al. (1989)	CPA	15	47	6.6	20	8
Yasargil et al. (1989)	CPA	22	97	0	0	5.7
De Souza et al. (1989)	CPA	27	18	3	14.8	15 (max)
Lunardi et al. (1990)	CPA	17	35	12	30	9
Samii et al. (1996)	CPA	40	75	2.5	7.5	5.7
Doyle et al. (1996)	CPA	13	54	0	31	8.6
Brunori et al. (1997)	CPA	12	33	0	17	6.5
Mohanty et al. (1997)	CPA	25	48	8	0	3.5
Talacchi et al. (1998)	PF	28	57	3	30	8.6
Kobata et al. (2002)	CPA	30	57	0	10	11.5
Scheifer et al. (2006)	CPA	24	54.1	0	25	4.3
Safavi-abbasi et al. (2008)	CPA	12	75	0	25	2.25
Gopalakrishnan et al. (2014)	PF	50	62	0	44.7	9.4
Czernicki et al. (2015)	CPA	17	29.4	0	29.4	9
Hasegawa et al. (2016)	CPA	22	81.8 (total/near-total)	0	–	9
Yawn et al. (2016)	CPA	47	46	0	8	3.5

better understanding of these lesions has led to 0% perioperative mortality rate in the contemporary series (Table 12.1). On the other hand, postoperative morbidity—both worsening of pre-existing deficit or development of new neurological deficit—is common. The reported incidence approaches 60% in some studies, and the injuries are mainly related to sixth, seventh, and eighth nerve complex and lower cranial nerve deficits [7, 30, 37]. However, most of these deficits resolve completely or improve on long-term follow-up [7].

Management of Recurrence and Malignant Transformation

Recurrence rates for these cysts vary depending on the follow-up periods; they have been reported to be 8–29.4% in the series published between 2002 and 2016 over a follow-up period ranging from 2.25 to 11.5 years [7, 14, 17, 28, 30, 37]. One recently published study including 50 patients with CPA epidermoid cysts reported a 44.5% recurrence rate over 9.3 years of follow-up, a high rate attributed to the long follow-up period [11]. Some authors have found that the recurrence rate is not influenced by the extent of resection [30, 37]; however, the follow-up periods for these studies were less than 5 years, and it is important to remember that these cysts are benign and slowly growing. Thus, a follow-up period longer than 5 years is necessary to reflect the true recurrence rate.

Recurrent cysts are managed based on the clinical status of the patients. Recurrent epidermoid on imaging with no evidence of a new neurological deficit or worsening of a baseline neurological deficit can be monitored with serial imaging. A second surgery for symptomatic recurrent epidermoid cysts in the CPA is unlikely to result in complete removal, but the postoperative result is generally comparable to that of the first surgery, with no increased mortality or morbidity [11].

Malignant transformation in epidermoid cysts is rare phenomena. Degeneration of the epidermoid cyst into squamous cell carcinoma, primary malignant epidermoid carcinoma, and leptomeningeal carcinomatosis with malignant epidermoid carcinoma has been reported [25]. Containment of the tumor within the intracranial and intradural compartment, evidence of benign squamous cell epithelium, and exclusion of metastasis or extension from a nasopharyngeal carcinoma are the criteria to diagnose malignant epidermoid [10, 13]. Metastasis occurs more commonly in male patients than in females, with a reported 4:3 male-to-female ratio [21]. Management options for this rare type of epidermoid cyst may include palliative treatment, surgery, stereotactic radiosurgery (SRS), chemotherapy, or a combination of these. In a systematic review of 58 patients with malignant epidermoids, the average survival was 5.3 months with palliative treatment, 29.5 months with SRS, and 25.7 months with chemotherapy (alone, combined with surgery, radiation, or SRS) [21]. When surgical resection is combined with radiation, SRS, or chemotherapy, the average survival was 36.3 months [21]. For leptomeningeal carcinomatosis associated with malignant epidermoids, the average survival was 9.1 months without treatment and 14.5 months with multimodality treatment [21].

Conclusion

Posterior fossa epidermoid cysts including those in the CPA and the fourth ventricle are typically benign and slow-growing lesions. When discovered incidentally and causing no significant mass effect or hydrocephalus, they can be managed conservatively. However, when symptomatic, surgery is the mainstay of treatment. Most of these cysts are amenable to surgical resection through a standard retrosigmoid or midline suboccipital craniotomy/craniotomy approach. These cysts are soft and often a small craniotomy will suffice to obtain access. The goal of treatment is safe gross total resection; however, epidermoid cysts wall can be very adherent to the surrounding neurovascular structure, and attempts to remove these parts of the wall should be resisted. Long-term follow-up with serial imaging postoperatively for completely removed or residual epidermoid cysts is recommended, especially in young patients. Recurrent epidermoid cysts can be observed clinically and radiologically when asymptomatic, but surgery should be offered when they become symptomatic without increased mortality or morbidity.

References

1. Akar Z, Tanriover N, Tuzgen S, Kafadar AM, Kuday C. Surgical treatment of intracranial epidermoid tumors. Neurol Med Chir (Tokyo). 2003;43:275–280.; discussion 281.
2. Alvord EC Jr. Growth rates of epidermoid tumors. Ann Neurol. 1977;2:367–70.
3. Baumann CH, Bucy PC. Paratrigeminal epidermoid tumors. J Neurosurg. 1956;13:455–68.
4. Berger MS, Wilson CB. Epidermoid cysts of the posterior fossa. J Neurosurg. 1985;62:214–9.
5. Braun IF, Naidich TP, Leeds NE, Koslow M, Zimmerman HM, Chase NE. Dense intracranial epidermoid tumors. Computed tomographic observations. Radiology. 1977;122:717–9.
6. Chen S, Ikawa F, Kurisu K, Arita K, Takaba J, Kanou Y. Quantitative MR evaluation of intracranial epidermoid tumors by fast fluid-attenuated inversion recovery imaging and echo-planar diffusion-weighted imaging. AJNR Am J Neuroradiol. 2001;22:1089–96.
7. Czernicki T, Kunert P, Nowak A, Wojciechowski J, Marchel A. Epidermoid cysts of the cerebellopontine angle: clinical features and treatment outcomes. Neurol Neurochir Pol. 2016;50:75–82.
8. de Souza CE, de Souza R, da Costa S, Sperling N, Yoon TH, Abdelhamid MM, et al. Cerebellopontine angle epidermoid cysts: a report on 30 cases. J Neurol Neurosurg Psychiatry. 1989;52:986–90.
9. Forghani R, Farb RI, Kiehl TR, Bernstein M. Fourth ventricle epidermoid tumor: radiologic, intraoperative, and pathologic findings. Radiographics. 2007;27:1489–94.
10. Garcia CA, McGarry PA, Rodriguez F. Primary intracranial squamous cell carcinoma of the right cerebellopontine angle. J Neurosurg. 1981;54:824–8.
11. Gopalakrishnan CV, Ansari KA, Nair S, Menon G. Long term outcome in surgically treated posterior fossa epidermoids. Clin Neurol Neurosurg. 2014;117:93–9.
12. Halcrow SJ, Crawford PJ, Craft AW. Epidermoid spinal cord tumour after lumbar puncture. Arch Dis Child. 1985;60:978–9.
13. Hamlat A, Hua ZF, Saikali S, Laurent JF, Gedouin D, Ben-Hassel M, et al. Malignant transformation of intra-cranial epithelial cysts: systematic article review. J Neuro-Oncol. 2005;74:187–94.
14. Hasegawa M, Nouri M, Nagahisa S, Yoshida K, Adachi K, Inamasu J, et al. Cerebellopontine angle epidermoid cysts: clinical presentations and surgical outcome. Neurosurg Rev. 2016;39:259–266; discussion 266–267.
15. Kallmes DF, Provenzale JM, Cloft HJ, McClendon RE. Typical and atypical MR imaging features of intracranial epidermoid tumors. AJR Am J Roentgenol. 1997;169:883–7.
16. Karantanas AH. MR imaging of intracranial epidermoid tumors: specific diagnosis with Turbo-FLAIR pulse sequence. Comput Med Imaging Graph. 2001;25:249–55.
17. Kobata H, Kondo A, Iwasaki K. Cerebellopontine angle epidermoids presenting with cranial nerve hyperactive dysfunction: pathogenesis and long-term surgical results in 30 patients. Neurosurgery. 2002;50:276–285; discussion 285–286.
18. Li F, Zhu S, Liu Y, Chen G, Chi L, Qu F. Hyperdense intracranial epidermoid cysts: a study of 15 cases. Acta Neurochir. 2007;149:31–39; discussion 39.
19. Long JM, Kier EL, Schechter MM. The radiology of epidermoid tumors of the cerebellopontine angle. Neuroradiology. 1973;6:188–92.
20. Lunardi P, Missori P, Gagliardi FM, Fortuna A. Long-term results of the surgical treatment of spinal dermoid and epidermoid tumors. Neurosurgery. 1989;25:860–4.
21. Nagasawa DT, Choy W, Spasic M, Yew A, Trang A, Garcia HM, et al. An analysis of intracranial epidermoid tumors with malignant transformation: treatment and outcomes. Clin Neurol Neurosurg. 2013;115:1071–8.
22. Nagashima C, Takahama M, Sakaguchi A. Dense cerebellopontine epidermoid cyst. Surg Neurol. 1982;17:172–7.
23. Osborn AG, Preece MT. Intracranial cysts: radiologic-pathologic correlation and imaging approach. Radiology. 2006;239:650–64.
24. Peng Y, Yu L, Li Y, Fan J, Qiu M, Qi S. Pure endoscopic removal of epidermoid tumors of the cerebellopontine angle. Childs Nerv Syst. 2014;30:1261–7.
25. Raheja A, Eli IM, Bowers CA, Palmer CA, Couldwell WT. Primary intracranial epidermoid carcinoma with diffuse leptomeningeal carcinomatosis: report of two cases. World Neurosurg. 2016;88:692 e699–16.
26. Ravindran K, Rogers TW, Yuen T, Gaillard F. Intracranial white epidermoid cyst with dystrophic calcification – a case report and literature review. J Clin Neurosci. 2017;42:43–7.
27. Rosenbluth PR, Lichtenstein BW. Pearly tumor (epidermoid cholesteatoma) of the brain. Clinicopathologic study of two cases. J Neurosurg. 1960;17:35–42.
28. Safavi-Abbasi S, Di Rocco F, Bambakidis N, Talley MC, Gharabaghi A, Luedemann W, et al. Has management of epidermoid tumors of the cerebellopon-

tine angle improved? Surg Synop Past Present Skull Base. 2008;18:85–98.

29. Sano K. Intracranial dysembryogenetic tumors: pathogenesis and their order of malignancy. Neurosurg Rev. 2001;24:162–167; discussion 168–170.

30. Schiefer TK, Link MJ. Epidermoids of the cerebellopontine angle: a 20-year experience. Surg Neurol. 2008;70:584–590; discussion 590.

31. Sirin S, Gonul E, Kahraman S, Timurkaynak E. Imaging of posterior fossa epidermoid tumors. Clin Neurol Neurosurg. 2005;107:461–7.

32. Smith CM, Timperley WR. Multiple intraspinal and intracranial epidermoids and lipomata following gunshot injury. Neuropathol Appl Neurobiol. 1984;10:235–9.

33. Talacchi A, Sala F, Alessandrini F, Turazzi S, Bricolo A. Assessment and surgical management of pos-

terior fossa epidermoid tumors: report of 28 cases. Neurosurgery. 1998;42:242–251; discussion 251–252.

34. Tancredi A, Fiume D, Gazzeri G. Epidermoid cysts of the fourth ventricle: very long follow up in 9 cases and review of the literature. Acta Neurochir. 2003;145:905–10.

35. Tancredi A, Fiume D, Gazzeri G. Epidermoid cysts of the fourth ventricle: very long follow up in 9 cases and review of the literature. Acta Neurochir. 2003;145:905–11.

36. Tekkok IH, Cataltepe O, Saglam S. Dense epidermoid cyst of the cerebellopontine angle. Neuroradiology. 1991;33:255–7.

37. Yawn RJ, Patel NS, Driscoll CL, Link MJ, Haynes DS, Wanna GB, et al. Primary epidermoid tumors of the cerebellopontine angle: a review of 47 cases. Otol Neurotol. 2016;37:951–5.

Metastasis to the Posterior Fossa

13

Bradley D. Weaver and Randy L. Jensen

Abbreviations

C1	First cervical vertebra
CSF	Cerebrospinal fluid
CT	Computed tomography
EGFR	Epidermal growth factor receptor
EVD	Extraventricular drain
GTR	Gross total resection
iMRI	Intraoperative MRI
KPS	Karnofsky performance scale
LINAC	Linear accelerator
LMD	Leptomeningeal disease/dissemination
MRI	Magnetic resonance imaging
PFS	Posterior fossa syndrome
RPA	Recursive partitioning analysis
SRS	Stereotactic radiosurgery
WBRT	Whole-brain radiotherapy

B.D. Weaver, BS (✉)
University of Utah School of Medicine,
Salt Lake City, UT, USA

Department of Oncological Sciences, Huntsman
Cancer Institute, Salt Lake City, UT, USA
e-mail: Bradley.weaver@hci.utah.edu

R.L. Jensen, MD, PhD
Department of Oncological Sciences, Huntsman
Cancer Institute, Salt Lake City, UT, USA

Department of Radiation Oncology, Huntsman
Cancer Institute, Salt Lake City, UT, USA

Department of Neurosurgery, Clinical Neurosciences
Center, University of Utah, Salt Lake City, UT, USA
e-mail: randy.jensen@hsc.utah.edu

Introduction

Retrospective analyses have estimated the incidence of brain metastasis among all cancer patients at or over 30% [1–3]. The discovery of brain metastasis in patients with previously diagnosed or as-yet-undiagnosed cancer significantly changes the prognosis and treatment options for these patients. If the metastasis is left untreated, the patient's survival is often measured in months; however, in many cases, life span can be significantly extended with treatment. Ultimately, brain metastases represent a far more common disease than primary brain tumors, and their incidence is increasing [1]. This increase is thought to be largely due to greater therapeutic control of extracranial disease, which allows more time and opportunity for metastatic spread from marginally controlled sites [4]. Improved brain imaging with expanded availability is also increasing discovery of solitary and multiple metastases. The problem of metastatic disease of the brain is thus one of the growing interests to the neurosurgeon and neuro-oncological teams, as improving therapies create larger numbers of long-term survivors.

Metastasis to the Cerebellum

The most common cancers that spread to the central nervous system parenchyma are the lung, melanoma, genitourinary, and breast. Approximately 10–15% of all brain metastases are located in the cerebellum or posterior

© Springer International Publishing AG 2018
W.T. Couldwell (ed.), *Skull Base Surgery of the Posterior Fossa*,
https://doi.org/10.1007/978-3-319-67038-6_13

fossa of the brain. This is generally explained as being due to the proportionally higher intracranial blood flow (15%), which is consistent with hematogenous spread of embolic, metastatic tumor cells [5]. Others have discussed that the retrograde dissemination via the paravertebral venous plexus may best explain posterior fossa metastasis from retroperitoneal organs, which are particularly overrepresented in the frequency of posterior fossa metastasis [6].

The genomic landscape of brain metastases also differs from the parental tumor in many instances. Recent reports highlight correlations between particular KRAS and epidermal growth factor receptor (EGFR) mutations and organotropic metastasis [7, 8]. Tumor exosome data also point toward metastatic specificity driven by expression patterns of key extracellular matrix proteins, such as integrins, and likely others [9]. Ultimately, the question of organotropic metastasis remains open for investigation, and as new technologies become available for assessing the biological underpinnings of metastasis, patterns and distributions of metastatic brain lesions will become increasingly clear. Nevertheless, the prevalence of brain metastasis demands that neurosurgeons understand the individualized interventions suitable for each patient, the surgical anatomy of the posterior fossa, the nonsurgical options such as stereotactic radiosurgery (SRS), and the importance of coordination with other neuro-oncological team members.

Metastasis to the Base of Skull

Skull base metastasis (SBM) represents a distinct, challenging, and relatively rare clinical entity. These metastatic lesions may cause significant morbidity when interfering with important neurovascular structures. Most data regarding patients with SBM comes from case reports, small case series, and retrospective analyses comparing treatment modalities. SBMs are estimated to occur in a small percentage of the general population, with up to 3% incidence of temporal bone metastatic lesions [10]. However, SBM is most commonly diagnosed in patients who have a known history of metastatic cancer, especially when osseous metastasis is already confirmed [11]. SBMs to the base of the frontal, ethmoidal, sphenoidal, temporal, and occipital bones are inherently more challenging to detect than calvarial metastases because of their variable clinical presentations and sequestered anatomy. This difficulty likely leads to an underestimation of their true incidence [12].

The three most common cancers contributing to skull base metastases are the breast, lung, and prostate, whose rate of metastasis were estimated at 40%, 14%, and 12%, respectively, in a cohort of 43 patients [11]. Prostate carcinoma represents the most frequent culprit in men, while carcinoma of the breast is the most frequent skull base metastasis found in women [13]; however, many other cancers, such as colon, melanoma, and lymphoma, may metastasize to the skull [14–16]. A large fraction of the time—28% in one meta-analysis [17]—SBM may incite the initial presentation of previously undiagnosed cancer. Further, as patients harboring widely metastatic lesions live longer because of improved current therapies, the prevalence of SBM is undoubtedly increasing, and modern neurosurgeons should be aware of the presentation and challenges presented by patients harboring these lesions.

The pathophysiology of SBM is relatively understudied, yet it is widely accepted that hematogenous spread directly (as from primary tumors of the lung or other tumors) or retrograde venous seeding through Batson's plexus likely account for the vast majority of SBM [17, 18].

Patient Presentation

Patients with metastasis to the cerebellum may have varied and dramatic clinical presentations. Metastases within the cerebellum may cause dysmetria, dysdiadochokinesia, dysarthria, truncal instability, and ataxia. Symptoms related to brainstem or fourth ventricular compression are also common in patients with infratentorial metastasis, often producing nausea and vomiting, headache, and other lower cranial nerve deficits [19]. Hydrocephalus may ensue via compression or blockage of the aqueduct of Sylvius or fourth ventricular outflow channels. Clinical presentation is ultimately determined by tumor location. Highly vascular metastatic tumors may have apoplectic onset of symptoms with associated hemorrhage, compression, and brainstem herniation. Rapidly decompensating and lethargic patients exhibiting signs of hydrocephalus may require urgent placement of an extraventricular drain (EVD) before preoperative planning or operative intervention. In fact, some patients with multiple metastatic lesions and hydrocephalus may require placement of ventriculoperitoneal shunt before undergoing radiosurgery or whole-brain radiotherapy (WBRT) (Fig. 13.1).

The most common overall presentation of patients with SBM includes a worsening, ipsilateral cranial nerve deficit, or craniofacial pain, depending on the extent and location of the lesion. Physicians and neurosurgeons should have a high index of suspicion for SBM in a patient with known metastatic disease presenting with progressive cranial nerve deficits or facial pain. Greenberg et al. [11], and others since, have described as many as five clinically distinct syndromes in patients that occur at different frequencies: orbital, parasellar, middle fossa, jugular foramen, and occipital condyle syndromes. Middle fossa syndrome predominated (35%) in one cohort of 43 patients [11], whereas parasellar and sellar syndromes predominated (29%) in the meta-analysis by Laigle-Donadey et al. [17], although up to 33% of patients in that review had an undefined clinical syndrome. In this chapter, we will focus our discussion on the two syndromes stereotypically affecting patients with posterior fossa SBM: the jugular foramen syndrome and the occipital condyle syndrome.

The jugular foramen syndrome is characterized by a lesion compressing cranial nerves IX, X, XI, and occasionally XII, depending on the size and exact location of the tumor. Patients may

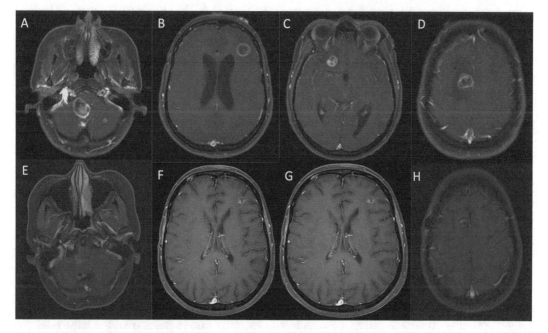

Fig. 13.1 Images of a breast cancer patient with multiple metastatic lesions. (**a–d**) Preoperative axial T1-weighted, contrast-enhanced MRIs demonstrating posterior fossa lesions and multiple supratentorial lesions. This patient had mild ventriculomegaly on imaging but severe nausea and vomiting requiring placement of ventriculoperitoneal shunt before further treatment. (**e–h**) Axial T1-weighted MRIs with gadolinium enhancement obtained at 6-month follow-up after patient underwent ventriculoperitoneal shunt placement and WBRT

describe this as a dull ache behind the ear or in the occipital region. The clinical picture of these patients often reveals dysphagia and weakness of the palate, hoarseness, and weakness of the ipsilateral sternocleidomastoid and trapezius muscles. Horner's syndrome has been reported [20], as has Collet-Sicard syndrome [11, 21, 22]. Jugular venous or transverse sinus compression may result in increased intracranial pressure and papilledema [11, 21, 22].

The occipital condyle syndrome is defined by unilateral, often superficial, pain in the occipital region. If the pain initially occurs in the absence of neurological deficits, it often progresses within a short period of time to dysphagia and dysarthria. Unilateral cranial nerve XII palsy is also often present, and patients often complain of a stiff neck [22–24] and pain exacerbated upon flexion or contralateral rotation. The extent of cranial nerve involvement and occipital and neck pain is undoubtedly a function of size and location of the offending tumor.

Diagnosis and Selection for Surgical Intervention

Increased surveillance imaging using computed tomography (CT) and magnetic resonance imaging (MRI) of patients with known cancer has allowed an increase in the detection of asymptomatic intracranial lesions [25, 26]. However, a large number (~30%) of patients who are ultimately found to have brain metastases have had no previous diagnosis of cancer [27]. In these patients, a thorough workup is mandatory during treatment planning and should include extensive imaging, using CT or MRI of the chest, abdomen, pelvis, and even radionucleotide bone scans and positron emission tomography scans. For the neurosurgeon, MRI with and without contrast is the modality of choice and is mandatory before surgical planning, unless it cannot be obtained because of an MRI contraindication. Metastases to the brain are typically found at the "gray-white" junction and have abnormal vascular permeability. Therefore, extensive vasogenic edema is common, and administration of contrast agent

typically produces enhancement of the metastases of interest, as nearly all metastases disrupt the blood–brain tumor barrier. Patterns of MRI signal intensity are currently not robust enough to use for diagnosis of specific metastatic tumors, yet many important distinctions can be made. Most brain metastases will show high T2 signal intensity [28]. Necrotic and cystic lesions may demonstrate sharp lesional demarcation but can have variable T1 and T2 signals. T1 rim enhancement is often noted [29]. Hemorrhagic metastases may have heterogeneous enhancement patterns and incomplete rim enhancement and can cause difficulty in diagnostic imaging. Identification of the tumor body is usually sufficient to diagnose a hemorrhaging metastasis versus an arteriovenous malformation or parenchymal hematoma [30]. Notably, MRI offers superior sensitivity to contrast-enhanced CT for detection of metastases in the posterior fossa as well as other small metastases throughout the brain [31].

Imaging studies obtained for a patient with suspected SBM include standard T1- and T2-weighted MRI with and without contrast. It may be helpful to rely on fat-suppressed images in the context of gadolinium administration to pick out enhancing lesions near bone and soft tissue junctions [17]. Skull base CT scan bone windows may provide confirmatory imaging or may substitute for MRI only when absolutely necessary. Radionuclide bone scans or positron emission tomography may be helpful in diagnosis of bony SBM (Fig. 13.2). Laboratory tests should include cerebrospinal fluid cytology to exclude meningeal carcinomatosis [32].

The number and location of metastases, as well as the overall clinical picture of each patient, must be used to guide the decision to intervene surgically. Single or solitary lesions, >3 cm in diameter, and close to the surface of the brain are most accessible to the neurosurgeon. This is especially true in patients with a large posterior fossa lesion causing mass effect, fourth ventricular compromise, and neurological symptoms (Fig. 13.4). In patients with stable, or relatively stable, metastatic disease, removal of these lesions surgically has been shown to provide sub-

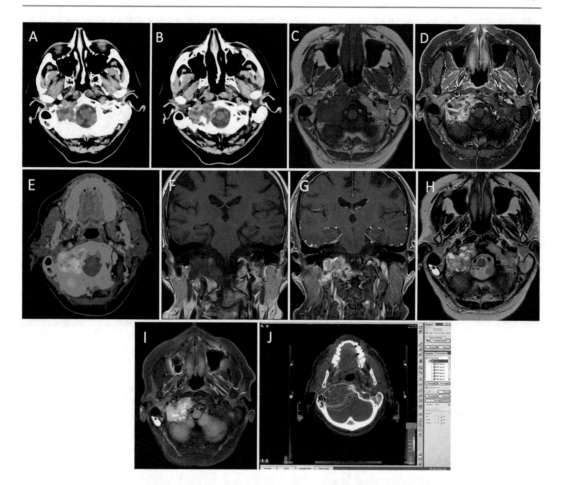

Fig. 13.2 (**a**, **b**) Axial CT images of right occipital condyle lesion initially thought to be a paraganglioma but confirmed a metastatic lung adenocarcinoma by needle biopsy. (**c**, **d**) T1-weighted axial MRI with and without gadolinium enhancement. (**e**) Positron emission tomography image consistent with active tumor. (**f**, **g**) Coronal T1-weighted MRI with and without gadolinium enhancement. (**h**) FLAIR imaging. (**i**) T2-weighted axial MRI. (**j**) Radiosurgical isodose treatment planning lines for this lesion treated with stereotactic radiosurgery

stantial survival benefits [33]. Alternatively, having more than three or four small metastases in eloquent brain or in a patient with rampant extracranial disease would be a relative contraindication for surgical intervention, and WBRT or SRS coupled with chemotherapy may be considered. In cases of asymptomatic patients with lesions in the posterior fossa, SRS is an excellent treatment choice (Figs. 13.3 and 13.4). This approach is even more attractive if multiple metastatic lesions are present in both the supratentorial and the infratentorial compartments in asymptomatic patients (Fig. 13.5). Even tumors thought to be moderately or highly "radioresistant" (i.e., melanoma, renal cell carcinoma, thyroid, non-small-cell lung cancer, colon) may benefit from SRS when WBRT might otherwise not prove to be efficacious. There is good evidence to suggest that the mechanism of SRS-induced cell death may be different than that of WBRT [34]. This is discussed later in this chapter. Nevertheless, SRS has been shown to be equivalent to surgical intervention in up to four metastatic lesions, but some surgeons contend that safe, effective radiosurgery can be performed for patients with up to ten metastases [35].

Tumors of the posterior fossa represent a unique challenge for the neurosurgeon. Normally a contraindication to surgical intervention, multiple metastases or single, relatively inaccessible

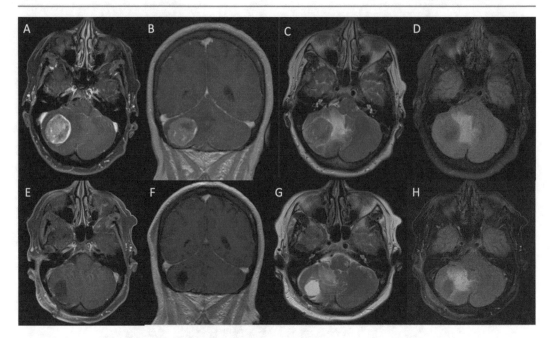

Fig. 13.3 Images of a patient with newly diagnosed lung cancer and solitary posterior fossa metastatic lesion. (**a, b**) Preoperative MRIs demonstrate (**a**) large enhancing mass on axial T1-weighted gadolinium-enhanced image; (**b**) coronal section of the same sequence both demonstrate significant mass effect and fourth ventricular compression. (**c, d**) Preoperative (**c**) T2-weighted and (**d**) FLAIR images demonstrate peritumoral edema. (**e–h**) Immediate postoperative (**e**) axial T1-weighted, gadolinium-enhanced, (**f**) coronal and (**g**) axial T2-weighted, and (**h**) FLAIR images demonstrate resection of the lesion, resolution of mass effect, and improving peritumoral edema

metastases may produce debilitating neurological symptoms that warrant surgical intervention despite no increase in patient survival and a greater chance of postoperative morbidity [36]. These cases should be approached judiciously; however, the opportunity to offer recourse from debilitating neurological impairment for a patient who has months to live cannot be overstated. A neurosurgeon must weigh all aspects of a patient's condition, as well as his or her own technical abilities, and exercise the appropriate clinical judgment.

For treatment of brain metastases, management algorithms seek to provide evidence-based prognostic indicators to inform treatment decisions. The recursive partitioning analysis (RPA) classification scale devised by Gaspar and associates within the Radiation Therapy Oncology Group is a well-known prognostication tool [37]. Notably, the RPA for brain metastasis is divided into three prognostic categories, incorporating Karnofsky performance scale (KPS) metrics as well as age and systemic disease state (Table 13.1). Class I patients appear to benefit the most from any therapeutic modalities, such as surgery, SRS, or WBRT, and tend to have KPS ≥70, controlled extracranial disease, and an age of <65 years. Most patients fall into Class II, with ambiguous benefit depending on the patient, disease, and therapeutic options available. Class III patients (KPS <70) do not consistently benefit from therapy, no matter the modality, and have a median survival of approximately 2 months [37]. Therefore, the decision to operate must be considered within the context of the systemic disease, and more advanced systemic disease often predicts short-term survival regardless of intracranial tumor burden [38, 39].

Because of the short overall median survival times often seen in patients with brain metastasis (8–12 months), much of a neurosurgeon's efforts may be palliative and short; however, with appropriate patient selection, instances of long-term survivors will continue to increase. For patients with high tumor burdens and multiple metastases, SRS

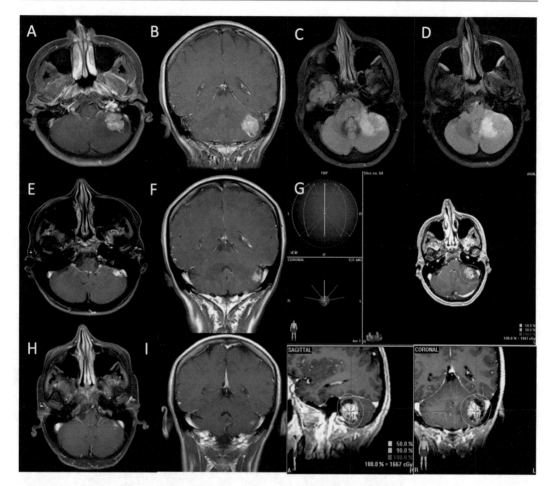

Fig. 13.4 Images of a patient with an asymptomatic ovarian cancer metastatic lesion to the left cerebellopontine angle. (**a**, **d**) Preoperative axial (**a**) and coronal (**b**) T1-weighted, gadolinium-enhanced MRIs demonstrating moderately sized lesion, with mild edema visible on axial (**c**) FLAIR and (**d**) T2-weighted images. Radiosurgery was performed to 1800 cGy to the 90% isodose line using dynamic conformal arc linear accelerator therapy (**g**). (**e**, **f**) Three-month posttreatment axial (**e**) and coronal (**f**) MRIs demonstrate significant decrease in size of the lesion. (**h**–**i**) Two-year follow-up axial (**h**) and coronal (**i**) MRIs demonstrate continued tumor control

or WBRT may provide palliation of symptoms in sync with the medical or neuro-oncological team approach. Aggressive cytoreductive surgeries are often contraindicated in the context of the broader health of these patients, especially if they are neurologically compromised and have short life expectancy at the time of presentation [40].

Treatment options for patients with SBM include conventional chemotherapeutics (i.e., cytotoxic or hormonal) targeted at the specific type of tumor. Surgical resection is typically reserved for solitary or rapidly enlarging tumors that are causing a high degree of morbidity and decreased quality of life, although total resection of these lesions is often precluded by involvement of critical neurovascular structures. Radiation therapy, or SRS, is often the treatment modality of choice in these patients.

SRS is now a frequently used, precise method for addressing local tumor control and SBM-related symptom management. Most reports of SRS used for SBM are positive, often citing patient symptom improvement until time of death [41–43].

Fig. 13.5 Images of a patient with metastatic colon cancer with controlled systemic disease and no neurological complaints or symptoms. Preoperative (**a**) axial and (**b**) coronal T1-weighted, gadolinium-enhanced MRIs demonstrate one small cerebellar lesion and one high parietal lesion. (**c**, **d**) Radiosurgical treatment of both lesions was performed. (**e**, **f**) MRI 3 years later demonstrate no new lesions and only small enhancing scar tissue with no evidence of tumor growth over this time period

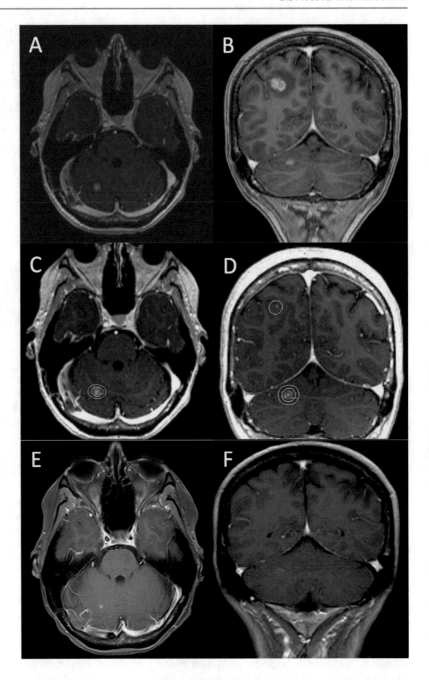

Perioperative Care and Surgical Techniques for Metastasis to the Posterior Fossa

Prior to the work of Harvey Cushing, tumor resection of posterior fossa lesions was seldom attempted because of the high morbidity and mortality associated with the procedure. Through meticulous documentation and perioperative care, coupled with new cautery instrumentation, Cushing added the practice of posterior fossa surgery into the neurosurgical armamentarium [44]. Much of today's surgical decision making is influenced by understanding the precise three-dimensional location of a tumor and the posterior fossa.

Table 13.1 Recursive partitioning analysis classification scale for brain metastasis

Class	Patient characteristics	Proportion of patients
I	KPS ≥70	20%
	Controlled primary disease	
	Age <65 years	
	No evidence of extracranial metastases	
II	KPS ≥70	65%
	Uncontrolled primary disease	
	Age ≥65 years	
	Other extracranial metastases present	
III	KPS <70	15%

Data from Gaspar et al. 1997, 2000 [37, 86]
Note that the majority of patients fall into Class II, where the prognostic benefit of any given form of therapeutic modality is more ambiguous.
KPS Karnofsky performance scale

The posterior fossa is a special surgical situation where space is limited, and vital structures such lower cranial nerves and the brainstem are in close proximity. Successful surgical resection of metastatic tumors in the posterior fossa requires careful study and examination of tumor volume, location, and neighboring structures. The primary surgical objective should be safe gross total resection (GTR) for any metastatic lesion without incurring new neurological deficits.

Preoperative Care

Preoperatively, patients with posterior fossa metastatic lesions are started on dexamethasone to control vasogenic edema and brain swelling. Intraoperatively, mannitol, 3% saline, and mild hyperventilation may be required to relax the cerebellum during the dural opening. Patients who present with features of hydrocephalus and ventricular obstruction may have received an EVD preoperatively. Alternatively, a prophylactic burr hole can be placed intraoperatively 7 cm superior and 3 cm lateral to the inion to aid in placement of a ventricular drain for intracranial fluid management throughout the case. Surgical neuronavigation can aid in this process as necessary.

Surgical Approaches to the Posterior Fossa

Many surgical corridors to posterior fossa lesions have been described [45–51]. For the purposes of this chapter, we describe approaches that can be applied to metastatic lesions of the vermis, cerebellar hemispheres, and often deeper anatomy including the cerebellar peduncles, depending on the use of stereotactic guidance as necessary to define acceptable boundaries of resection. Approaches to the midline vermis, as well as the cerebellar hemispheres, can follow standard practices of suboccipital craniotomy and exposure. Lateral lesions, such as those near the cerebellopontine angle or jugular foramen, as well as deeper or anteriorly distributed metastases are accessed via retrosigmoid or skull base approaches. Frameless stereotaxis guided by thin-sliced MRI for real-time image guidance is used to avoid damaging important structures during approach and to ensure efficient and thorough tumor resection.

Posterior fossa craniectomy or craniotomy may be appropriate for single or multiple metastatic lesions that are surgically resectable. A recent retrospective, multivariate analysis of 88 patients undergoing surgical removal of metastatic posterior fossa lesions highlights a potential difference in patient outcome resulting from choice of surgical approach. The authors report a lower incidence of postoperative complications (12.5%) in patients receiving a craniotomy rather than craniectomy (34.6% overall complication rate). However, the relatively small number of patients and single-institution analysis precludes any strong conclusions based on this work. Importantly, mortality was unaffected by surgical approach [52]. Another group arrived at a similar conclusion in the pediatric population [53].

Proper patient positioning for posterior fossa craniotomies is important to provide clear working space, microscope visibility, and maneuverability of surgical instrumentation. Historically, three major positions have been used for surgical access to the posterior fossa: a park bench (lateral oblique), prone (or modified prone), or sitting position. Although the latter provides excellent exposure, a clear operative field, and venous drainage, it is associated with a risk of air emboli and surgeon fatigue after operating with out-stretched arms. This approach has largely been abandoned by the senior surgeon and will not be further discussed in this chapter. A 3/4 prone posi-tion or lateral oblique position is preferred by the senior author for lateral hemispheric cerebellar lesions; however, in cases in which intraoperative MRI (iMRI) is used, this position is difficult because of limitations on the size of the MR bore (especially in larger patients), and a straight prone position has been adopted as a compromise. iMRI is an excellent adjunct to compensate for "brain shift," a common phenomenon in posterior fossa surgery where cerebrospinal fluid (CSF) drainage, retraction, lesion excision, and brain edema are frequent occurrences. iMRI can compensate for these factors and ensure that complete removal of the lesion has been achieved [54].

Midline Approach for Vermial or Medial Hemispheric Lesions

For midline lesions, the patients are positioned straight prone on the operating table. Special atten-tion must be given so that the skull is securely placed in the head-holding fixation device. Military flexion (axial distraction and head flexion) is obtained by allowing at least a finger's breadth spacing between chin and chest. The venous jugu-lar drainage and endotracheal tube are checked for any kinking, and the surgeon and anesthesiologist together confirm that ventilation and venous out-flow are intact. For prone cases, a rigid or the so-called "armored" endotracheal tube may help with airway patency throughout the case. The table is elevated 10–15° above horizontal; with the patient's head in about 20° of military flexion, there is a clear line of sight for midline approaches including C1 and foramen magnum anatomy when working under the operating microscopes. The patient's legs may be flexed and supported with pillows under the shins. All extremities are padded, and the patient is securely belted or taped to the bed to allow for table rotation during the case for more avenues of visual-ization into the posterior fossa.

For medial lesions of the vermis or medial cer-ebellar hemispheres, a linear, medial incision is made beginning 2 cm superior and extending 6 cm inferior to the inion. Dissection of the soft tissue should occur along the nuchal line, care-fully dividing it in the midline. Skin hemostasis is obtained with Raney clips, and the incision is retracted to provide access to the skull base for bony opening. The periosteum is reflected off of the bone with a periosteal elevator, and bone wax is used to occlude bridging and epiploic veins. The craniotomy or craniectomy (preferred by the senior author) is then performed, with special attention to remove all bone up to the venous sinuses (Fig. 13.6a). Neuronavigation can be used in these instances to verify vascular anat-omy, especially if placing burr holes for a crani-otomy; however, most of the time, with careful drilling and dural visualization, injury to the sinuses can be avoided. Small amounts of Surgicel or other hemostatic agents can be placed on any small areas of venous bleeding and with gentle pressure usually are sufficient to obtain hemostasis.

The exposed dura is carefully examined for venous lakes and divided in a "Y"-shaped inci-sion as possible to avoid these areas. The depth of the tumor will dictate its visibility at this stage, but careful surgical planning and extensive knowledge of posterior fossa anatomy often pre-cludes excessive use of stereotactic navigation in many cases. For a deeper, midline lesions affect-ing the fourth ventricle, the inferior vermis may be divided at the midline, permitting resection of the tumor. The major concern with this approach is the risk of cerebellar mutism. Alternatively, a telovelar approach can be adopted to avoid split-ting the vermis during resection of a fourth ven-tricular lesion. For deeper hemispheric lesions, the cerebellar cortex should be divided with a small corticectomy parallel to the cerebellar folia, and the tumor may then be visualized and resected. Neuronavigational tools may be useful here to define acceptable boundaries of resection, and intraoperative ultrasound can be used to localize tumors that are not easily visible at the surface. In select cases, iMRI can confirm ade-quate removal of tumor.

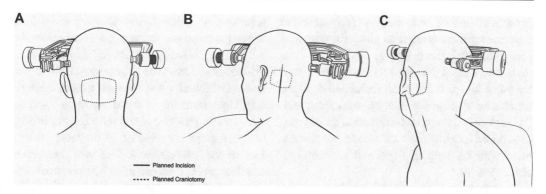

Fig. 13.6 Patient positioning and surgical approaches for lesions of the posterior fossa. *Solid lines* represent planned incision points. *Dashed lines* represent planned craniotomy/craniectomy areas. (**a**) Positioning, incision, and craniotomy/craniectomy for straight prone positioning for a midline or medial hemispheric lesion. Deeper midline lesions can be accessed through this approach, and the craniectomy may be extended inferiorly as far as the foramen magnum, often including C1 laminectomy for greater inferior exposure. Superior lesions of the cerebellar hemispheres may be accessible through this approach as well but necessitate tentorial retraction or transtentorial dissection. The incision in these cases may be moved progressively farther off of the midline to provide access to more anteriorly oriented lesions. (**b**) Park bench positioning for a lateralized lesion of the cerebellar hemisphere. Incision and craniotomy/craniectomy are made in relation to the mastoid notch but should be modified depending on the exact location of the lesion. (**c**) Modified supine positioning is useful for retrosigmoid approaches to far lateralized or anterior lesions of the cerebellum and/or brainstem. Incision and craniectomy are made in relation to the mastoid notch. A linear or curved (*black line*) incision can be made, depending on surgeon preference. Craniotomy/craniectomy can follow a similar path, using transverse and sigmoid sinuses as boundaries when possible. Importantly, the approach can be altered slightly depending on the anterolateral positioning of the lesion for maximal tumor exposure

Paramedian and Retrosigmoid Approaches for Lateral and Far Anterolateral Lesions

For lateral lesions, a retrosigmoid or paramedian bony exposure will provide maximum access to the tumor, allow sufficient working space for resection, and reduce unnecessary retraction on the cerebellum. Patients are positioned in the lateral oblique position for paramedian and retrosigmoidal approaches. If iMRI will be needed for successful completion of the tumor removal, a prone position with mild head turn might be a reasonable compromise and still allow for paramedian approach.

In the lateral oblique position, axillary rolls are used to support the downward arm. The upward arm is supported with pillows, and the superior portion of the table should be elevated 10–15° above horizontal. The head is then rotated into a flexed position with the vertex shifted toward the floor. Again, attention to the placement of the Mayfield pins—with the single pin placed on the superior side and the double pins placed in the most dependent area of the cranium—to securely stabilize the patient is critical. Careful thought about pin placement and Mayfield attachment is necessary to avoid line-of-sight or instrument interference during the microsurgical portion of the procedure.

For a paramedian approach to a lateralized, hemispheric lesion, a vertical, linear incision is made beginning approximately 5 cm above and 2 cm medial to the mastoid notch. The incision is extended inferiorly approximately 4 cm below the level of the mastoid notch (Fig. 13.6b). Soft-tissue dissection should preserve the paraspinal musculature as much as possible, while hemostasis is maintained by using cautery. Depending on the level of the planned craniotomy, the vertebral artery may be identified and carefully avoided. The craniotomy can be extended above, or situated below, the transverse sinus, and care should be taken to avoid injury to these structures during approach. The dura is opened such that the bases of the dural flaps are on the transverse and/or sigmoid sinuses. CSF is then carefully aspirated from the adjacent cisterns to allow for a relaxed cerebellar hemisphere. Taking a little extra time to remove CSF at this point will make the rest of the procedure proceed much easier and decrease the chance of retraction injury to the cerebellum. For surface lesions, en bloc resection should proceed after identification of tumor boundaries, often with the help of registered neuronavigational systems.

Patient positioning in retrosigmoid approaches may be modified depending on tumor location. Modified supine positions may be appropriate for far anterior lesions bordering the cerebellopontine angle and brainstem. In these approaches, the patient is positioned supine, with a large roll placed under the shoulder on the same side as the lesion. The patient is thus rotated away from the neurosurgeon, and the head may be further rotated approximately 45° to the contralateral side. Depending on surgeon preference and tumor size, the skin incision may be positioned linearly over or slightly lateral to the mastoid notch, following a path beginning 5 cm superior and terminating 4 cm inferior to the notch. Other surgeons may prefer a C-shaped incision beginning 2 cm above the ear, proceeding to its vertex at the mastoid notch and terminating 2 cm posterior to the pinna. The craniotomy can be planned following a similar arc; the transverse sinus may be used as the upper border and the mastoid process as the lower border (Fig. 13.6c). Mastoid air cells exposed during the procedure should be plugged with bone wax. After bone flap removal, the dura is divided, exposing the lateral border of the cerebellar hemisphere. Once again, aspiration of CSF from the cerebellopontine angle cistern is key to obtaining relaxation of the cerebellum, which is then progressively and gently retracted posteriorly using small cottonoids, exposing the lateralized or anteriorly extending tumor.

Superior Cerebellar Approach

Far anterior or superior cerebellar lesions can be accessed by modifying the standard suboccipital craniotomy via a supracerebellar, infratentorial approach. A vertical, linear incision is made 2 cm above the inion and extending 6–8 cm below the inion. The preferred craniotomy in these cases extends from above the torcula superiorly to just above or including the foramen magnum inferiorly. Upon bone flap removal and dural opening, the tentorium may be gently retracted superiorly, allowing clear visualization of the tentorial surface of the cerebellum. Resection of the tumor can then proceed according to best practices outlined below. This approach can be moved progressively further lateral, allowing greater access to more anterior lesions. A transtentorial dissection after occipital craniotomy may provide better viewing of the cerebellar peduncles and anterosuperior anatomy of the posterior fossa. These approaches should employ stereotactic navigation to aid in tumor resection and definition of acceptable boundaries of resection.

Excision of Metastatic Lesions

The technique for excision of metastatic lesions is an important consideration. The senior author favors an en bloc resection whenever possible. This minimizes disruption to the tumor body and at least theoretically reduces the incidence of local and regional recurrence [55, 56]. Dissection just outside of the glial pseudocapsule of the tumor allows for excellent hemostatic control of interfacing and feeding vessels and provides the surgeon with an opportunity for thorough GTR. Some tumors may be too large for en bloc resection, and an ultrasonic aspirator may be used initially to debulk the tumor in these cases. The gliotic pseudocapsule should be targeted thereafter, ensuring a safe and efficient resection. Recent retrospective analyses have examined the extent to which resection technique influences leptomeningeal disease (LMD) after posterior fossa metastasis as well as local and regional tumor recurrence. LMD is a known risk after resection of metastases to the posterior fossa [57–61] and confers a shortened survival time and dismal prognosis once discovered. Suki and colleagues discovered that piecemeal tumor resection was associated with a significantly higher incidence of LMD than en bloc resection, but there was no significant increase in LMD in the SRS treatment arm versus the surgical resection arm of the analysis [55]. Finally, the neurosurgical oncologist must be aware of the varying tumor biologies posed by metastatic lesions to the brain. Vascular tumors such as renal cell carcinoma, thyroid cancer, and melanoma are probably best devascularized externally before attempting removal, and an en bloc approach is preferred for these lesions, if feasible. Other lesions such as breast cancer and lung cancer can be very friable, making en bloc resection difficult. After the tumor is resected, hemostasis should be a priority within the tumor cavity. Gelfoam and Surgicel may be applied to the cavity, initiating hemostatic cascades and reducing oozing of blood into the subarachnoid space. CSF flow pathways should be examined and cleared of debris. The dura can then be closed in a watertight fashion, and a Valsalva maneuver should be performed to assess the seal. A dural patch is a norm rather than an exception. The bone flap is replaced if a craniotomy has been performed. Muscle is closed in multiple layers to ensure a tight, secure, postoperative surgical site.

Postoperative Care and Complications

The postoperative period is critical after posterior fossa surgery. Patients should receive an immediate postoperative CT scan if there are any new neurological deficits. Otherwise, unless the iMRI has been used for the case, a postoperative MRI with and without contrast should occur within 72 h of surgery to define the extent of resection and guide future care. Patients who have EVDs placed preoperatively will be gradually weaned as tolerated or converted to a permanent shunt.

Common complications during the postoperative period after posterior fossa surgery include double vision, hearing loss, facial nerve weakness, and swallowing difficulty. Respiratory depression and hydrocephalus are the leading causes of rapid patient deterioration. The constricted space of the posterior fossa allows for neurological decompensation to occur much more quickly and without attendant supratentorial signs (confusion, etc.), which typically signal a progressively deteriorating clinical picture in most brain surgery. Loss of brainstem function secondary to surgical injury or hydrocephalic compression may preclude spontaneous respiration and prevent weaning from ventilation after surgery. Cranial nerves should be meticulously monitored in the postoperative period. A rare, but particularly troublesome, complication of posterior fossa tumor resection is the so-called posterior fossa syndrome (PFS). PFS is described as a collection of symptoms including cranial nerve deficits, nausea, transient mutism, emotional lability, and other cerebellar signs such as imbalance and ataxia. These symptoms appear to be most common after radical and aggressive resection of tumors adjacent to the lateral fourth ventricular borders [62]. Not surprisingly, these symptoms may cause patients and their families great anguish throughout the postoperative and follow-up period. An early rehabilitation medicine consultation, and immediate initiation of physical therapy, may speed recovery if a patient begins to manifest PFS. However, with time, most symptoms tend to resolve on their own.

Late common complications in the postoperative period after posterior fossa surgery include wound infection and pseudomeningocele. A pseudomeningocele, by definition, is a collection of CSF outside the dura. This may occur after posterior fossa surgery because of a failure of dural closure but in many cases is due to hydrocephalus/increased intracranial pressure. This once again calls to mind the attention to detail necessary for dural closure in the posterior fossa. Pseudomeningoceles must be identified early, and many can resolve over time or with placement of a lumbar drain. Rarely, the CSF leakage can transgress the wound closure, with the potential for meningitis. These leaks need to be treated emergently to wash out and close the wound to prevent further infectious complications.

Stereotactic Radiosurgery for Treatment of Posterior Fossa Metastasis

Traditionally, most brain metastases were treated with fractionated radiotherapy, in which patients receive small, fractionated doses of radiation daily for 10–15 days to the whole brain (WBRT). Within the last few decades, there has been a trend to move to newer models of radiation delivery focused on higher doses delivered to smaller target volumes. SRS defines the application of one to five doses of radiation to a precise location, with high-dose delivery to the site of interest, yet minimal dose toxicity in the surrounding tissue. Today this is achieved through a number of different systems. The first was the Gamma Knife system, which was introduced in 1967 by Leksell [63]. This system utilizes a series of 192 or 201 cobalt (60) decay sources whose beams of radiation are mechanically focused at a single site to achieve high-dose delivery with good precision and rapid falloff of radiation dosage in the adjacent tissues [64]. Newer methods of delivery have been developed that rely on the use of a linear accelerator (LINAC) and the robot-based delivery LINAC system called the CyberKnife. LINAC systems function through the same basic principle as Gamma Knife and rotate around a patient's head to deliver "arcs" of radiation at varying, nonoverlapping points of incidence—all targeting a defined site to produce high-dose delivery to the tumor with minimal extralesional tissue toxicity and necrosis. These methods have proven to have similar complications and tumor-treating efficacy [65, 66].

The first cases of SRS for cerebral metastasis were described in 1987 by Sturm et al., who used a LINAC system [67]. Gamma Knife therapy has been demonstrated in numerous studies to provide an average local tumor control rate ranging from 84% to 97% [68]. There have been numerous prospective and retrospective studies examining the clinical utility of SRS versus WBRT versus surgical resection [69–72]. An exhaustive review of this literature is outside the scope of this chapter but we review a few key studies and summarize the use of SRS in the context of pos-

terior fossa metastasis. This first began with the demonstration that WBRT in addition to surgical resection was superior to WBRT alone. Patients had better functional outcomes as well as better median survival rates [33]. Follow-up studies confirmed these findings [73].

Subsequently, a number of studies compared the efficacy of SRS with that of surgery. In these studies, surgery with postoperative WBRT was compared with SRS with follow-up WBRT, and the authors found no difference between the SRS or surgical resection arms of the studies [74–76]. These data suggest that surgery and SRS have equal efficacy for lesions with little to no mass effect. It is not clear whether this is always the case in the posterior fossa, where smaller volume tumors can cause more mass effect than within the supratentorial space. The biggest limitation of SRS is that although local control rates are very good, distant brain metastasis control is not included. This is overcome in studies that demonstrate SRS + WBRT offers a better 1-year local and distant tumor control and survival when compared with SRS-only treatments but at the expense of neurocognitive decline [77, 78]. There are a couple of tumor biological considerations associated with radiosurgery treatment. The relative radiosensitivity of metastatic lesions is an important caveat when considering the results of these trials. Many tumors that are relatively radioresistant to WBRT (such as renal cell carcinoma or melanoma) may be treated successfully with SRS [79, 80].

Although radiotherapy and radiosurgery have been appreciated as a cytotoxic therapy historically, recently uncovered molecular mechanisms of cell death after radiotherapy point toward an intersecting role with the tumor immune response. Immune evasion is necessary for clinically significant tumors [81]. Ionizing radiation has a demonstrated ability to increase proinflammatory cascades such as interferon gamma release and to promote recruitment of effector and helper T-cells [82–84]. Current data support the hypothesis that radiation treatments can create novel epitopes to be leveraged for immune cell activation, in essence creating an in vivo vaccine.

Metastatic lesions of the posterior fossa are often well suited for SRS intervention, yet SRS is not without complications. Brain edema after SRS is a well-described phenomenon, and the small space of the posterior fossa amplifies these effects. Judicious use of steroid therapy and a slow wean over a couple of weeks can overcome most brain edema issues. Post-SRS contrast-enhanced MRI often demonstrates an apparent increase in tumor size and surrounding edema, but this increase often does not truly represent tumor progression [85]. Tumor "pseudoprogression" on radiographic imaging is a complicating factor for predicting patient prognosis and planning future therapies after initial intervention. We tend to ignore early small increases in enhancing volume, especially those clearly within the treated field. Persistent increasing volume or development of symptoms not relieved with steroids leads to surgical resection if possible or stereotactic biopsy if the lesion is not amenable to open resection. Despite these complicating factors, SRS is used to treat small metastatic lesions to the posterior fossa, especially those that are deemed unresectable because of their proximity to vital structures. We propose that SRS can be used for metastatic lesions to the posterior fossa in the following situations:

1. Lesions deemed unresectable due to their proximity to eloquent brain
2. Lesions <3 cm or without any mass effect
3. Up to three lesions in the posterior fossa (or five total including lesions in supratentorial compartment) in the absence of mass effect

Relative contraindications for SRS include space-occupying lesions and symptoms of brainstem or aqueductal compression and hydrocephalus. Resection of the offending lesions in these cases should be expedited, and SRS may be considered as an adjunct therapy or for locally recurrent lesions. When multiple lesions are present, WBRT should always be considered. If the known cancer is melanoma, renal cell carcinoma, or sarcoma, we tend to favor SRS for up to five or six lesions. For other cancers, our threshold is typically three lesions but can be up to five

lesions. Radiosurgical treatments have become a mainstay in the neurosurgical oncologist's practice. The indications for these therapies appear to be increasing, and future clinical analyses teasing apart optimal integration of SRS with other chemotherapeutics will undoubtedly advance the field of neuro-oncology.

Conclusions

Metastatic lesions to the posterior fossa present complex clinical and surgical challenges for the neurosurgical oncologist. With a ratio of metastases to primary brain tumors of approximately 10:1, these lesions represent a large volume of the neurosurgeon's caseload. Despite the progress made in the past decades, devising optimal treatment strategy paradigms that incorporate a patient's overall disease state, the tumor's location, and tumor biology remains a central problem.

Surgical approaches to the posterior fossa necessitate specialized care and perioperative consideration for hydrocephalus, cerebellar mutism, and leptomeningeal spread of metastatic lesions. The neurosurgical oncologist needs to be well versed in posterior fossa anatomy, standard cranial base approaches, and indications and contraindications for these procedures in the context of metastatic neoplasms. Tumors should be removed en bloc whenever possible, paying respect to the varying tumor biologies that are encountered. Many lesions can be targeted with SRS, and often SRS and surgical approaches are combined for optimal therapy. Moving forward, the optimization of SRS promises to influence therapeutic decision making well into the future.

In the past, surgical intervention of lesions in the posterior fossa was often deemed futile, owing to the often-devastating outcomes of surgery. Today, techniques marrying MRI and real-time neuronavigational software allow tumors to be removed in previously inoperable regions of the brain. SRS has further reduced the invasiveness of treating brain metastases, yet evidence supports the superiority of surgical excision in many instances. Detailed knowledge of the clinical picture, surgical approaches, and therapeutic decision making regarding metastasis to the posterior fossa is important background for the modern neurosurgical oncologist, and this knowledge will only increase in utility throughout the coming decades.

Acknowledgments We thank Kristin Kraus, MSc, for editorial assistance and Jennie Williams, MA, for illustrations.

References

1. Gavrilovic IT, Posner JB. Brain metastases: epidemiology and pathophysiology. J Neuro-Oncol. 2005;75(1):5–14.
2. Lassman AB, DeAngelis LM. Brain metastases. Neurol Clin. 2003;21(1):1–23.
3. Landis SH, Murray T, Bolden S, Wingo PA. Cancer statistics, 1999. CA Cancer J Clin. 1999;49(1):8–31.
4. McDonald MW, McMullen KP. A new paradigm in treatment of brain metastases. Curr Probl Cancer. 2015;39(2):70–88.
5. Delattre JY, Krol G, Thaler HT, Posner JB. Distribution of brain metastases. Arch Neurol. 1988;45(7):741–4.
6. Batson OV. The function of the vertebral veins and their role in the spread of metastases. Ann Surg. 1940;112(1):138.
7. Renaud S, Seitlinger J, Falcoz P-E, Schaeffer M, Voegeli A-C, Legrain M, et al. Specific KRAS amino acid substitutions and EGFR mutations predict site-specific recurrence and metastasis following non-small-cell lung cancer surgery. Br J Cancer. 2016;115:346–53.
8. Kim M-J, Lee HS, Kim JH, Kim YJ, Kwon JH, Lee J-O, et al. Different metastatic pattern according to the KRAS mutational status and site-specific discordance of KRAS status in patients with colorectal cancer. BMC Cancer. 2012;12(1):347.
9. Hoshino A, Costa-Silva B, Shen T-L, Rodrigues G, Hashimoto A, Mark MT, et al. Tumour exosome integrins determine organotropic metastasis. Nature. 2015;527(7578):329–35.
10. Belal A Jr. Metastatic tumours of the temporal bone. A histopathological report. J Laryngol Otol. 1985;99(9):839–46.
11. Greenberg HS, Deck MD, Vikram B, Chu FC, Posner JB. Metastasis to the base of the skull: clinical findings in 43 patients. Neurology. 1981;31(5):530–7.
12. Stark AM, Eichmann T, Mehdorn HM. Skull metastases: clinical features, differential diagnosis, and review of the literature. Surg Neurol. 2003;60(3):219–25. discussion 25–6
13. Vikram B, Chu FC. Radiation therapy for metastases to the base of the skull. Radiology. 1979;130(2):465–8.
14. Bairey O, Kremer I, Rakowsky E, Hadar H, Shaklai M. Orbital and adnexal involvement in systemic non-Hodgkin's lymphoma. Cancer. 1994;73(9):2395–9.
15. Harada S, Toya S, Iisaka Y, Ohtani M, Nakamura Y. Basal skull metastasis of stomach cancer presenting with Garcin's syndrome – a case report. No Shinkei Geka. 1987;15(7):765–9.
16. Weisenthal R, Frayer WC, Nichols CW, Eagle RC. Bilateral ocular disease as the initial presentation of malignant lymphoma. Br J Ophthalmol. 1988;72(4):248–52.
17. Laigle-Donadey F, Taillibert S, Martin-Duverneuil N, Hildebrand J, Delattre JY. Skull-base metastases. J Neuro-Oncol. 2005;75(1):63–9.
18. Svare A, Fossa SD, Heier MS. Cranial nerve dysfunction in metastatic cancer of the prostate. Br J Urol. 1988;61(5):441–4.
19. Morreale VM, Ebersold MJ, Quast LM, Parisi JE. Cerebellar astrocytoma: experience with 54 cases surgically treated at the Mayo Clinic, Rochester, Minnesota, from 1978 to 1990. J Neurosurg. 1997;87(2):257–61.
20. Svien HJ, Baker HL, Rivers MH. Jugular foramen syndrome and allied syndromes. Neurology. 1963;13:797–809.
21. Graus F, Walker RW, Allen JC. Brain metastases in children. J Pediatr. 1983;103(4):558–61.
22. Posner JB. Brain metastases: 1995. A brief review. J Neuro-Oncol. 1996;27(3):287–93.
23. Moris G, Roig C, Misiego M, Alvarez A, Berciano J, Pascual J. The distinctive headache of the occipital condyle syndrome: a report of four cases. Headache. 1998;38(4):308–11.
24. Pascual J, Gutierrez A, Polo JM, Berciano J. Occipital condyle syndrome: presentation of a case. Neurologia. 1989;4(8):293–5.
25. Seaman EK, Ross S, Sawczuk IS. High incidence of asymptomatic brain lesions in metastatic renal cell carcinoma. J Neuro-Oncol. 1995;23(3):253–6.
26. Hochstenbag M, Twijnstra A, Wilmink J, Wouters E, Ten Velde G. Asymptomatic brain metastases (BM) in small cell lung cancer (SCLC): MR-imaging is useful at initial diagnosis. J Neuro-Oncol. 2000;48(3):243–8.
27. Merchut MP. Brain metastases from undiagnosed systemic neoplasms. Arch Int Med. 1989;149(5):1076–80.
28. Komiyama M, Yagura H, Baba M, Yasui T, Hakuba A, Nishimura S, et al. MR imaging: possibility of tissue characterization of brain tumors using T1 and T2 values. AJNR Am J Neuroradiol. 1987;8(1):65–70.
29. Lignelli A, Khandji AG. Review of imaging techniques in the diagnosis and management of brain metastases. Neurosurg Clin N Am. 2011;22(1):15–25.
30. Destian S, Sze G, Krol G, Zimmerman R, Deck M. MR imaging of hemorrhagic intracranial neoplasms. AJR Am J Roentgenol. 1989;152(1):137–44.
31. Mintz AP, Cairncross JG. Treatment of a single brain metastasis: the role of radiation following surgical resection. JAMA. 1998;280(17):1527–9.
32. Brillman J, Valeriano J, Adatepe MH. The diagnosis of skull base metastases by radionuclide bone scan. Cancer. 1987;59(11):1887–91.

33. Patchell RA, Tibbs PA, Walsh JW, Dempsey RJ, Maruyama Y, Kryscio RJ, et al. A randomized trial of surgery in the treatment of single metastases to the brain. New Engl J Med. 1990;322(8):494–500.

34. Brown PD, Brown CA, Pollock BE, Gorman DA, Foote RL. Stereotactic radiosurgery for patients with "radioresistant" brain metastases. Neurosurgery. 2002;51(3):656–67.

35. Morton R, Holland E. Brain metastasis. In: Sekhar L, Fessler R, editors. Atlas of neurosurgical techniques. 2nd ed. New York: Thieme; 2016. p. 33–7.

36. Bindal RK, Sawaya R, Leavens ME, Lee JJ. Surgical treatment of multiple brain metastases. J Neurosurg. 1993;79(2):210–6.

37. Gaspar L, Scott C, Rotman M, Asbell S, Phillips T, Wasserman T, et al. Recursive partitioning analysis (RPA) of prognostic factors in three Radiation Therapy Oncology Group (RTOG) brain metastases trials. Int J Radiat Oncol Biol Phys. 1997;37(4):745–51.

38. Bindal RK, Sawaya R, Leavens ME, Hess KR, Taylor SH. Reoperation for recurrent metastatic brain tumors. J Neurosurg. 1995;83(4):600–4.

39. Galicich JH, Sundaresan N, Arbit E, Passe S. Surgical treatment of single brain metastasis: factors associated with survival. Cancer. 1980;45(2):381–6.

40. Sundaresan N, Galicich JH. Surgical treatment of brain metastases. Clinical and computerized tomography evaluation of the results of treatment. Cancer. 1985;55(6):1382–8.

41. Miller RC, Foote RL, Coffey RJ, Gorman DA, Earle JD, Schomberg PJ, et al. The role of stereotactic radiosurgery in the treatment of malignant skull base tumors. Int J Radiat Oncol Biol Phys. 1997;39(5):977–81.

42. Mori Y, Hashizume C, Kobayashi T, Shibamoto Y, Kosaki K, Nagai A. Stereotactic radiotherapy using Novalis for skull base metastases developing with cranial nerve symptoms. J Neuro-Oncol. 2010;98(2):213–9.

43. Pan H, Cervino LI, Pawlicki T, Jiang SB, Alksne J, Detorie N, et al. Frameless, real-time, surface imaging-guided radiosurgery: clinical outcomes for brain metastases. Neurosurgery. 2012;71(4):844–52.

44. Malekpour M, Cohen-Gadol AA. Making the "inoperable" tumors "operable": Harvey Cushing's contributions to the surgery of posterior fossa tumors. Neurosurg Focus. 2014;36(4):E15.

45. Rhoton AL Jr. The posterior cranial fossa: microsurgical anatomy and surgical approaches. Neurosurgery. 2000;47(3):S5–6.

46. Rhoton AL Jr. The cerebellopontine angle and posterior fossa cranial nerves by the retrosigmoid approach. Neurosurgery. 2000;47(3):S93–S129.

47. Kurokawa Y, Uede T, Hashi K. Operative approach to mediosuperior cerebellar tumors: occipital interhemispheric transtentorial approach. Surg Neurol. 1999;51(4):421–5.

48. François P, Ismail MB, Hamel O, Bataille B, Jan M, Velut S. Anterior transpetrosal and subtemporal trans-tentorial approaches for pontine cavernomas. Acta Neurochir. 2010;152(8):1321–9.

49. Shirane R, Kumabe T, Yoshida Y, Su C-C, Jokura H, Umezawa K, et al. Surgical treatment of posterior fossa tumors via the occipital transtentorial approach: evaluation of operative safety and results in 14 patients with anterosuperior cerebellar tumors. J Neurosurg. 2001;94(6):927–35.

50. Heros RC. Lateral suboccipital approach for vertebral and vertebrobasilar artery lesions. J Neurosurg. 1986;64(4):559–62.

51. Wen D, Heros R. Surgical approaches to the brain stem. Neurosurg Clin N Am. 1993;4(3):457–68.

52. Hadanny A, Rozovski U, Nossek E, Shapira Y, Strauss I, Kanner AA, et al. Craniectomy versus craniotomy for posterior fossa metastases: complication profile. World Neurosurg. 2016;89:193–8.

53. Gnanalingham KK, Lafuente J, Thompson D, Harkness W, Hayward R. Surgical procedures for posterior fossa tumors in children: does craniotomy lead to fewer complications than craniectomy? J Neurosurg. 2002;97(4):821–6.

54. Bergsneider M, Sehati N, Villablanca P, McArthur DL, Becker DP, Liau LM. Extent of glioma resection using low-field (0.2 T) versus high-field (1.5 T) intraoperative MRI and image-guided frameless neuronavigation. Clin Neurosurg. 2005;52:389–99.

55. Suki D, Abouassi H, Patel AJ, Sawaya R, Weinberg JS, Groves MD. Comparative risk of leptomeningeal disease after resection or stereotactic radiosurgery for solid tumor metastasis to the posterior fossa. J Neurosurg. 2008;108(2):248–57.

56. Suki D, Hatiboglu MA, Patel AJ, Weinberg JS, Groves MD, Mahajan A, et al. Comparative risk of leptomeningeal dissemination of cancer after surgery or stereotactic radiosurgery for a single supratentorial solid tumor metastasis. Neurosurgery. 2009;64(4):664–76.

57. DeAngelis LM, Mandell LR, Thaler TH, Kimmel DW, Galicich JH, Fuks Z, et al. The role of postoperative radiotherapy after resection of single brain metastases. Neurosurgery. 1989;24(6):798–805.

58. Kitaoka K, Abe H, Aida T, Satoh M, Itoh T, Nakagawa Y. Follow-up study on metastatic cerebellar tumor surgery. Neurol Med Chir (Tokyo). 1990;30(8):591–8.

59. Mahajan A, Borden J. Tsai J-s. Carcinomatous meningitis: are surgery or gamma knife radiosurgery treatment risk factors? J Neurosurg. 2002;97:441–4.

60. Siomin VE, Vogelbaum MA, Kanner AA, Lee S-Y, Suh JH, Barnett GH. Posterior fossa metastases: risk of leptomeningeal disease when treated with stereotactic radiosurgery compared to surgery. J Neuro-Oncol. 2004;67(1–2):115–21.

61. Norris LK, Grossman SA, Olivi A. Neoplastic meningitis following surgical resection of isolated cerebellar metastasis: a potentially preventable complication. J Neuro-Oncol. 1997;32(3):215–23.

62. Ojemann JG, Partridge SC, Poliakov AV, Niazi TN, Shaw DW, Ishak GE, et al. Diffusion tensor imaging

of the superior cerebellar peduncle identifies patients with posterior fossa syndrome. Childs Nerv Syst. 2013;29(11):2071–7.

63. Leksell L. Stereotactic radiosurgery. J Neurol Neurosurg Psychiatry. 1983;46(9):797–803.

64. Kihlström L, Karlsson B, Lindquist C. Gamma Knife surgery for cerebral metastases. Implications for survival based on 16 years experience. Stereotact Funct Neurosurg. 1993;61(Suppl. 1):45–50.

65. Kondziolka D, Martin JJ, Flickinger JC, Friedland DM, Brufsky AM, Baar J, et al. Long-term survivors after gamma knife radiosurgery for brain metastases. Cancer. 2005;104(12):2784–91.

66. Niranjan A, Lunsford LD. Radiosurgery: where we were, are, and may be in the third millennium. Neurosurgery. 2000;46(3):531.

67. Sturm V, Kober B, Hover K-H, Schlegel W, Boesecke R, Pastyr O, et al. Stereotactic percutaneous single dose irradiation of brain metastases with a linear accelerator. Int J Radiat Oncol Biol Phys. 1987;13(2):279–82.

68. Lippitz B, Lindquist C, Paddick I, Peterson D, O'Neill K, Beaney R. Stereotactic radiosurgery in the treatment of brain metastases: the current evidence. Cancer Treat Rev. 2014;40(1):48–59.

69. Muacevic A, Wowra B, Siefert A, Tonn J-C, Steiger H-J, Kreth FW. Microsurgery plus whole brain irradiation versus gamma knife surgery alone for treatment of single metastases to the brain: a randomized controlled multicentre phase III trial. J Neuro-Oncol. 2008;87(3):299–307.

70. Rades D, Bohlen G, Pluemer A, Veninga T, Hanssens P, Dunst J, et al. Stereotactic radiosurgery alone versus resection plus whole-brain radiotherapy for 1 or 2 brain metastases in recursive partitioning analysis class 1 and 2 patients. Cancer. 2007;109(12):2515–21.

71. Datta R, Jawahar A, Ampil FL, Shi R, Nanda A, D'Agostino H. Survival in relation to radiotherapeutic modality for brain metastasis: whole brain irradiation vs. gamma knife radiosurgery. Am J Clin Oncol. 2004;27(4):420–4.

72. Aoyama H, Shirato H, Tago M, Nakagawa K, Toyoda T, Hatano K, et al. Stereotactic radiosurgery plus whole-brain radiation therapy vs stereotactic radiosurgery alone for treatment of brain metastases: a randomized controlled trial. JAMA. 2006;295(21):2483–91.

73. Patchell RA, Tibbs PA, Regine WF, Dempsey RJ, Mohiuddin M, Kryscio RJ, et al. Postoperative radiotherapy in the treatment of single metastases to the brain: a randomized trial. JAMA. 1998;280(17):1485–9.

74. Schöggl A, Kitz K, Reddy M, Schneider B, Dieckmann K, Ungersböck K. Defining the role of stereotactic radiosurgery versus microsurgery in the treatment of single brain metastases. Acta Neurochir. 2000;142(6):621–6.

75. O'Neill BP, Iturria NJ, Link MJ, Pollock BE, Ballman KV, O'Fallon JR. A comparison of surgical resection and stereotactic radiosurgery in the treatment of solitary brain metastases. Int J Radiat Oncol Biol Phys. 2003;55(5):1169–76.

76. Rades D, Kueter J-D, Veninga T, Gliemroth J, Schild SE. Whole brain radiotherapy plus stereotactic radiosurgery (WBRT+ SRS) versus surgery plus whole brain radiotherapy (OP+ WBRT) for 1–3 brain metastases: results of a matched pair analysis. Eur J Cancer. 2009;45(3):400–4.

77. Chang EL, Wefel JS, Hess KR, Allen PK, Lang FF, Kornguth DG, et al. Neurocognition in patients with brain metastases treated with radiosurgery or radiosurgery plus whole-brain irradiation: a randomised controlled trial. Lancet Oncol. 2009;10(11):1037–44.

78. Brown PD, Jaeckle K, Ballman KV, Farace E, Cerhan JH, Anderson SK, et al. Effect of radiosurgery alone vs radiosurgery with whole brain radiation therapy on cognitive function in patients with 1 to 3 brain metastases: a randomized clinical trial. JAMA. 2016;316(4):401–9.

79. Mathieu D, Kondziolka D, Cooper PB, Flickinger JC, Niranjan A, Agarwala S, et al. Gamma knife radiosurgery for malignant melanoma brain metastases. Clin Neurosurg. 2007;54:241.

80. Brown W, Wu X, Fowler J, Garcia S, Fayad F, Amendola B, et al. Lung metastases treated by CyberKnife (R) image-guided robotic stereotactic radiosurgery at 41 months. South Med J. 2008;101(4):376–82.

81. Hanahan D, Weinberg RA. Hallmarks of cancer: the next generation. Cell. 2011;144(5):646–74.

82. Demaria S, Formenti SC. Sensors of ionizing radiation effects on the immunological microenvironment of cancer. Int J Radiat Biol. 2007;83(11–12):819–25.

83. Matsumura S, Demaria S. Up-regulation of the pro-inflammatory chemokine CXCL16 is a common response of tumor cells to ionizing radiation. Radiat Res. 2010;173(4):418–25.

84. Lugade AA, Sorensen EW, Gerber SA, Moran JP, Frelinger JG, Lord EM. Radiation-induced IFN-γ production within the tumor microenvironment influences antitumor immunity. J Immunol. 2008;180(5):3132–9.

85. Jensen RL. Brain tumor hypoxia: tumorigenesis, angiogenesis, imaging, pseudoprogression, and as a therapeutic target. J Neuro-Oncol. 2009;92(3):317–35.

86. Gaspar LE, Scott C, Murray K, Curran W. Validation of the RTOG recursive partitioning analysis (RPA) classification for brain metastases. Int J Radiat Oncol Biol Phys. 2000;47(4):1001–6.

Microsurgical Management of Posterior Fossa Vascular Lesions

14

M. Yashar S. Kalani and Robert F. Spetzler

Abbreviations

AICA	Anterior inferior cerebellar artery
ARUBA	A Randomized Trial of Unruptured Brain AVMs
AVM	Arteriovenous malformation
BA	Basilar artery
CT	Computed tomography
CTA	Computed tomography angiography
DSA	Digital subtraction angiography
ICG	Indocyanine green angiography
ISUIA	International Study of Unruptured Intracranial Aneurysms
MRA	Magnetic resonance angiography
MRI	Magnetic resonance imaging
PCA	Posterior cerebral artery
PCoA	Posterior communicating artery
PICA	Posterior inferior cerebellar artery
SAH	Subarachnoid hemorrhage
SCA	Superior cerebral artery
SCIT	Supracerebellar infratentorial
VA	Vertebral artery

M.Y.S. Kalani, MD, PhD • R.F. Spetzler, MD (✉)
Department of Neurosurgery, Barrow Neurological Institute, St. Joseph's Hospital and Medical Center, 350 W. Thomas Rd., Phoenix, AZ 85013, USA
e-mail: Neuropub@dignityhealth.org

Introduction

Microsurgical management of lesions in the posterior fossa is complicated by the labyrinth of critical neurovascular structures that reside in a confined corridor encased by a dense fortress of bone. The complexity of the anatomy and the unforgiving nature of the neurovascular bundle in the posterior fossa have resulted in reluctance on the part of many practitioners to surgically treat lesions in this region. The past two decades have seen a gradual decline in reliance on surgical treatment of lesions in the posterior fossa and a greater dependence on other treatment modalities, such as endovascular treatment for vascular lesions and radiosurgery for tumors and vascular malformations. Nonetheless, surgical competence and excellence remains essential for treating select posterior fossa lesions, including those vascular lesions that cannot be treated optimally using other modalities [1]. In this chapter, we review the microsurgical treatment of posterior circulation vascular lesions, focusing on the treatment of aneurysms, arteriovenous malformations (AVMs), and cavernous malformations.

Surgical Vascular Anatomy of the Posterior Circulation

The vascular anatomy of the posterior circulation consists of the paired vertebral arteries (VAs), the basilar artery (BA), the posterior inferior cerebellar arteries (PICAs), the anterior inferior cerebellar arteries (AICAs), the superior cerebellar arteries (SCAs), and the posterior cerebral arteries (PCAs) [2].

The VA consists of four segments (Fig. 14.1). The V1 segment originates from the subclavian artery and enters into the transverse foramina of the cervical vertebrae, most commonly at C6. The V2 segment of the vessel begins as the VA enters the transverse foramina and continues

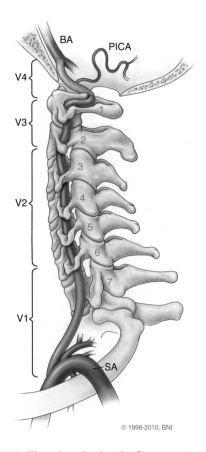

Fig. 14.1 Illustration showing the four segments of the vertebral artery (V1-V4) as well as its relationship to adjacent structures. *BA* basilar artery, *PICA* posterior inferior cerebellar artery, *SA* subclavian artery (Used with permission from Barrow Neurological Institute, Phoenix, Arizona)

until C1. The V3 segment of the VA is the portion of the vessel from its emergence from the C1 transverse foramen to the point that it penetrates the dura of the posterior fossa at the level of the foramen magnum. The V4 segment of the VA constitutes its intracranial course until its union with the opposite VA at the vertebrobasilar junction to form the BA. The intracranial VAs give rise to medullary perforators before joining to form the BA. The first intracranial branch of the VA is the posterior spinal artery, although this vessel may arise from the V3 segment of the VA in exceptional cases. The anterior spinal artery is another major branch of the VA that is responsible for supplying the spinal cord. It is the third major branch of the VA before it joins the contralateral VA at the vertebrobasilar junction.

The PICA is the second branch vessel to arise from the VA (Fig. 14.2) [3]. This vessel is divided into five segments, designated p1 through p5. The p1 segment (the anterior medullary segment) arises from the VA and travels anterior to the medulla to the hypoglossal rootlets at the medial edge of the olive. The p2 segment (the lateral medullary segment) courses from the medial edge of the olive to the rootlets of the lower cranial nerves at the lateral edge of the olive. The p3 segment (the tonsillomedullary segment) begins at the lateral edge of the olive and extends to the inferior extent of the cerebellar tonsil, coursing rostrally to the midpoint of the medial tonsil. The p4 segment (the telovelotonsillar segment) begins at the midpoint of the medial tonsil, courses past the roof of the fourth ventricle, and extends to the tonsillobiventral fissure. The p5 segment (the cortical segment) is the remainder of the artery distal from the tonsillobiventral fissure and is responsible for irrigating the cerebellar hemispheres.

At the pontomedullary junction, the VAs join to form the BA (Fig. 14.3) [4]. The BA extends from the pontomedullary junction to the mesencephalopontine junction where it bifurcates to form the PCAs. In addition to a rich array of perforating vessels arising from the dorsal surface of the basilar apex, the BA gives rise to large pontine vessels, including the pontomedullary arteries, the posterolateral arteries, and the long lateral pontine branches that supply the brainstem. The

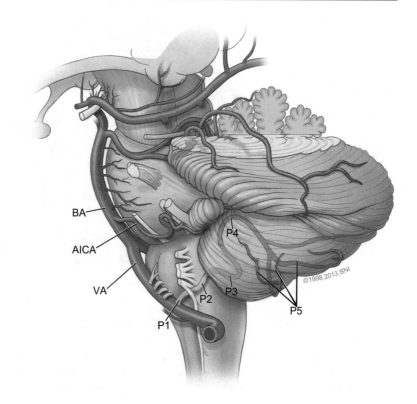

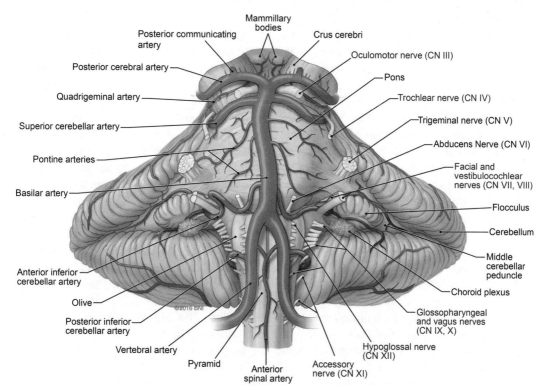

Fig. 14.3   Illustration showing the anatomy of the basilar artery and its relationship to adjacent neural structures (Used with permission from Barrow Neurological Institute, Phoenix, Arizona)

Fig. 14.4 Illustration
showing the anatomy of
the anterior inferior
cerebellar artery
(segments a1-a4) and its
relationship to adjacent
neural structures (Used
with permission from
Barrow Neurological
Institute, Phoenix,
Arizona)

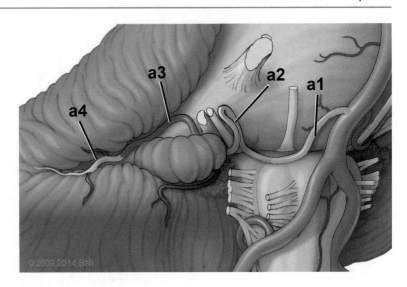

height of the basilar bifurcation relative to the bony anatomy of the clivus is of important clinical consideration because the level of the bifurcation can render approaches to the basilar apex challenging in some cases.

The BA gives rise to three paired vessels: these include the AICAs, SCAs, and PCAs.

The AICAs arise from the lower half of the BA, most commonly from a single trunk (Fig. 14.4) [5]. There are four segments to the AICA: the anterior pontine (a1), the lateral pontine (a2), the flocculopeduncular (a3), and the cortical (a4) segments. The a1 extends from its origin to the midpoint of the inferior olive. The a2 extends from the inferior olive to the flocculus and consists of multiple named branches, including the labyrinthine, the subarcuate, the cerebellosubarcuate, and recurrent perforating arteries. The a3 extends from the flocculus to the cerebellopontine fissure. The a4 constitutes the vessel distal to the cerebellopontine fissure.

The SCAs originate from the BA proximal to or within 2.5 mm of the PCAs (Fig. 14.5) [6]. The SCA is divided into four segments: the anterior pontomesencephalic (s1), the lateral pontomesencephalic (s2), the cerebellomesencephalic (s3), and the cortical (s4) segments. The s1 extends from the origin to the anterolateral margin of the brainstem. The s2 extends

from the anterolateral margin of the brainstem to the cerebellomesencephalic fissure. The s3 is the portion that resides within the cerebellomesencephalic fissure. The s4 is the portion of the vessel distal to the cerebellomesencephalic fissure.

The PCAs constitute the termination of the BA (Fig. 14.6) [7]. The PCAs have complementary calibers with their associated posterior communicating arteries (PCoA), a remnant of their development in the embryo (i.e., the caliber of the PCA and PCoA will vary but complement each other to serve the vascular territory). The PCA also consists of four named segments, with branches of clinical importance. The P1 segment is the portion of the vessel from where it branches from the BA to its point of insertion on the PCoA. This portion of the PCA is rich in thalamoperforating arteries, which if injured can result in devastating effects, particularly during surgical treatment of basilar apex aneurysms. The P2 segment is further divided into an anterior (P2a) and a posterior (P2p) segment. The P2a segment is the portion of the PCA from the insertion of the PCoA to the posterior border of the peduncle. It gives rise to the peduncular perforating arteries, the thalamogeniculate arteries, the medial posterior choroidal artery, the anterior temporal artery, and the hippocampal arteries. The

Fig. 14.5 Illustration showing the segments of the superior cerebellar artery (SCA, segments s1-s4) and its relationship to adjacent neural structures. *PCA* posterior cerebral artery (Used with permission from Barrow Neurological Institute, Phoenix, Arizona)

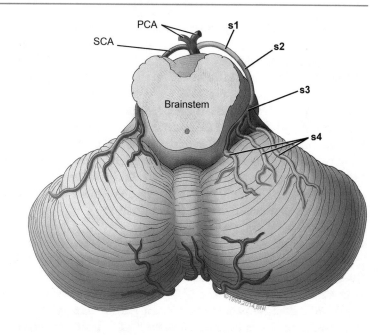

Fig. 14.6 Illustration showing the segments (P1-P4) of the posterior cerebral artery (PCA) and its relationship to adjacent neural structures. *a* artery, *aa* arteries, *CN* cranial nerve, *SCA* superior cerebellar artery (Used with permission from Barrow Neurological Institute, Phoenix, Arizona)

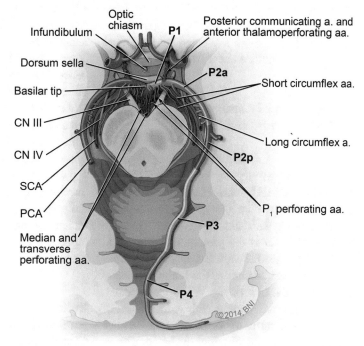

P2p is the portion of the vessel from the posterior peduncle to the calcarine fissure. It gives rise to thalamogeniculate arteries, the lateral posterior choroidal artery, and the middle and posterior temporal arteries. The P3 segment is the portion of the PCA from the posterior border of the midbrain to the calcarine fissure. Many cortical arteries branch from the P3 and P4 segments, including the parieto-occipital, calcarine, and splenial arteries.

Posterior Circulation Aneurysms

Incidence of Aneurysms of the Posterior Circulation

One to five percent of individuals harbor cerebral aneurysms [8]. Aneurysms of the posterior circulation constitute 15–20% of all intracranial aneurysms [9]. The most common location of posterior circulation aneurysms is the BA apex (49–72% of cases), followed by aneurysms of the VA and PICA (which constitute 18–20% of all infratentorial aneurysms). Less commonly, aneurysms arise from the SCA (7–9%), the basilar trunk (2–8%), or the vertebrobasilar junction (9–13%) [10–16]. The mean age of patients harboring aneurysms is between 50.5 and 53.9 years old, and 60–70% of these patients are women [10–16]. Most posterior circulation aneurysms are small (≤11 mm; 47–63%), followed by large aneurysms (12–24 mm; 25–40%) and giant aneurysms (≥25 mm; 6–9%). Women are also more likely to have multiple aneurysms [17].

Presentation of Aneurysms of the Posterior Circulation

The three most common presentations of posterior circulation aneurysms include subarachnoid hemorrhage (SAH), mass effect, and ischemia [18, 19]. Posterior circulation aneurysms commonly present with sudden onset of headache from SAH. SAH is the presenting symptom in 55–81% of cases [18–20]. Because of the proximity of the vasculature to the brainstem, especially the proximity of the VA to the medulla, these patients may present with sudden onset of loss of consciousness, respiratory or cardiac arrest, or lower cranial nerve dysfunction from aneurysm rupture [20]. Large or giant aneurysms may become symptomatic due to mass effect on the brainstem or the lower cranial nerves or due to hydrocephalus caused by compression of the fourth ventricle. Fusiform or dissecting aneurysms can present with ischemic episodes, likely caused by thromboembolic phenomena resulting in hemiparesis. Smaller aneurysms can be discovered incidentally during imaging workup for other symptoms. In general, 22–45% of posterior circulation aneurysms are unruptured when discovered [10–16]. Due to the proximity of the PCA and SCA to the third cranial nerve, patients with aneurysms arising from these vessels may present with a partial or complete third cranial nerve palsy. Alternatively, the proximity of the SCA to the fifth cranial nerve may result in trigeminal neuralgia as a presenting symptom. Patients with AICA aneurysms may present with facial weakness or hearing loss.

Natural History of Aneurysms of the Posterior Circulation

Aneurysms of the posterior circulation have a more aggressive course and natural history than their counterparts in the anterior circulation [21, 22]. The International Study of Unruptured Intracranial Aneurysms (ISUIA) found that regardless of size, aneurysms of the posterior circulation had a higher rate of rupture over a 5-year period than aneurysms of the cavernous sinus or other anterior circulation locations [21] (Table 14.1). The outcomes for patients with ruptured aneurysms treated conservatively are poor, with rebleeding rates approaching 40% at 4 weeks and mortality from a repeat hemorrhage approaching 50% [23–25]. The common risk factors for development and rupture of aneurysms in the posterior circulation include female sex, increasing age, family history of aneurysms, tobacco use, connective tissue disorders, hypertension, and prior history of SAH.

Indications for Interventions for Aneurysms of the Posterior Circulation

The decision to intervene and treat any lesion depends on the natural history of the lesion, the risk associated with treatment versus observation, the experience of the surgeon, intrinsic patient factors (such as health and life expectancy), and the wishes of the patient and family. Because of the aggressive nature of posterior circulation aneurysms compared to anterior

Table 14.1 Relationship between size and location of aneurysms and the annual and cumulative risk of rupture after 5 years

Aneurysm location	Aneurysm size (% of aneurysms)				
	<7 mm group 1[a]	<7 mm group 2[b]	7–12 mm	13–24 mm	≥25 mm
Cavernous carotid artery (n = 210)	0	0	0	3.0	6.4
AC/MC/IC (n = 1037)	0	1.5	2.6	14.5	40
Post-P comm (n = 445)	2.5	3.4	14.5	18.4	50

Data from International Study of Unruptured Intracranial Aneurysms Investigators [21]
AC/MC/IC, anterior communicating artery or anterior cerebral artery, middle cerebral artery, internal carotid artery (not cavernous carotid artery); Post-P comm, posterior cerebral arterial system, vertebrobasilar, or posterior communicating artery.
[a]Group 1, no history of SAH; group 2, previous SAH from another aneurysm
[b]The data were not provided in the original article because for lesions larger than 7 mm the presence of previous SAH made no difference in bleeding rate
Adapted from *Lancet* 2003;362:103–110

circulation aneurysms, posterior circulation aneurysms should be considered for treatment if they occur in patients with a history of SAH, if they exhibit growth, if they are present in a patient with a family history of SAH, if the patient is symptomatic and the symptoms could be attributed to the aneurysm, and if they are of a size that place them at significant risk for rupture based on the ISUIA data. Factors such as patient age, sex, comorbidities, patient wishes, and other risk factors should be taken into account when deciding whether the patient should undergo treatment and the type of treatment that would best suit the patient.

Posterior Fossa Arteriovenous Malformations

Incidence of Arteriovenous Malformations of the Posterior Fossa

AVMs constitute 2% of all hemorrhagic strokes [26]. They are ten times less common than aneurysms but cause 38% of all intracerebral hemorrhages in patients between 15 and 45 years old, and they are a disproportionate cause of morbidity and mortality [27–29]. Posterior fossa AVMs represent 7–15% of all intracranial AVMs, with cerebellar AVMs being the most common subtype (75–82%) [30, 31]. Brainstem AVMs constitute 12.5–23% of cases [30, 31]. The mean age at

presentation for all AVMs is 32.8 ± 15 years, and the mean age of patients with AVMs in the posterior fossa is 42 years [32, 33]. There is no gender predilection.

Presentation of Arteriovenous Malformations of the Posterior Fossa

Unlike supratentorial AVMs, AVMs in the posterior fossa rarely present with seizures. Instead, these lesions are more likely to present with hemorrhage (60–86% of cases compared to 34–55% for supratentorial AVMs) [33–35]. Hemorrhage from AVMs in the posterior fossa may be subarachnoid, intraventricular, or intraparenchymal. Hemorrhage into the ventricular space can result in hydrocephalus.

The second most common presentation of posterior fossa AVMs is progressive neurological deficit (seen in nearly 1/3 of cases) [34]. These symptoms may be due to ischemia, mass effect, or hydrocephalus. Less common presentations include cranial nerve palsies, gait instability, cerebellar symptoms, hemiparesis, and headache.

Natural History of Arteriovenous Malformations of the Posterior Fossa

As discussed above, posterior fossa AVMs are more likely to present with hemorrhage than their intracranial counterparts [36–38]. The annual risk of hemorrhage for all AVMs is estimated to be between 2% and 4%, but rates as low as 1% have been reported [32, 36, 37, 39–44]. Each episode of hemorrhage is associated with a 15–20% risk of significant morbidity and mortality [32, 38, 42–44]. Mortality associated with hemorrhage has been reported to be as high as 67% for patients with posterior fossa AVMs [45]. In one of the largest data sets on the natural history of AVMs, Hernesniemi et al. determined that posterior fossa AVMs have a relative rupture risk of 3.07 compared to supratentorial AVMs [32]. The risk of hemorrhage increases in patients with a history of a prior hemorrhage. Ruptured AVMs have an annual rerupture rate of 6–7%, compared to a rate of 2–3% for previously unruptured AVMs. The 5-year risk of rupture of a previously ruptured AVM can approach 26%, while that of an unruptured AVM is 10% [32]. Other features that could increase the likelihood of hemorrhage include the presence of flow-related and intranidal aneurysms [46–48], venous outflow stenosis [49], and high feeding artery pressures [50, 51].

Indications for Interventions for Arteriovenous Malformations of the Posterior Fossa

Patient selection is critical in order to optimize outcomes for AVM treatment. Although a full discussion of patient selection is beyond the scope of this chapter, we refer the reader to the excellent reviews on patient selection and considerations in AVM surgery that are available [52–56]. The Spetzler-Martin grading scale provides a paradigm for selecting an appropriate treatment algorithm and ascertaining the likely risk of morbidity from surgical treatment [57]. In general, patients with low-grade AVMs (Spetzler-Martin grade I and grade II lesions) should be considered for treatment with surgery, regardless of presentation. Patients with high-grade lesions (Spetzler-Martin grade IV and grade V lesions) whose lesions are identified incidentally should be monitored closely, although a subset may undergo multimodality treatment with good outcomes

[58]. Patients with intermediate-grade AVMs (Spetzler-Martin grade III lesions) should be considered on a case-by-case basis [57, 59, 60]. In patients who present with hemorrhage, the surgeon may be forced to intervene, despite a high-grade lesion, in order to prevent devastating consequences from the hemorrhage [61]. In many cases, the surgeon may evacuate the hematoma in the acute setting to ameliorate symptoms caused by mass effect until definitive treatment can be considered. Patients who present with incidental lesions that demonstrate high-grade features may undergo selective treatment of the high-risk component of their AVM, but selective treatment, especially with endovascular techniques, is not without risk [62, 63]. Although rare, patients with posterior fossa AVMs may present with seizures due to vascular steal. In this cohort with high-grade lesions, selective embolization may relieve the symptoms caused by steal [64].

Brainstem and Cerebellar Cavernous Malformations

Incidence of Cavernous Malformations of the Brainstem and Cerebellum

The incidence of cavernous malformations in the general population is estimated to be on the order of 0.5%, meaning that 1 in 200 individuals harbor a cavernous malformation [65]. Cavernous malformations are distributed in the supratentorial and infratentorial compartments in proportions roughly equal to the volume of the brain. Supratentorial lesions constitute 60–90% [66, 67] of all cavernous malformations, while infratentorial lesions account for 8–36% of all cases [68–72]. In the posterior fossa, the brainstem [73] is the involved site in 4–35% of cases [67]. Brainstem cavernous malformations account for 13% of all vascular malformations of the posterior fossa [73]. The remainder of the cavernous malformations of the posterior fossa are located in the cerebellum, and cerebellar cavernous malformations account for 1–12% of all intracranial cavernous malformations and 9.3–52.9% of all infratentorial lesions [67, 74].

Presentation of Cavernous Malformations of the Brainstem and Cerebellum

The mean age of patients who present with symptomatic cavernous malformations ranges between 32 and 38 years [66, 75, 76]. In patients who present with bleeding from a posterior fossa cavernous malformation, the most common symptoms are headache, nausea, vomiting, gait disturbances, and symptoms attributable to various cranial nerve palsies. The site of the hemorrhage determines the type of neurological deficit. These deficits can include hemiparesis, facial and abducens nerve palsies, internuclear ophthalmoplegia, and sensory disturbances, among others [66, 71, 76]. Fatal hemorrhage from brainstem cavernous malformations is rare, and with few exceptions, most patients experience improvement of their symptoms after hemorrhage, making the decision on the timing of surgery a rather complicated point of discussion with patients.

Natural History of Cavernous Malformations of the Brainstem and Cerebellum

A discussion of the natural history of cavernous malformations is beyond the scope of this chapter. Readers are referred to other recent sources for an extensive discussion [77]. In short, the annual risk of hemorrhage from a cavernous malformation without a previous history of hemorrhage ranges between 0.6% and 1.1% per year [72, 78]. This rate increases significantly in patients who have had a previous episode of hemorrhage, and in the posterior fossa, this risk may be as high as 25% per year in the year immediately after hemorrhage [79]. Evidence also exists for clustering of hemorrhagic events, which may explain this rather high rate in the year immediately after the initial hemorrhage

[65, 77, 80, 81]. Although patients may suffer from neurological deficits after a hemorrhage, it is important to remember that neurological recovery is the rule rather than the exception after a hemorrhage, and this fact should be considered when advising patients regarding surgery. Samii et al. [82] reported that 16.7% of the patients in their series of surgically treated brainstem cavernous malformations had completely recovered before surgery. Kupersmith et al. [83] reported that 37% of patients in their series had recovered completely, while Li et al. [84] reported complete recovery in more than a quarter of their patients (28.7%).

Indications for Intervention for Cavernous Malformations of the Brainstem and Cerebellum

Because of the more aggressive natural history of posterior fossa cavernous malformations, surgical resection is indicated in patients whose lesions abut a pial or ependymal surface or in patients with fixed and permanent deficits [85]. The goal of surgery is to eliminate repeated episodes of hemorrhage that may cause the patient to suffer additional morbidity or even death; therefore, resection should be complete when possible. In patients in which the lesion does not abut a pial or ependymal surface or in patients in which the lesion is identified incidentally, conservative monitoring is a perfectly reasonable approach. However, we do recommend resection for lesions that may not abut a pial plane but that can be accessed using a safe-entry zone [86] with acceptable morbidity or for lesions that have undergone repeated episodes of hemorrhage. For surgical timing, there is no consensus regarding when lesions should be resected after a hemorrhage. As previously stated, most patients improve and recover most of their neurological function after a hemorrhage, so the decision may be made to follow the patient after a hemorrhage to see how much function is regained. Alternatively, surgery immediately after a hemorrhage may relieve mass effect caused by the hemorrhage and may allow a patient to recover more readily from the bleed by removing blood and toxic blood products from the eloquent structures of the brainstem.

Preoperative Evaluation

Patient History and General Considerations

The preoperative evaluation of patients with posterior circulation vascular lesions should begin with a thorough history and physical examination [87]. The history should consist of family history of aneurysms or vascular malformation, personal history of prior hemorrhage, predisposing factors such as hypertension, fibromuscular, and collagen vascular disorders, and disorders such as Osler-Weber-Rendu syndrome. The patient's social history, specifically smoking and illicit drug use, should be obtained. History of recent infection, trauma, cancer, or immunosuppression should also be obtained, as these can predispose patients to the risk of rare aneurysm types, such as infectious or traumatic aneurysm formation. The patient should be asked to describe symptoms and durations because some patients may have experienced a sentinel bleed, a forbearer of a larger eventual hemorrhage from an aneurysm or vascular malformation. The patient should also be questioned regarding nausea, vomiting, or a history of transient weakness, which may be indicative of compressive or ischemic etiology. A review of patient medications often reveals much about other underlying conditions that could predispose the patient to the formation of aneurysms or ischemic lesions in the posterior circulation. Additionally, medications such as antiplatelet and antithrombotic medications should be noted. Allergies to medications can also reveal much about patient physiology. Specifically, any allergy to common antiplatelet medications should be noted.

A detailed physical examination, including a thorough neurological examination, should be performed to evaluate for alterations in mood, cognition, new onset or progressive weakness, gait instability, evidence of cerebellar dysfunction, brainstem symptoms, and cranial nerve deficits.

Patients undergoing microsurgical treatment of vascular pathologies should undergo routine laboratory testing including a basic metabolic panel, a complete blood count, coagulation status, and a chest x-ray. Patients with a history of cardiac disease should be evaluated and cleared by a cardiologist for surgery. An additional group of patients who require close medical workup are those who will undergo surgery in a sitting position because the presence of a patent foramen ovale in this position can result in preventable complications.

Diagnostic Imaging

In patients who present with sudden onset neurological alterations, the initial evaluation should include computed tomography (CT). CT has a sensitivity of nearly 100% for detecting SAH immediately after ictus [88]. When hemorrhage is not shown on CT but the patient has a history concerning for hemorrhage, a lumbar puncture should be performed to evaluate the presence of any blood cells. All patients who are suspected of having vascular lesions in the posterior circulation should undergo a CT angiography (CTA) study. CTA with three-dimensional reconstruction protocols can evaluate the vascular tree, including collateral circulation and can identify aneurysms, dissections, vascular malformations, and vascular malignancies. CTA has a sensitivity of 96% for aneurysms as small as 3 mm, but may underestimate the size of partially thrombosed aneurysms [89, 90]. For cases of suspected vascular lesions, we favor obtaining imaging of the vasculature of the head and neck.

An alternative to CT is magnetic resonance imaging (MRI) and magnetic resonance angiography (MRA). These modalities permit improved visualization of soft tissues and better assessment of aneurysm size compared to CT. MRI can help delineate the proximity of the vascular malformations to eloquent brain regions. Because blood of various ages has different signal intensities, MRI can help identify the age of any hemorrhage from cavernous malformations. Fluid-attenuated inversion recovery (FLAIR) MRI sequences have a sensitivity approaching that of CT for detecting acute hemorrhage [91]. Fine-cut fast imaging employing steady-state acquisition (FIESTA) MRI sequences can help identify vascular compression syndromes in the confines of the posterior fossa [92, 93].

The gold standard for workup of vascular pathologies in the posterior fossa is digital subtraction angiography (DSA). Biplane rotational DSA with three-dimensional reconstruction provides dynamic views of blood flow, which can assist surgeons with surgical planning. DSA can evaluate collateral circulation, and by applying selective and sequential compression or temporary occlusion of inflow vessels to the brain, by using the Alcock's test, for example, can provide essential information for planning treatment. In patients with AVMs, DSA can provide important information regarding the extent of shunting, flow-related aneurysms, and evidence of venous outflow obstruction. In some cases, DSA can be combined with endovascular intervention as a part of a multimodality treatment strategy [62], for example, combined endovascular and microsurgical treatment of AVMs and aneurysms.

Operative Adjuncts

Neuromonitoring and Mapping

We routinely use intraoperative neuromonitoring for neurovascular surgery in the posterior fossa, including monitoring of somatosensory evoked potentials, motor evoked potentials, and cranial nerve-specific monitoring, depending on the location of the lesion in the posterior fossa [94, 95]. Intraoperative neuromonitoring provides real-time output of the function of pathways that may be injured during the operation. Caution should be used, however, because of the dependence of these techniques on the type and depth of anesthesia. A neuroanesthesia team that is proficient with the use of monitoring is critical to properly perform the operation. In addition to monitoring the function of pathways, electrophysiological mapping of critical nuclei is possi-

ble, especially during operations on the brainstem for intrinsic lesions.

Intraoperative Evaluation of Blood Flow

Several well-accepted adjuncts exist for evaluating intraoperative blood flow. The most common modalities include intraoperative angiography, which provides similar information to traditional DSA, indocyanine green angiography (ICG), and intraoperative ultrasonography. ICG is now widely used in operating theaters and has replaced the need for intraoperative angiography in many cases [96–98]. In this technique, a fluorescent dye is administered that allows the blood flow in vessels to be visualized in real time. ICG can be used to confirm the patency of vessels and occlusion of flow from an aneurysm dome during aneurysm surgery. ICG can help identify inflow arteries and draining veins during AVM surgery (although ICG is most useful for superficial lesions, and its application for deep AVM surgery is debated). Quantitative ICG can provide flow measurements [99, 100]. Alternatively, handheld Doppler ultrasonography probes can be used to evaluate blood flow measurement in the operating room. The best application of this technology is for the selection of donor and recipient vessels during bypass surgery and for confirming patency of inflow and outflow vessels before and after aneurysm clipping [101, 102].

Cerebral Protection and Hypothermia

Cerebrovascular surgical procedures have the potential for significant injury to neural structures. Hypotension, retraction, excessive blood loss, iatrogenic injury, hemodilution, hypo- and hyperglycemia, and hypoxia can all cause ischemic injury. Maneuvers that decrease cerebral metabolism greatly prolong the amount of time that the brain can tolerate ischemia. For that reason, all operations should be performed under pharmacological cerebral protection (using barbiturates or propofol) with mild hypothermia (33 °C) [103–105].

Pharmacological Cardiac Arrest

Circulatory arrest is an important adjunct for the treatment of cerebrovascular lesions. In properly selected patients, circulatory arrest greatly facilitates the surgical treatment of aneurysms and AVMs, but it is associated with a high risk of complications [106]. As a result, the use of hypothermic circulatory arrest has largely been abandoned, particularly due to the introduction of well-tolerated pharmacological alternatives. The introduction of adenosine has transformed circulatory arrest from an invasive procedure to one that is much better tolerated, safer, and more transient than hypothermic circulatory arrest. Moreover, adenosine produces reliably reproducible arrest durations. Adenosine allows the surgeon to decrease flow into an aneurysm (or a ruptured AVM), allowing for vascular control and final intervention for the lesion [107]. In aneurysms, the use of adenosine allows the surgeon to obtain proximal and distal control, or it provides the relaxation necessary to allow proper placement of the clip across the neck of the aneurysm. In AVMs, the use of adenosine allows the rupture point to be identified and controlled. Akin to other methods of cardiac arrest, rapid ventricular pacing allows for a reproducible period of cardiac arrest, necessary for the final steps of aneurysm dissection or for identification of bleeding points, especially in the confines of the posterior fossa. Unlike adenosine arrest, rapid ventricular pacing is titratable, and controlled periods of arrest can be obtained with this technique.

Approaches and Approach Selection to Posterior Fossa Vascular Lesions

The choice of approach for any lesion should take certain basic parameters into consideration. These parameters include the shortest approach (when possible), an approach that allows the surgeon to readily visualize the lesion or lesions while minimally disturbing other eloquent neurovascular structures, thereby limiting patient morbidity, and the approach that is most convenient to the surgeon due to handedness and experience. For intrinsic lesions, such as cavernous malformations of the brainstem, the two-point method is an excellent starting point for approach selection but must be combined with knowledge of safe-entry zones for optimal approach selection [86]. The judicious use of skull base approaches allows for adequate visualization of the contents of the posterior fossa, without undue risk of injury to the critical structures (Fig. 14.7). An important tenet of skull base surgery is the removal of bone and minimization of tissue and brain retraction to achieve the necessary visualization and working trajectory. Some general approach-related considerations are presented below; however, the specific steps of the various surgical approaches are not outlined, and the reader is referred to other material for details of the approaches [85, 86, 108–110].

Approaches to the Ventral Midbrain/ Posterior Fossa

Approaches to the ventral midbrain include the pterional, orbitozygomatic, and anterior petrosectomy approach and their variants. Aneurysms of the basilar apex, proximal PCA, and SCA can be readily exposed using the pterional, subtemporal, supraorbital, modified orbitozygomatic, and full orbitozygomatic approaches (Fig. 14.8) [111]. These ventrolateral approaches allow the surgeon to release cerebrospinal fluid from the basal cisterns and develop working corridors between the carotid artery, optic nerve, and oculomotor nerve to arrive at the region of the basilar apex. These approaches are also well suited for intrinsic lesions that lie in the ventral midbrain. Exposure using these surgical corridors leads the surgeon to two safe-entry zones on the ventral midbrain, the anterior mesencephalic and the interpeduncular safe-entry zones, which can be accessed to remove lesions from the lateral and

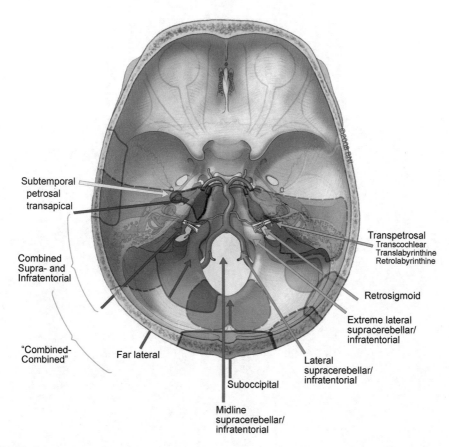

Subtemporal
petrosal
transapical

Transpetrosal
Transcochlear
Translabyrinthine
Retrolabyrinthine

Combined
Supra- and
Infratentorial

Retrosigmoid

Extreme lateral
supracerebellar/
infratentorial

"Combined-
Combined"

Far lateral

Lateral
supracerebellar/
infratentorial

Suboccipital

Midline
supracerebellar/
infratentorial

Fig. 14.7 Skull base approaches to the posterior fossa (Used with permission from Barrow Neurological Institute, Phoenix, Arizona)

centeromedian mesencephalon [85, 86, 112]. The addition of an anterior petrosectomy [113] allows the surgeon to expose the basilar trunk down to the level of the sixth cranial nerve. This additional exposure can be used to treat aneurysms of the BA or the AICA, as well as cavernous malformations located at the mesencephalic-pontine junction on the ventral surface of the brainstem.

Approaches to the Lateral Midbrain

The lateral midbrain surface can be approached using a posterior petrosal approach [114], a retrosigmoid approach, or a lateral (or extreme lateral) supracerebellar infratentorial (SCIT) [115] approach. These approaches afford the surgeon

exposure of the lateral PCA and SCA that may be used for the surgical treatment of aneurysms or AVMs that involve these vessels. They also allow the surgeon to visualize the lateral midbrain surface, thereby facilitating removal of intrinsic lesions, such as cavernous malformations. The lateral brainstem contains the lateral mesencephalic sulcus safe-entry zone, which is readily exposed using a lateral or extreme lateral SCIT approach to resect lateral mesencephalic lesions [85, 86]. At our institution, we have moved away from the use of the posterior petrosal approaches due to the added morbidity associated with their use. In lieu of the posterior petrosal approaches, we prefer to approach lesions in the lateral midbrain using the retrosigmoid approach or the SCIT approach (and its variants).

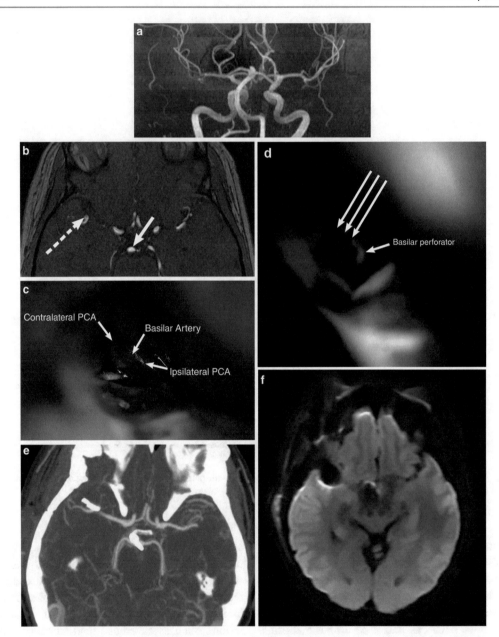

Fig. 14.8 Orbitozygomatic approach to a basilar apex aneurysm. A 61-year-old woman with history of more than 40 pack-years of smoking presented for evaluation after workup for headaches. (**a**, **b**) Magnetic resonance angiography revealed two aneurysms, a right middle cerebral artery (MCA) aneurysm (dashed arrow) and a basilar apex aneurysm (solid arrow). The lesions were approached using a right orbitozygomatic craniotomy. After the Sylvian fissure was widely split, three operative corridors to the basilar apex were explored. These included the supracarotid, carotico-oculomotor, and optico-carotid working corridors. Next, the arachnoid on the medial surface of the third nerve was dissected to allow it to fall away with the temporal lobe. (**c**) After Liliequist's membrane was opened, the contents of the posterior fossa, including the basilar apex aneurysm, were identified. The basilar perforators, emanating from the posterior surface of the basilar artery, were carefully dissected prior to application of the clip. (**d**) Indocyanine green angiography revealed occlusion of the basilar apex aneurysm (long arrows) and preservation of the flow in the perforator. Postoperatively, the patient was neurologically intact. (**e**) Postoperative computed tomography angiography demonstrated complete occlusion of the aneurysm, and (**f**) postoperative magnetic resonance imaging revealed no infarction (**a**, **b**, **e**, **f** are used with permission from *Journal of Neurosurgery*, and **c**, **d** are used with permission from Barrow Neurological Institute, Phoenix, Arizona)

Approaches to the Dorsal Midbrain

The dorsal midbrain can be approached using the midline SCIT approach or the posterior interhemispheric transtentorial approach [116]. These approaches expose the distal most aspect of the PCA and SCA and can be used to approach aneurysms involving these vessels, to perform technically challenging occipital artery-to-PCA or -SCA bypasses, to remove AVMs involving the incisura, cerebellar hemisphere, and posterior midbrain, and to remove cavernous malformations at the level of the colliculi, using the intercollicular safe-entry zone. We prefer to use the SCIT approach over the posterior interhemispheric transtentorial approach to avoid the scenario where there may be a rich venous network draining into the superior sagittal sinus posteriorly.

Approaches to the Ventral Pons

The ventral pons is encased by the clivus, and ventral pontine lesions are usually not approached using a direct anterior route but rather by a ventrolateral approach. More recently, endonasal endoscopic, transclival approaches have been reported for resecting ventral pontine/posterior fossa lesions. Care must be selected when approaching vascular lesions using this approach, and the use of these approaches should be limited to surgeons with extensive experience [117–120].

Approaches to the Lateral Pons

The posterior petrosal and retrosigmoid approaches are the workhorses for exposure of the lateral pons [121]. These approaches allow the surgeon to release cerebrospinal fluid from the cerebellopontine angle, thereby allowing for cerebellar relaxation and exposure of the entire lateral surface of the pons. These exposures allow for visualization of the lateral SCA, the AICA, and the entire BA for treating aneurysms involving these vessels (Fig. 14.9). The additional exposure of the lateral pons allows for surgical removal of AVMs and fistulas on this lateral surface (Fig. 14.10). These exposures also allow the surgeon to enter the pons at three safe-entry zones: the peritrigeminal, the supratrigeminal, and the lateral pontine or middle cerebellar peduncle safe-entry zones (Fig. 14.11). These safe-entry zones permit safe entry into the lateral pons for resecting intrinsic lesions. At our institution, we rarely use petrosal approaches and instead most often use the retrosigmoid approach and the middle cerebellar peduncle safe-entry zone to remove lateral pontine cavernous malformations [121].

Approaches to the Dorsal Pons

The dorsal pons is approached using a suboccipital craniotomy. The suboccipital craniotomy can be used for resecting posterior pontine/cerebellar AVMs and cavernous malformations in this region. When combined with opening of the tela and the velum interpositum, the suboccipital telovelar approach permits the dorsal pons to be visualized to the level of the foramen of Luschka. The telovelar approach allows the surgeon to expose the superior fovea safe-entry zone to resect lesions at the level of the facial colliculus (Fig. 14.12) [122]. In addition to this safe-entry zone, the surgeon may use the suboccipital approach to expose the median sulcus of the fourth ventricle, as well as the suprafacial colliculus and infrafacial colliculus safe-entry zones [86]. In general, we prefer to avoid incising the floor of the fourth ventricle in the midline when possible to avoid injury to the calamus scriptorius.

Approaches to the Ventral Medulla

Similar to the ventral pons, direct approaches to the ventral medulla are seldom necessary. Lesions at the level of the ventral medulla can be readily exposed laterally or dorsolaterally.

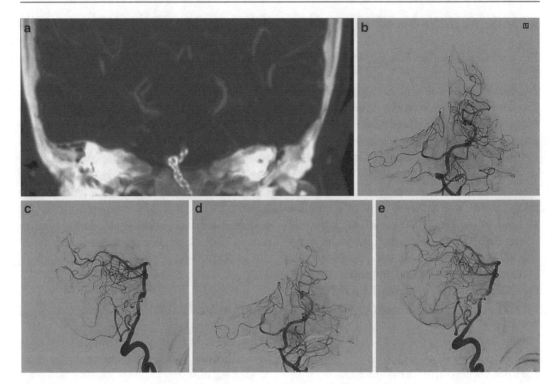

Fig. 14.9 Retrosigmoid approach to an anterior inferior cerebellar artery (AICA) aneurysm. A 68-year-old woman presented who had a history of aneurysmal subarachnoid hemorrhage 4 years previously caused by rupture of an AICA aneurysm, which was treated by a flow-diverting device. Upon presentation to our institute, the aneurysm exhibited (**a**) continued growth on computed tomography angiography. (**b**) Anteroposterior and (**c**) lateral vertebral artery angiography better delineates the anatomy of the recurrent right AICA aneurysm. The aneurysm was approached using a right retrosigmoid craniotomy. The aneurysm was occluded using a stacking clipping strategy. Postoperative (**d**) anteroposterior and (**e**) lateral vertebral artery angiography demonstrates complete occlusion of the aneurysm with preservation of the parent artery (Used with permission from Barrow Neurological Institute, Phoenix, Arizona)

Approaches to the Lateral Medulla

The lateral medulla can be exposed using a low retrosigmoid or a far lateral approach [85, 86, 123]. These approaches allow for visualization of the lower BA, the vertebrobasilar junction, the VA, the PICA, and the lateral medullary surface. Aneurysms involving these arteries can be surgically treated using these approaches with excellent proximal control and exposure for treatment. Additionally, AVMs of the lateral cerebellar hemisphere and lateral medulla can be resected using these approaches. These approaches also expose the anterior medullary sulcus, the olive, and the lateral medullary zone (or the inferior cerebellar peduncle), all of which can be used as safe-entry zones to resect intrinsic medullary lesions.

Approaches to the Dorsal Medulla and Cervicomedullary Junction

The posterior medulla and the cervicomedullary junction can be exposed using a suboccipital craniotomy. In addition to pontine lesions, the suboc-

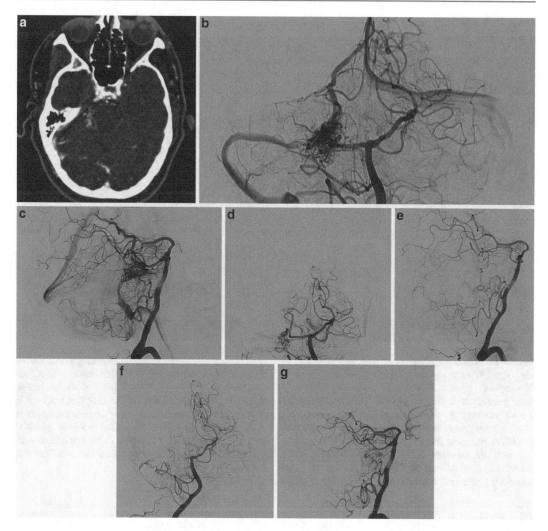

Fig. 14.10 Retrosigmoid approach to a brainstem AVM. A 58-year-old man suffered from a sudden onset ptosis of the right eye. (**a**) Axial computed tomography angiography demonstrates a tangle of vessels in the right cerebellopontine angle. (**b**) Anteroposterior (AP) and (**c**) lateral vertebral artery angiography demonstrates an AVM of the lateral brainstem that is exophytic into the right cerebellopontine angle cistern. Preoperative angiography demonstrated two branches of the SCA and a single feeder from AICA. The lesion was preoperatively embolized using n-butyl cyanoacrylate glue. (**d**) AP and (**e**) lateral angiograms demonstrate partial devascularization of the AVM after embolization. The lesion was approached using a right retrosigmoid craniotomy and resected in a gross-total fashion. (**f**) AP and (**g**) lateral postoperative vertebral artery angiography demonstrates complete removal of the lesion. The patient was at his baseline postoperatively (Used with permission from Barrow Neurological Institute, Phoenix, Arizona)

cipital craniotomy exposes the posterior sulci of the medulla, which can be used as a safe-entry zone for resection of intrinsic medullary lesions. When combined with resection of the posterior arch of C1 and ligation of the dentate ligaments, the suboccipital (or far lateral craniotomies) may be used to approach more ventrally located lesions.

Outcomes of Microsurgery

Posterior Circulation Aneurysms

The treatment of posterior circulation aneurysms has evolved greatly over the past two decades, in large part due to the publication of two random-

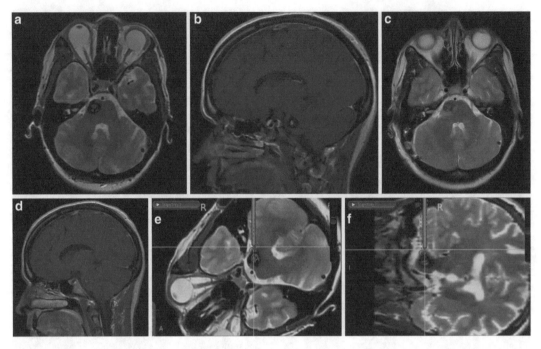

Fig. 14.11 Retrosigmoid, trans-middle cerebellar peduncle approach to a pontine cavernous malformation. A 38-year-old woman with a pontine cavernous malformation presents for evaluation. (**a**) Preoperative axial T2-weighted and (**b**) sagittal T1-weighted magnetic resonance imaging scans demonstrate the lesion. The middle cerebellar peduncle (MCP) safe-entry zone was used to approach this pontine lesion. (**c**) Postoperative axial T2-weighted and (**d**) sagittal T1-weighted magnetic resonance imaging scans demonstrate the complete removal of the lesion. (**e**) Intraoperative neuronavigation trajectories in axial and (**f**) coronal views demonstrate the trajectory of surgical approach without (*vertical dashed line at right*) and with (*vertical dashed line at left*) the dissection of the petrosal fissure. Dissection of the petrosal fissure is an important step for dissection and exposure of the MCP during a transpeduncular approach to the pons (Used with permission from Barrow Neurological Institute, Phoenix, Arizona)

ized controlled trials, the International Subarachnoid Aneurysm Trial (ISAT) [124] and the Barrow Ruptured Aneurysm Trial (BRAT) [17]. A shortcoming of ISAT, in particular, is the relatively small number of posterior circulation aneurysms that were treated in this trial, 3%, yet the results of the trial were widely applied to all posterior circulation aneurysms. In the BRAT study, endovascular coil embolization did seem to confer an improved outcome, with results that were sustained at both 3- and 6-year follow-ups [125, 126]. Based on this data, and many smaller case series, the current treatment recommendation for most posterior circulation aneurysms is an endovascular first approach. This recommendation does not preclude scenarios in which surgical treatment can be an alternative and, at times, a better alternative to endovascular therapy.

With regard to surgical outcomes of posterior circulation aneurysms for each specific vascular territory, several studies warrant discussion and are described below.

Basilar and Vertebral Artery Aneurysms

Peerless et al. [127] reviewed their extensive experience with microsurgical clipping of BA aneurysms and reported a morbidity of 25% and mortality rate of 8% for all basilar aneurysms treated. In their series, the rate of morbidity was related to the size of the aneurysm. The morbidity and mortality was 13% for small aneurysms and increased to 42% for giant aneurysms. Samson et al. [128] reviewed their results with surgical treatment of basilar apex aneurysms and noted a rate of morbidity of 17% and a rate of mortality of 7% at the time of

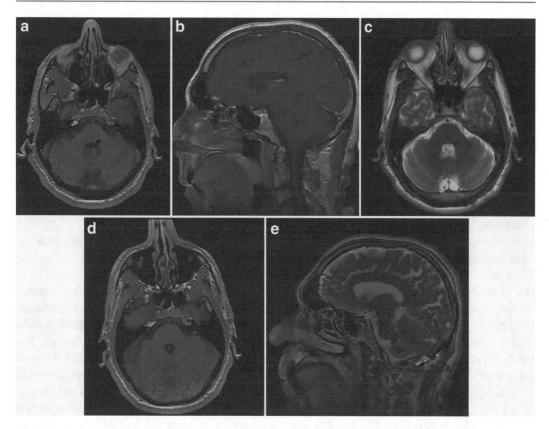

Fig. 14.12 Suboccipital, trans-superior fovea approach to a dorsal pontine cavernous malformation. A 68-year-old man presented with acute-onset facial paralysis. (**a**) Preoperative axial T1-weighted, (**b**) sagittal T1-weighted and (**c**) axial T1-weighted, magnetic resonance imaging studies demonstrate a dorsal pontine cavernous malformation at the level of the facial colliculus. The lesion was approached using a midline suboccipital telovelar approach and through the superior fovea safe-entry zone. (**d**) Postoperative axial T1-weighted and (**e**) sagittal T2-weighted magnetic resonance imaging studies demonstrate complete resection of the lesion. The patient exhibited transient worsening of his facial weakness but improved to baseline at follow-up (Used with permission from the *Journal of Neurosurgery*)

discharge after basilar aneurysm surgery. Krisht et al. [129] reported a more recent experience with the surgical treatment of basilar apex aneurysms, of which half presented with SAH. In this cohort, 98% of aneurysms were successfully clipped. The authors report that 88% of patients had a Glasgow Outcome Scale score of 4 or 5.

Posterior Inferior Cerebellar Artery Aneurysms

D'Ambrosio et al. [130] reviewed a series of 20 patients with PICA aneurysms who were treated using microsurgery. Most of these patients (16 patients; 80%) presented with SAH. In this cohort, 93% of patients had a good outcome, and there were no mortalities. Al-Khayat et al. [131] reviewed their experience with 52 aneurysms and reported good outcomes in 90% of patients, with a mortality rate of 2%. Williamson et al. [132] reported a series of 22 patients with PICA aneurysms from the BRAT cohort. In this group, 19 patients were treated with clipping, 1 died before treatment, and 2 were treated using an endovascular technique. The authors reported that although the demographics of patients harboring PICA aneurysms were not significantly different than patients who harbored aneurysms at other locations, these patients had a higher incidence of poor outcome compared to all other patients included in the BRAT study at discharge (91% versus 67%), at the 1-year follow-up (63% versus 29%), and at the 3-year follow-up (63% versus 32%). They attributed these outcomes to the location of the aneurysm and hemorrhage relative to the lower cranial nerves and medulla.

Posterior Cerebral Artery, Superior Cerebral Artery, and Anterior Inferior Cerebellar Artery Aneurysms

Aneurysms of the PCA, SCA, and AICA are less common than their counterparts in the posterior circulation, and, as such, the results of microsurgical treatment involving these aneurysms arise from smaller case series, most of which include fewer than 20 patients. For PCA aneurysms, the results of good outcomes after microsurgical treatment ranges from 57.1% to 90.9% with mortality rates ranging from 0% to 20% [20, 133–139]. The treatment of SCA aneurysms similarly result in good outcomes in 67% to 90% of pateints, with mortality rates ranging from 0% to 10% [20, 140, 141]. For patients with AICA aneurysms, good outcomes were achieved in 65% to 100% of patients, with mortality rates ranging from 0% to 6% [20, 142–144].

Posterior Fossa Arteriovenous Malformations

Any discussion of treatment outcomes of cerebral AVMs must take into account the recent results of A Randomized Trial of Unruptured Brain AVMs (ARUBA), its impact on patient selection and referral, and its shortcomings [145–147]. A full discussion of the shortcomings of the ARUBA trial is beyond the scope of this chapter, but an important point is that, of the 1740 patients screened, only 726 were deemed eligible and 323 refused enrollment in the trial. Another 177 chose to have treatment outside of the trial randomization process. In addition, the study looked at all treatments and compared them against medical management. The widely accepted standard of treatment for low-grade AVMs, surgery, was used in only five cases, although 76 patients in the trial had grade I or II AVMs. When combined with the very short follow-up of the trial, the results of

ARUBA and its recommendations must be taken into consideration with great caution.

Drake et al. [31] reported a series of surgical treatment of posterior fossa AVMs and demonstrated that complete resection can be achieved in most cases (92% in this series), and good outcomes can be achieved in 71%. The morbidity and mortality rates in this series were 21% and 15%, respectively. Other series report good outcomes in 80–91% of patients, morbidity rates of 9–17%, and mortality rates of 4.1–8.3% [30, 45, 148].

Brainstem and Cerebellar Cavernous Malformations

With improvements in microsurgical techniques and surgical tools, including neuronavigation and microinstruments, surgical resection of cavernous malformations in eloquent regions has become possible. In a recent report [80] from our institution, 260 adults with brainstem cavernous malformations underwent microsurgical resection. These patients suffered a new or transient worsening of their existing deficits in 53% of cases and permanent deficits were noted in 36% of patients. More than one-quarter of the patients (28%) experienced perioperative deficits. The rate of rehemorrhage after resection was 2% at an average follow-up of 51 months, and the average Glasgow Outcome Scale score was 4.6. In this cohort, 12 patients required reoperation for recurrence or residual lesion. The Stanford group [149] reported their experience with 176 deepseated cavernous malformations that included those in the brainstem and thalamus. Of these, 136 cavernous malformations were in the brainstem. They reported new postoperative deficits in 31.2% of patients. At follow-up, however, the majority (61.8%) had improved, and 11.2% had worsened. Li et al. [150] reviewed their experience with 242 cavernous malformations of the brainstem. They noted that 95% of patients achieved complete resection, and 46.3% of patients suffered postoperative deficits. At a mean of 89.4 months of follow-up, the majority of patients (60.7%) had improved. They calculated a postoperative annual hemorrhage rate of 0.4%. The mean modified Rankin Scale score at last follow-up was 1.8, whereas the mean score at the time of discharge was 2.6.

Microsurgical resection of cerebellar cavernous malformations is associated with good outcomes in the majority of cases. Because cerebellar cavernous malformations are often grouped with cavernous malformations in the brainstem, a few reports have looked at the outcome of these lesions independent of others in the posterior fossa. Wu et al. [151] recently reported a series of 58 patients with cerebellar cavernous malformations treated using microsurgery. They found that complete resection could be achieved in every case and that the mean postoperative modified Rankin Scale score was 0.5.

Conclusions

Despite advances in endovascular techniques and chemoradiotherapy, many lesions in the posterior fossa are best treated by microsurgery. Continued developments in interventional tools and techniques, as well as better chemotherapeutic, radiosurgical, and radiotherapy regimens, are likely to continue to help shrink lesions in the posterior fossa so that they may be treated using open surgery. However, for the foreseeable future, continued training in microsurgery in this confined space is necessary and essential.

References

1. Kalani MYS, Wanebo JE, Martirosyan NL, Nakaji P, Zabramski JM, Spetzler RF. A raised bar for aneurysm surgery in the endovascular era. J Neurosurg. 2017;126(5):1731–1739. Epub 2017/02/24.
2. Bruneau M, Pouleau HB. Cranial vascular anatomy of the posterior circulation. In: Spetzler RF, Kalani MYS, Nakaji P, editors. Neurovascular surgery. 2nd ed. New York: Thieme; 2015. p. 49–70.
3. Lister JR, Rhoton AL Jr, Matsushima T, Peace DA. Microsurgical anatomy of the posterior inferior cerebellar artery. Neurosurgery. 1982;10(2):170–99. Epub 1982/02/01.
4. Saeki N, Rhoton AL Jr. Microsurgical anatomy of the upper basilar artery and the posterior circle of Willis. J Neurosurg. 1977;46(5):563–78. Epub 1977/05/01.
5. Martin RG, Grant JL, Peace D, Theiss C, Rhoton AL Jr. Microsurgical relationships of the anterior inferior cerebellar artery and the facial-vestibulocochlear nerve complex. Neurosurgery. 1980;6(5):483–507. Epub 1980/05/01.
6. Hardy DG, Peace DA, Rhoton AL Jr. Microsurgical anatomy of the superior cerebellar artery. Neurosurgery. 1980;6(1):10–28. Epub 1980/01/01.
7. Seoane ER, Tedeschi H, de Oliveira E, Siqueira MG, Calderon GA, Rhoton AL Jr. Management strategies for posterior cerebral artery aneurysms: a proposed new surgical classification. Acta Neurochir. 1997;139(4):325–31. Epub 1997/01/01.
8. Lehecka M, Frösen J, Korja M, et al. Intracranial aneurysms. In: Spetzler RF, Kalani MYS, Nakaji P, editors. Neurovascular surgery. 2nd ed. New York: Thieme; 2015. p. 457–67.
9. Ogilvy CS, Quinones-Hinojosa A. Surgical treatment of vertebral and posterior inferior cerebellar artery aneurysms. Neurosurg Clin N Am. 1998;9(4):851–60. Epub 1998/09/17.
10. Bavinzski G, Killer M, Gruber A, Reinprecht A, Gross CE, Richling B. Treatment of basilar artery bifurcation aneurysms by using Guglielmi detachable coils: a 6-year experience. J Neurosurg. 1999;90(5):843–52. Epub 1999/05/01.
11. Eskridge JM, Song JK. Endovascular embolization of 150 basilar tip aneurysms with Guglielmi detachable coils: results of the Food and Drug Administration multicenter clinical trial. J Neurosurg. 1998;89(1):81–6. Epub 1998/07/01.
12. Guglielmi G, Vinuela F, Duckwiler G, et al. Endovascular treatment of posterior circulation aneurysms by electrothrombosis using electrically detachable coils. J Neurosurg. 1992;77(4):515–24. Epub 1992/10/01.
13. Lempert TE, Malek AM, Halbach VV, et al. Endovascular treatment of ruptured posterior circulation cerebral aneurysms. Clinical and angiographic outcomes. Stroke. 2000;31(1):100–10. Epub 2000/01/08.
14. Lozier AP, Connolly ES Jr, Lavine SD, Solomon RA. Guglielmi detachable coil embolization of posterior circulation aneurysms: a systematic review of the literature. Stroke. 2002;33(10):2509–18. Epub 2002/10/05.
15. Mordasini P, Schroth G, Guzman R, Barth A, Seiler RW, Remonda L. Endovascular treatment of posterior circulation cerebral aneurysms by using Guglielmi detachable coils: a 10-year single-center experience with special regard to technical development. AJNR Am J Neuroradiol. 2005;26(7):1732–8. Epub 2005/08/11.
16. Pandey AS, Koebbe C, Rosenwasser RH, Veznedaroglu E. Endovascular coil embolization of ruptured and unruptured posterior circulation aneurysms: review of a 10-year experience. Neurosurgery. 2007;60(4):626–36. Discussion 36–37. Epub 2007/04/07.
17. McDougall CG, Spetzler RF, Zabramski JM, et al. The Barrow Ruptured Aneurysm Trial. J Neurosurg. 2012;116(1):135–44. Epub 2011/11/08.
18. Anson JA, Lawton MT, Spetzler RF. Characteristics and surgical treatment of dolichoectatic and fusiform aneurysms. J Neurosurg. 1996;84(2):185–93. Epub 1996/02/01.

19. Kalani MY, Zabramski JM, Nakaji P, Spetzler RF. Bypass and flow reduction for complex basilar and vertebrobasilar junction aneurysms. Neurosurgery. 2013;72(5):763–75. Discussion 75–76. Epub 2013/01/22.

20. Sanai N, Tarapore P, Lee AC, Lawton MT. The current role of microsurgery for posterior circulation aneurysms: a selective approach in the endovascular era. Neurosurgery. 2008;62(6):1236–49. Discussion 49–53. Epub 2008/10/01.

21. International Study of Unruptured Intracranial Aneurysms Investigators. Unruptured intracranial aneurysms – risk of rupture and risks of surgical intervention. N Engl J Med. 1998;339(24):1725–33. Epub 1998/12/29.

22. Ucas Japan Investigators, Morita A, Kirino T, et al. The natural course of unruptured cerebral aneurysms in a Japanese cohort. N Engl J Med. 2012;366(26):2474–82. Epub 2012/06/29.

23. Naidech AM, Janjua N, Kreiter KT, et al. Predictors and impact of aneurysm rebleeding after subarachnoid hemorrhage. Arch Neurol. 2005;62(3):410–6. Epub 2005/03/16.

24. Phillips TJ, Dowling RJ, Yan B, Laidlaw JD, Mitchell PJ. Does treatment of ruptured intracranial aneurysms within 24 hours improve clinical outcome? Stroke. 2011;42(7):1936–45. Epub 2011/06/18.

25. Schievink WI, Wijdicks EF, Piepgras DG, Chu CP, O'Fallon WM, Whisnant JP. The poor prognosis of ruptured intracranial aneurysms of the posterior circulation. J Neurosurg. 1995;82(5):791–5. Epub 1995/05/01.

26. Choi JH, Mohr JP. Brain arteriovenous malformations in adults. Lancet Neurol. 2005;4(5):299–308. Epub 2005/04/26.

27. Perret G, Nishioka H. Report on the cooperative study of intracranial aneurysms and subarachnoid hemorrhage. Section VI. Arteriovenous malformations. An analysis of 545 cases of cranio-cerebral arteriovenous malformations and fistulae reported to the cooperative study. J Neurosurg. 1966;25(4):467–90. Epub 1966/10/01.

28. Gross CR, Kase CS, Mohr JP, Cunningham SC, Baker WE. Stroke in south Alabama: incidence and diagnostic features – a population based study. Stroke. 1984;15(2):249–55. Epub 1984/03/01.

29. Toffol GJ, Biller J, Adams HP Jr. Nontraumatic intracerebral hemorrhage in young adults. Arch Neurol. 1987;44(5):483–5. Epub 1987/05/01.

30. Batjer H, Samson D. Arteriovenous malformations of the posterior fossa. Clinical presentation, diagnostic evaluation, and surgical treatment. J Neurosurg. 1986;64(6):849–56. Epub 1986/06/01.

31. Drake CG, Friedman AH, Peerless SJ. Posterior fossa arteriovenous malformations. J Neurosurg. 1986;64(1):1–10. Epub 1986/01/01.

32. Hernesniemi JA, Dashti R, Juvela S, Vaart K, Niemela M, Laakso A. Natural history of brain arteriovenous malformations: a long-term follow-up study of risk of hemorrhage in 238 patients.

Neurosurgery. 2008;63(5):823–9. Discussion 9–31. Epub 2008/11/14.

33. Khaw AV, Mohr JP, Sciacca RR, et al. Association of infratentorial brain arteriovenous malformations with hemorrhage at initial presentation. Stroke. 2004;35(3):660–3. Epub 2004/01/31.

34. Arnaout OM, Gross BA, Eddleman CS, Bendok BR, Getch CC, Batjer HH. Posterior fossa arteriovenous malformations. Neurosurg Focus. 2009;26(5):E12. Epub 2009/05/05.

35. Kader A, Young WL, Pile-Spellman J, et al. The influence of hemodynamic and anatomic factors on hemorrhage from cerebral arteriovenous malformations. Neurosurgery. 1994;34(5):801–7. Discussion 7–8. Epub 1994/05/01.

36. da Costa L, Wallace MC, Ter Brugge KG, O'Kelly C, Willinsky RA, Tymianski M. The natural history and predictive features of hemorrhage from brain arteriovenous malformations. Stroke. 2009;40(1):100–5. Epub 2008/11/15.

37. Kim H, Sidney S, McCulloch CE, et al. Racial/ethnic differences in longitudinal risk of intracranial hemorrhage in brain arteriovenous malformation patients. Stroke. 2007;38(9):2430–7. Epub 2007/08/04.

38. Yamada S, Takagi Y, Nozaki K, Kikuta K, Hashimoto N. Risk factors for subsequent hemorrhage in patients with cerebral arteriovenous malformations. J Neurosurg. 2007;107(5):965–72. Epub 2007/11/06.

39. Yang W, Anderson-Keightly H, Westbroek EM, et al. Long-term hemorrhagic risk in pediatric patients with arteriovenous malformations. J Neurosurg Pediatr. 2016;18(3):329-38. Epub 2016/05/07.

40. Gross BA, Du R. Natural history of cerebral arteriovenous malformations: a meta-analysis. J Neurosurg. 2013;118(2):437–43. Epub 2012/12/04.

41. Brown RD Jr, Wiebers DO, Forbes GS. Unruptured intracranial aneurysms and arteriovenous malformations: frequency of intracranial hemorrhage and relationship of lesions. J Neurosurg. 1990;73(6):859–63. Epub 1990/12/01.

42. Crawford PM, West CR, Chadwick DW, Shaw MD. Arteriovenous malformations of the brain: natural history in unoperated patients. J Neurol Neurosurg Psychiatry. 1986;49(1):1–10. Epub 1986/01/01.

43. Graf CJ, Perret GE, Torner JC. Bleeding from cerebral arteriovenous malformations as part of their natural history. J Neurosurg. 1983;58(3):331–7. Epub 1983/03/01.

44. Stapf C, Mast H, Sciacca RR, et al. Predictors of hemorrhage in patients with untreated brain arteriovenous malformation. Neurology. 2006;66(9):1350–5. Epub 2006/05/10.

45. Symon L, Tacconi L, Mendoza N, Nakaji P. Arteriovenous malformations of the posterior fossa: a report on 28 cases and review of the literature. Br J Neurosurg. 1995;9(6):721–32. Epub 1995/01/01.

46. Stein KP, Wanke I, Forsting M, et al. Associated aneurysms in infratentorial arteriovenous malforma-

tions: role of aneurysm size and comparison with supratentorial lesions. Cerebrovasc Dis. 2016;41 (5–6):219–25. Epub 2016/01/23.

47. Platz J, Berkefeld J, Singer OC, et al. Frequency, risk of hemorrhage and treatment considerations for cerebral arteriovenous malformations with associated aneurysms. Acta Neurochir. 2014;156(11):2025–34. Epub 2014/09/24.

48. Lv X, Wu Z, Li Y, Jiang C, Yang X, Zhang J. Cerebral arteriovenous malformations associated with flow-related and circle of Willis aneurysms. World Neurosurg. 2011;76(5):455–8. Epub 2011/12/14.

49. Kim BS, Sarma D, Lee SK, ter Brugge KG. Brain edema associated with unruptured brain arteriovenous malformations. Neuroradiology. 2009;51(5): 327–35. Epub 2009/02/17.

50. Spetzler RF, Hargraves RW, McCormick PW, Zabramski JM, Flom RA, Zimmerman RS. Relationship of perfusion pressure and size to risk of hemorrhage from arteriovenous malformations. J Neurosurg. 1992;76(6):918–23. Epub 1992/06/01.

51. Young WL, Kader A, Pile-Spellman J, Ornstein E, Stein BM. Arteriovenous malformation draining vein physiology and determinants of transnidal pressure gradients. The Columbia University AVM Study Project. Neurosurgery. 1994;35(3):389–95. discussion 95–96. Epub 1994/09/01.

52. Barr JC, Ogilvy CS. Selection of treatment modalities or observation of arteriovenous malformations. Neurosurg Clin N Am. 2012;23(1):63–75. Epub 2011/11/24.

53. Pradilla G, Coon AL, Huang J, Tamargo RJ. Surgical treatment of cranial arteriovenous malformations and dural arteriovenous fistulas. Neurosurg Clin N Am. 2012;23(1):105–22. Epub 2011/11/24.

54. van Beijnum J, van der Worp HB, Buis DR, et al. Treatment of brain arteriovenous malformations: a systematic review and meta-analysis. JAMA. 2011;306(18):2011–9. Epub 2011/11/10.

55. Aziz-Sultan MA, Elhammady MS, Heros RC. Surgical approaches and nuances for supratentorial arteriovenous malformations. In: Spetzler RF, Kondziolka DS, Higashida RT, Kalani MYS, editors. Comprehensive management of arteriovenous malformations of the brain and spine. Cambridge, UK: Cambridge University Press; 2015, p. 113–129.

56. El Tecle NE, Bendok BR, El Ahmadieh TY, et al. Surgical approaches and nuances for arteriovenous malformations in the posterior fossa. In: Spetzler RF, Kondziolka DS, Higashida RT, Kalani MYS, editors. Comprehensive management of arteriovenous malformations of the brain and spine. Cambridge, UK: Cambridge University Press; 2015, p. 130–143.

57. Spetzler RF, Martin NA. A proposed grading system for arteriovenous malformations. J Neurosurg. 1986;65(4):476–83. Epub 1986/10/01.

58. Chang SD, Marcellus ML, Marks MP, Levy RP, Do HM, Steinberg GK. Multimodality treatment of giant intracranial arteriovenous malformations.

Neurosurgery. 2007;61(1 Suppl):432–42. Discussion 42–4. Epub 2008/09/25.

59. Spetzler RF, Ponce FA. A 3-tier classification of cerebral arteriovenous malformations. Clinical Article J Neurosurg. 2011;114(3):842–9. Epub 2010/10/12.

60. Pandey P, Marks MP, Harraher CD, et al. Multimodality management of Spetzler-Martin grade III arteriovenous malformations. J Neurosurg. 2012;116(6):1279–88. Epub 2012/04/10.

61. Rammos SK, Gardenghi B, Bortolotti C, Cloft HJ, Lanzino G. Aneurysms associated with brain arteriovenous malformations. AJNR Am J Neuroradiol. 2016;37(11):1966-1971. Epub 2016/06/25.

62. Kalani MY, Albuquerque FC, Fiorella D, McDougall CG. Endovascular treatment of cerebral arteriovenous malformations. Neuroimaging Clin N Am. 2013;23(4):605–24. Epub 2013/10/26.

63. Crowley RW, Ducruet AF, Kalani MY, Kim LJ, Albuquerque FC, McDougall CG. Neurological morbidity and mortality associated with the endovascular treatment of cerebral arteriovenous malformations before and during the Onyx era. J Neurosurg. 2015;122(6):1492–7. Epub 2015/03/31.

64. Hoh BL, Chapman PH, Loeffler JS, Carter BS, Ogilvy CS. Results of multimodality treatment for 141 patients with brain arteriovenous malformations and seizures: factors associated with seizure incidence and seizure outcomes. Neurosurgery. 2002;51(2):303–9. Discussion 9–11. Epub 2002/08/17.

65. Kalani MY, Zabramski JM. Risk for symptomatic hemorrhage of cerebral cavernous malformations during pregnancy. J Neurosurg. 2013;118(1):50–5. Epub 2012/10/09.

66. Bertalanffy H, Benes L, Miyazawa T, Alberti O, Siegel AM, Sure U. Cerebral cavernomas in the adult. Review of the literature and analysis of 72 surgically treated patients. Neurosurg Rev. 2002;25(1–2):1–53. discussion 4–5. Epub 2002/04/17.

67. de Oliveira JG, Rassi-Neto A, Ferraz FA, Braga FM. Neurosurgical management of cerebellar cavernous malformations. Neurosurg Focus. 2006;21(1):e11. Epub 2006/07/25.

68. Del Curling O Jr, Kelly DL Jr, Elster AD, Craven TE. An analysis of the natural history of cavernous angiomas. J Neurosurg. 1991;75(5):702–8. Epub 1991/11/11.

69. Kim DS, Park YG, Choi JU, Chung SS, Lee KC. An analysis of the natural history of cavernous malformations. Surg Neurol. 1997;48(1):9–17. Discussion 8. Epub 1997/07/01.

70. Moriarity JL, Wetzel M, Clatterbuck RE, et al. The natural history of cavernous malformations: a prospective study of 68 patients. Neurosurgery. 1999;44(6):1166–71. discussion 72–73. Epub 1999/06/17.

71. Porter RW, Detwiler PW, Spetzler RF, et al. Cavernous malformations of the brainstem: experience with 100 patients. J Neurosurg. 1999;90(1):50–8. Epub 1999/07/21.

72. Robinson JR, Awad IA, Little JR. Natural history of the cavernous angioma. J Neurosurg. 1991;75(5):709–14. Epub 1991/11/01.

73. Petr O, Lanzino G. Brainstem cavernous malformations. J Neurosurg Sci. 2015;59(3):271–82. Epub 2015/05/07.

74. Hasegawa T, McInerney J, Kondziolka D, Lee JY, Flickinger JC, Lunsford LD. Long-term results after stereotactic radiosurgery for patients with cavernous malformations. Neurosurgery. 2002;50(6):1190–7. Discussion 7–8. Epub 2002/05/23.

75. Porter PJ, Willinsky RA, Harper W, Wallace MC. Cerebral cavernous malformations: natural history and prognosis after clinical deterioration with or without hemorrhage. J Neurosurg. 1997;87(2):190–7. Epub 1997/08/01.

76. Fritschi JA, Reulen HJ, Spetzler RF, Zabramski JM. Cavernous malformations of the brain stem. A review of 139 cases. Acta Neurochir. 1994;130 (1–4):35–46. Epub 1994/01/01.

77. Zabramski JM, Kalani MYS. Natural history of cavernous malformations. In: Winn HR, editor. Youmans and Winn neurological surgery. 7th ed. New York: Elsevier; 2016.

78. Kondziolka D, Lunsford LD, Kestle JR. The natural history of cerebral cavernous malformations. J Neurosurg. 1995;83(5):820–4. Epub 1995/11/01.

79. Flemming KD, Link MJ, Christianson TJ, Brown RD Jr. Prospective hemorrhage risk of intracerebral cavernous malformations. Neurology. 2012;78(9):632–6. Epub 2012/02/04.

80. Abla AA, Lekovic GP, Turner JD, de Oliveira JG, Porter R, Spetzler RF. Advances in the treatment and outcome of brainstem cavernous malformation surgery: a single-center case series of 300 surgically treated patients. Neurosurgery. 2011;68(2):403–14. discussion 14–5. Epub 2011/06/10.

81. Gross BA, Du R. Hemorrhage from cerebral cavernous malformations: a systematic pooled analysis. J Neurosurg. 2017;126(4):1079–1087. Epub 2016/05/21.

82. Samii M, Eghbal R, Carvalho GA, Matthies C. Surgical management of brainstem cavernomas. J Neurosurg. 2001;95(5):825–32. Epub 2001/11/13.

83. Kupersmith MJ, Kalish H, Epstein F, et al. Natural history of brainstem cavernous malformations. Neurosurgery. 2001;48(1):47–53. Discussion 53–4 Epub 2001/01/11.

84. Li D, Hao SY, Jia GJ, Wu Z, Zhang LW, Zhang JT. Hemorrhage risks and functional outcomes of untreated brainstem cavernous malformations. J Neurosurg. 2014;121(1):32–41. Epub 2014/05/03.

85. Kalani MYS, Yagmurlu K, Martirosyan NL, Cavalcanti DD, Spetzler RF. Approach selection for intrinsic brainstem pathologies. J Neurosurg. 2016;125(6):1596–1607.

86. Cavalcanti DD, Preul MC, Kalani MY, Spetzler RF. Microsurgical anatomy of safe entry zones to the brainstem. J Neurosurg. 2016;124(5):1359–76. Epub 2015/10/10.

87. Kalani MYS, Perez-Orribo L, Bhardwaj G, Francis IC, Zabramski JM. Neurovascular history and examination. In: Spetzler RF, Kalani MYS, Nakaji P, editors. Neurovascular surgery. 2nd ed. New York: Thieme; 2015. p. 119–30.

88. Horstman P, Linn FH, Voorbij HA, Rinkel GJ. Chance of aneurysm in patients suspected of SAH who have a 'negative' CT scan but a 'positive' lumbar puncture. J Neurol. 2012;259(4):649–52. Epub 2011/09/09.

89. Miley JT, Taylor RA, Janardhan V, Tummala R, Lanzino G, Qureshi AI. The value of computed tomography angiography in determining treatment allocation for aneurysmal subarachnoid hemorrhage. Neurocrit Care. 2008;9(3):300–6. Epub 2008/05/29.

90. Xing W, Chen W, Sheng J, et al. Sixty-four-row multislice computed tomographic angiography in the diagnosis and characterization of intracranial aneurysms: comparison with 3D rotational angiography. World Neurosurg. 2011;76(1–2):105–13. Epub 2011/08/16.

91. Edjlali M, Rodriguez-Regent C, Hodel J, et al. Subarachnoid hemorrhage in ten questions. Diagn Interv Imaging. 2015;96(7–8):657–66. Epub 2015/07/05.

92. Gultekin S, Celik H, Akpek S, Oner Y, Gumus T, Tokgoz N. Vascular loops at the cerebellopontine angle: is there a correlation with tinnitus? AJNR Am J Neuroradiol. 2008;29(9):1746–9. Epub 2008/07/26.

93. Zhou Q, Liu ZL, Qu CC, Ni SL, Xue F, Zeng QS. Preoperative demonstration of neurovascular relationship in trigeminal neuralgia by using 3D FIESTA sequence. Magn Reson Imaging. 2012;30(5):666–71. Epub 2012/03/13.

94. Sanzenbacher KE. Intraoperative monitoring during aneurysm surgery as a neuroprotective activity with reference to evoked potential and microvascular Doppler techniques. Ann N Y Acad Sci. 2005;1053:28–9. Epub 2005/09/24.

95. Slotty PJ, Abdulazim A, Kodama K, et al. Intraoperative neurophysiological monitoring during resection of infratentorial lesions: the surgeon's view. J Neurosurg. 2017;126(1):281–288. Epub 2016/02/27.

96. Thind H, Hardesty DA, Zabramski JM, Spetzler RF, Nakaji P. The role of microscope-integrated near-infrared indocyanine green videoangiography in the surgical treatment of intracranial dural arteriovenous fistulas. J Neurosurg. 2015;122(4):876–82. Epub 2015/01/03.

97. Hardesty DA, Thind H, Zabramski JM, Spetzler RF, Nakaji P. Safety, efficacy, and cost of intraoperative indocyanine green angiography compared to intraoperative catheter angiography in cerebral aneurysm surgery. J Clin Neurosci. 2014;21(8):1377–82. Epub 2014/04/17.

98. Raabe A, Nakaji P, Beck J, et al. Prospective evaluation of surgical microscope-integrated intraoperative near-infrared indocyanine green videoangiography during aneurysm surgery. J Neurosurg. 2005;103(6):982–9. Epub 2005/12/31.

99. Fukuda K, Kataoka H, Nakajima N, Masuoka J, Satow T, Iihara K. Efficacy of FLOW 800 with indocyanine green videoangiography for the quantitative assessment of flow dynamics in cerebral arteriovenous malformation surgery. World Neurosurg. 2015;83(2):203–10. Epub 2014/07/22.

100. Jhawar SS, Kato Y, Oda J, Oguri D, Sano H, Hirose Y. FLOW 800-assisted surgery for arteriovenous malformation. J Clin Neurosci. 2011;18(11):1556–7. Epub 2011/09/17.

101. Amin-Hanjani S, Alaraj A, Charbel FT. Flow replacement bypass for aneurysms: decision-making using intraoperative blood flow measurements. Acta Neurochir. 2010;152(6):1021–32. Discussion 32. Epub 2010/04/08.

102. Amin-Hanjani S, Singh A, Rifai H, et al. Combined direct and indirect bypass for moyamoya: quantitative assessment of direct bypass flow over time. Neurosurgery. 2013;73(6):962–7. Discussion 7–8. Epub 2013/08/21.

103. Li LR, You C, Chaudhary B. Intraoperative mild hypothermia for postoperative neurological deficits in people with intracranial aneurysm. Cochrane Database Syst Rev. 2016;3:CD008445. Epub 2016/03/24.

104. Lavine SD, Masri LS, Levy ML, Giannotta SL. Temporary occlusion of the middle cerebral artery in intracranial aneurysm surgery: time limitation and advantage of brain protection. J Neurosurg. 1997;87(6):817–24. Epub 1997/12/31.

105. Hoffman WE, Charbel FT, Edelman G, Ausman JI. Thiopental and desflurane treatment for brain protection. Neurosurgery. 1998;43(5):1050–3. Epub 1998/11/05.

106. Ponce FA, Spetzler RF, Han PP, et al. Cardiac standstill for cerebral aneurysms in 103 patients: an update on the experience at the Barrow Neurological Institute. Clinical article. J Neurosurg. 2011;114(3):877–84. Epub 2010/10/19.

107. Bendok BR, Gupta DK, Rahme RJ, et al. Adenosine for temporary flow arrest during intracranial aneurysm surgery: a single-center retrospective review. Neurosurgery. 2011;69(4):815–20. Discussion 20–21. Epub 2011/06/04.

108. Almefty KK, Al-Mefty O. Skullbase approaches to the anterior and middle cranial fossa. In: Spetzler RF, Kalani MYS, Nakaji P, editors. Neurovascular surgery. 2nd ed. New York: Thieme; 2015. p. 1055–1068.

109. Sweeney JM, Youssef AS, Agazzi S, van Loveren HR. Surgical approaches to the posterior fossa. In: Spetzler RF, Kalani MYS, Nakaji P, editors. Neurovascular surgery. 2nd ed. New York: Thieme; 2015. p. 1069–1081.

110. George B, Bruneau M. Surgical exposure of the vertebral artery. In: Spetzler RF, Kalani MYS, Nakaji P,editors. Neurovascular surgery. 2nd ed. New York: Thieme; 2015. p. 1111–1123.

111. Lemole GM Jr, Henn JS, Zabramski JM, Spetzler RF. Modifications to the orbitozygomatic approach. Technical Note J Neurosurg. 2003;99(5):924–30. Epub 2003/11/12.

112. Kalani MY, Yagmurlu K, Spetzler RF. The interpeduncular fossa approach for resection of ventromedial midbrain lesions. J Neurosurg. Epub 2017/3/10 [Epub ahead of print].

113. Kawase T, Toya S, Shiobara R, Mine T. Transpetrosal approach for aneurysms of the lower basilar artery. J Neurosurg. 1985;63(6):857–61. Epub 1985/12/01.

114. Gross BA, Dunn IF, Du R, Al-Mefty O. Petrosal approaches to brainstem cavernous malformations. Neurosurg Focus. 2012;33(2):E10. Epub 2012/08/03.

115. de Oliveira JG, Lekovic GP, Safavi-Abbasi S, et al. Supracerebellar infratentorial approach to cavernous malformations of the brainstem: surgical variants and clinical experience with 45 patients. Neurosurgery. 2010;66(2):389–99. Epub 2010/01/01.

116. McLaughlin N, Martin NA. The occipital interhemispheric transtentorial approach for superior vermian, superomedian cerebellar, and tectal arteriovenous malformations: advantages, limitations, and alternatives. World Neurosurg. 2014;82(3–4):409–16. Epub 2013/07/31.

117. Gardner PA, Vaz-Guimaraes F, Jankowitz B, et al. Endoscopic endonasal clipping of intracranial aneurysms: surgical technique and results. World Neurosurg. 2015;84(5):1380–93. Epub 2015/06/29.

118. Drazin D, Zhuang L, Schievink WI, Mamelak AN. Expanded endonasal approach for the clipping of a ruptured basilar aneurysm and feeding artery to a cerebellar arteriovenous malformation. J Clin Neurosci. 2012;19(1):144–8. Epub 2011/11/18.

119. Kassam AB, Mintz AH, Gardner PA, Horowitz MB, Carrau RL, Snyderman CH. The expanded endonasal approach for an endoscopic transnasal clipping and aneurysmorrhaphy of a large vertebral artery aneurysm: technical case report. Neurosurgery. 2006;59(1 Suppl 1):ONSE162-5. Discussion ONSE-5. Epub 2006/08/05.

120. Sanborn MR, Kramarz MJ, Storm PB, Adappa ND, Palmer JN, Lee JY. Endoscopic, endonasal, transclival resection of a pontine cavernoma: case report. Neurosurgery. 2012;71(1 Suppl Operative):198–203. Epub 2012/05/11.

121. Kalani MY, Yagmurlu K, Martirosyan NL, Spetzler RF. The retrosigmoid petrosal fissure transpeduncular approach to central pontine lesions. World Neurosurg. 2016;87:235–41. Epub 2015/12/01.

122. Yagmurlu K, Kalani MYS, Preul MC, Spetzler RF. The superior fovea triangle approach: a novel safe entry zone to the brainstem. J Neurosurg. Epub 2016/12/23 [Epub ahead of print].

123. Deshmukh VR, Rangel-Castilla L, Spetzler RF. Lateral inferior cerebellar peduncle approach to dorsolateral medullary cavernous malformation. J Neurosurg. 2014;121(3):723–9. Epub 2014/06/28.

124. Molyneux AJ, Kerr RS, Yu LM, et al. International subarachnoid aneurysm trial (ISAT) of neurosurgical clipping versus endovascular coiling in 2143 patients with ruptured intracranial aneurysms: a randomised comparison of effects on survival, dependency, seizures, rebleeding, subgroups, and aneurysm

occlusion. Lancet. 2005;366(9488):809–17. Epub 2005/09/06.

125. Spetzler RF, McDougall CG, Zabramski JM, et al. The Barrow Ruptured Aneurysm Trial: 6-year results. J Neurosurg. 2015;123(3):609–17. Epub 2015/06/27.

126. Spetzler RF, McDougall CG, Albuquerque FC, et al. The Barrow Ruptured Aneurysm Trial: 3-year results. J Neurosurg. 2013;119(1):146–57. Epub 2013/04/30.

127. Peerless SJ, Hernesniemi JA, Gutman FB, Drake CG. Early surgery for ruptured vertebrobasilar aneurysms. J Neurosurg. 1994;80(4):643–9. Epub 1994/04/01.

128. Samson D, Batjer HH, Kopitnik TA Jr. Current results of the surgical management of aneurysms of the basilar apex. Neurosurgery. 1999;44(4):697–702. Discussion 702–4. Epub 1999/04/14.

129. Krisht AF, Krayenbuhl N, Sercl D, Bikmaz K, Kadri PA. Results of microsurgical clipping of 50 high complexity basilar apex aneurysms. Neurosurgery. 2007;60(2):242–50. Discussion 50–2. Epub 2007/02/10.

130. D'Ambrosio AL, Kreiter KT, Bush CA, et al. Far lateral suboccipital approach for the treatment of proximal posteroinferior cerebellar artery aneurysms: surgical results and long-term outcome. Neurosurgery. 2004;55(1):39–50. Discussion 50–4. Epub 2004/06/25.

131. Al-khayat H, Al-Khayat H, Beshay J, Manner D, White J. Vertebral artery-posteroinferior cerebellar artery aneurysms: clinical and lower cranial nerve outcomes in 52 patients. Neurosurgery. 2005;56(1):2–10. Discussion 1. Epub 2004/12/25.

132. Williamson RW, Wilson DA, Abla AA, et al. Clinical characteristics and long-term outcomes in patients with ruptured posterior inferior cerebellar artery aneurysms: a comparative analysis. J Neurosurg. 2015;123(2):441–5. Epub 2015/04/18.

133. Hamada J, Morioka M, Yano S, Todaka T, Kai Y, Kuratsu J. Clinical features of aneurysms of the posterior cerebral artery: a 15-year experience with 21 cases. Neurosurgery. 2005;56(4):662–70. Discussion 662–70. Epub 2005/03/29.

134. Drake CG, Amacher AL. Aneurysms of the posterior cerebral artery. J Neurosurg. 1969;30(4):468–74. Epub 1969/04/01.

135. Chang HS, Fukushima T, Takakura K, Shimizu T. Aneurysms of the posterior cerebral artery: report of ten cases. Neurosurgery. 1986;19(6):1006–11. Epub 1986/12/01.

136. Honda M, Tsutsumi K, Yokoyama H, Yonekura M, Nagata I. Aneurysms of the posterior cerebral artery: retrospective review of surgical treatment. Neurol Med Chir (Tokyo). 2004;44(4):164–8. Discussion 9. Epub 2004/06/10.

137. Taylor CL, Kopitnik TA Jr, Samson DS, Purdy PD. Treatment and outcome in 30 patients with posterior cerebral artery aneurysms. J Neurosurg. 2003;99(1):15–22. Epub 2003/07/12.

138. Sakata S, Fujii K, Matsushima T, et al. Aneurysm of the posterior cerebral artery: report of eleven cases – surgical approaches and procedures. Neurosurgery. 1993;32(2):163–7. discussion 7–8. Epub 1993/02/01.

139. Kitazawa K, Tanaka Y, Muraoka S, et al. Specific characteristics and management strategies of cerebral artery aneurysms: report of eleven cases. J Clin Neurosci. 2001;8(1):23–6. Epub 2001/04/27.

140. Jin SC, Park ES, Kwon do H, et al. Endovascular and microsurgical treatment of superior cerebellar artery aneurysms. J Cerebrovasc Endovasc Neurosurg. 2012;14(1):29–36. Epub 2012/12/05.

141. Peerless S, Hernesniemi JA, Drake CG. Posterior circulation aneurysms. In: Wilkins R, Rengachard SS, editors. Neurosurgery. New York: McGraw-Hill; 1996. p. 2341–56.

142. Tokimura H, Ishigami T, Yamahata H, et al. Clinical presentation and treatment of distal anterior inferior cerebellar artery aneurysms. Neurosurg Rev. 2012;35(4):497–503. Discussion 503–4. Epub 2012/05/11.

143. Gonzalez LF, Alexander MJ, McDougall CG, Spetzler RF. Anteroinferior cerebellar artery aneurysms: surgical approaches and outcomes – a review of 34 cases. Neurosurgery. 2004;55(5):1025–35. Epub 2004/10/29.

144. Li X, Zhang D, Zhao J. Anterior inferior cerebellar artery aneurysms: six cases and a review of the literature. Neurosurg Rev. 2012;35(1):111–9. discussion 9. Epub 2011/07/13.

145. Mohr JP, Parides MK, Stapf C, et al. Medical management with or without interventional therapy for unruptured brain arteriovenous malformations (ARUBA): a multicentre, non-blinded, randomised trial. Lancet. 2014;383(9917):614–21. Epub 2013/11/26.

146. Russin J, Spetzler R. Commentary: the ARUBA trial. Neurosurgery. 2014;75(1):E96–7. Epub 2014/03/29.

147. Lawton MT. The role of AVM microsurgery in the aftermath of a randomized trial of unruptured brain arteriovenous malformations. AJNR Am J Neuroradiol. 2015;36(4):617–9. Epub 2014/12/06.

148. Kelly ME, Guzman R, Sinclair J, et al. Multimodality treatment of posterior fossa arteriovenous malformations. J Neurosurg. 2008;108(6):1152–61. Epub 2008/06/04.

149. Pandey P, Westbroek EM, Gooderham PA, Steinberg GK. Cavernous malformation of brainstem, thalamus, and basal ganglia: a series of 176 patients. Neurosurgery. 2013;72(4):573–89. Discussion 88–9. Epub 2012/12/25.

150. Li D, Yang Y, Hao SY, et al. Hemorrhage risk, surgical management, and functional outcome of brainstem cavernous malformations. J Neurosurg. 2013;119(4):996–1008. Epub 2013/08/21.

151. Wu H, Yu T, Wang S, Zhao J, Zhao Y. Surgical treatment of cerebellar cavernous malformations: a single-center experience with 58 cases. World Neurosurg. 2015;84(4):1103–11. Epub 2015/06/14.

Index

A

AAO-HNS hearing classification, 39
Acoustic neuroma
    AAO-HNS, 39
    CPA, 39
    indications, 39
    middle fossa, 37
    patient counseling, 39
    preoperative evaluation, 38
    preoperative preparation, 40
Adjuvant therapy, 89
AICA, *see* Anterior inferior cerebellar artery (AICA)
AlloDerm, 149
American Academy of Otolaryngology-Head and Neck
    Surgery (AAO-HNS), 39
Anesthetic technique, far lateral, 65, 67
Aneurysms
    incidence, 200
    indications, 200
    risk factors, 200
    SAH, 200
    size and location, 201
Angiographic studies, 80
Anterior approach, 80
Anterior cerebellar arteries (AICAs), 198
Anterior foramen magnum, 73
Anterior inferior cerebellar artery (AICA), 11, 198, 210
Anterior petrous face meningiomas (APFM), 103–107
Anterior transpetrosal (Kawase's) approach, 116,
    117, 120
    complications and avoidance, 97
    indications and limitations, 96
    surgical technique and nuances, 96
Anteriorly based tumors, 137
Anterolateral approaches, 80, 94
Anteroposterior flexion, 66
Anterosuperior portion, 155
Arachnoidal fibers, 138
Arterial encasement, 82
Arterial narrowing, 80
Arteries, 9
Arteriovenous malformations (AVM)
    ARUBA trial, 214
    incidence, 201
    indications, 202
    natural history, 202
    neurological deficit, 201
Atlanto-occipital joint, 67
Atlanto-occipital variant, 70
Audiovestibular symptoms, 103

B

Balloon occlusion test, 92
Barrow Ruptured Aneurysm Trial (BRAT), 212
Basilar venous plexus, 77
Bill's bar, 151
Bipolar devascularization, 138, 139
Bony destruction, 80
Bony exposure, 152–155
Brainstem, 4, 6–8, 11, 15, 18, 19, 21, 178, 187, 188,
    191, 203
Brainstem auditory evoked responses (BAERs), 56, 149
Brainstem compression/displacement influenced
    functional outcome, 90
Burr hole placement, 58

C

Carotid compression test, 92
Cartilaginous tissue, 80
Cavernous malformations
    dorsal pontine, 213
    hemorrhage rate, 214
    incidence, 202
    indications, 203
    natural history, 203
    symptoms, 203
Cavernous sinus (CS), 11, 89, 94
Cerebellopontine angle (CPA), 37–39, 48, 145, 147, 149,
    157–159, 165, 183, 185, 188
    anatomic classification, 103–104
    APFM, 105, 106
    MPFM, 106, 107
    petrous face meningiomas, 112
    PPFM, 106–108
    preoperative preparation, 104
Cerebellum, 203

© Springer International Publishing AG 2018
W.T. Couldwell (ed.), *Skull Base Surgery of the Posterior Fossa*,
https://doi.org/10.1007/978-3-319-67038-6

Cerebral protection, 205–206
Cerebral revascularization, 92
Cerebrospinal fluid (CSF), 49, 90, 97–99, 105, 147
Cervicomedullary junction, 210–211
Chondrosarcomas, 75, 77–81
    axial and appendicular skeleton, 77
    EEA, total resection, 77, 78
    house cartilage, 77
    hypointense/isointense, 79
    nonsurgical management/observation, 79
    notochord remnants, 79
    radiologic investigation and preoperative planning,
        79–80
    recurrence-free survival, 79
    skull base, 77, 79
    slow-growing nature, 79
    treatment goals, 79
Chordomas, 81
    and chondrosarcomas, 77–81
Circumferential access, 70
Clival chordoma, 94
Clival meningiomas, 83, 89
Clivus, 12
Closure, 61
Combined petrosal approach
    craniotomy, 60
    patient positioning, 58
    skin incision, 58
Combined presigmoid approach, 128, 129
Combined transpetrosal approaches, 95, 116, 117, 122
    complications and avoidance, 99
    indications and limitations, 98–99
    surgical technique and nuances, 99
Complete transcondylar, 70
Computed tomography (CT), 79, 90
Computed tomography angiography (CTA), 82
Condylar emissary vein, 70
Condylar fossa, 68–69
Contralateral flexion, 66
Contralateral rotation, 66
Conventional angiography, 82
Cranial and extradural anatomy, 27, 28
Cranial nerves (CN), 3, 8, 11–15, 18, 135
    palsy, 90
    positioning, 82
Craniectomy, 147
Craniocervical junction, 135
Craniopharyngioma, 94
Craniotomy, 96, 147
Craniovertebral junction, 65, 70
CyberKnife, 190

D

Deficit-free survival, 89
Digital subtraction angiogram, 92
Digital subtraction angiography (DSA), 205
Dorsal medulla, 210–211
Dorsal midbrain, 209
Dorsal pons, 209

Dorsum sellae meningiomas, 84
3D reconstruction, 62
Dural opening techniques, 59, 155, 156

E

Electrocautery, 68
Endolymphatic sac, 103
Endoscopic endonasal approach (EEA), 81
    chordomas, 75–77
    development, 75
    extradural and intradural posterior fossa tumors, 75
    meningiomas, 75, 78
    microsurgical dissection, 75
    posterior fossa tumors (*see* Posterior fossa tumors)
    schwannomas, 75, 76
    skull base approaches, 75
    skull base reconstruction, 75, 84, 85
    and surgical tools, 75
    transnasal access, 76–77
Endoscopic endonasal route, 137
Endoscopic endonasal transclival approach, 76
Epidermoid cysts
    brain MRI, 167
    clinical presentation, 165, 166
    complication avoidance, 169, 172
    CPA, 167, 172
    differential diagnosis, 166
    imaging, 166
    long-term follow-up, 173
    malignant transformation, 173
    PF, 172
    recurrent cysts, 173
    SRS, 173
    surgical approach
        abducens and trochlear nerves, 168, 169
        asterion, 168
        bone window, 169
        dura, 168
        hydrocephalus, 168
        neuronavigation system, 168
        outcomes, 172, 173
        patient position, 168
Eustachian tube, 81, 150
External auditory canal (EAC), 18, 41
Extradural exposure, 68–72
    bone removal, 68, 69
    foramen magnum, 68, 69
    paracondylar variants, 71, 72
    suboccipital craniotomy, 68
    supracondylar variants, 70–72
    transcondylar variants, 69–70
Extradural posterior fossa tumors, 75
    anterior approach, 80
    anterolateral approach, 80
    chondrosarcomas, 77, 80
    chordomas, 77
    cranio-cervical junction stabilization/fusion, 80
    EEA role, 81
    lateral approach, 80

petroclival synchondrosis, 80
posterolateral approach, 80
surgical route, 80
Extraventricular drain (EVD), 179
Extreme-lateral approach, 136

F
Facial nerve function, 47, 48
Facial nerve preservation, 159
Falcotentorial junction, 117, 124, 125
posterior interhemispheric transtentorial approach,
125–127
surgical planning, 124–125
Falcotentorial meningioma, 124
Far/extreme lateral approaches, 95
Far-lateral approach, 15, 136, 138
anesthetic technique and positioning, 65–67
craniovertebral junction, 65
extradural exposure, 68–71
foramen magnum/craniovertebral junction region, 65
incision and muscle dissection, 66–68
intradural exposure, 72, 73
principles, 65
trans-tumor corridor, 65
variants, 72, 73
vascular lesions, 65
Fluid-attenuated inversion recover (FLAIR), 166
Foramen magnum, 89
Foramen magnum meningiomas (FMMs), 83, 89
arachnoidal fibers, 138
bipolar devascularization, 138, 139
classification, 136, 137
clinical presentation, 135
description, 135
EEA, 137
extreme-lateral approach, 136
far-lateral approach, 136, 138
monitoring, 138
outcomes and complications, 140–142
pathologic entity, 135
preoperative assessment, 136
radiosurgery, 136
resection, 139
rostrocaudal extent, 138
self-retaining retractors, 138
surgical approach, 135, 136
surgical factors, 136–140
tuberculum sella meningiomas, 138
ultrasonic aspirators, 140
vertebral artery, 138
Foramen magnum region, 65
Fourth ventricle, 165–167, 172, 173

G
Gadolinium-enhanced contrast imaging, 82
Gadolinium-enhanced MRI, 90
Gadolinium enhancement, 79
Galenic system, 124

Galenic venous system, 125
Gamma Knife therapy, 190
Garcia-Ibanez technique, 152
Gasserian ganglion (GG), 151
Gelatinous matrix, 80
Glasgow Outcome Scale score, 214
Greater superficial petrosal nerve (GSPN), 41, 60, 96, 97,
150–152, 155, 157
Gross total resection (GTR), 185

H
Hearing loss, 98
Hearing preservation, 47, 145, 146, 149, 150, 157–159
Hearing status, PC meningiomas, 92
Hemorrhage, 49
Hemostasis, 149
Honeycomb appearance, 79
Horner's syndrome, 180
Hydrocephalus, 179
Hypothermia, 205–206

I
Indocyanine green angiography (ICG), 205
Internal acoustic canal (IAC), 96
Internal auditory canal (IAC), 43, 46, 103, 145, 147,
149–152, 155–159, 161
Internal auditory meatus, 12, 13
Internal carotid arteries (ICA), 90, 97
International Study of Unruptured Intracranial
Aneurysms (ISUIA), 200
Intracanalicular tumors, 157
Intracanalicular VSs, 150
Intracranial meningiomas, 115
Intradural anatomy, 28
Intradural exposure, 72, 73
Intradural posterior fossa tumors, 75, 81–84
Intraoperative electrophysiological neuromonitoring, 93
Intraoperative lumbar drain, 96
Intraoperative monitoring, 56
Intraoperative MRI (iMRI), 186

J
Jugular foramen, 13, 89
Jugular foramen syndrome, 179

K
Karnofsky performance scale (KPS), 182
Kerrison rongeurs, 31

L
Labyrinthectomy, 44, 45, 55
Lamina cribrosa, 156
Lateral approach, 80
Lateral and far anterolateral lesions, 187, 188
Lateral medulla, 210

Lateral midbrain, 207
Lateral pons, 209
Lateral/posterolateral approaches, 95
Lateral tentorium
    combined presigmoid approach, 128, 129
    retrosigmoid approach, 125–129
    sigmoid sinus, 128, 129
    surgical planning, 125
Leptomeningeal disease (LMD), 188, 189
LINAC system, 190
Linear/curvilinear retromastoid incision, 66
Lower clivus, 76

M
Macewen's triangle, 97
Magnetic resonance imaging (MRI), 79, 82, 104
Malignant transformation, 173
Mastoidectomy, 15–18, 44, 97
Mayfield clamp, 66
Meckel's cave, 81, 89, 94
MEDPOR cranioplasty, 149, 154
Ménière's disease, 150
Meniere's syndrome, 103
Meningiomas, 75, 78, 82, 83, 89, 103, 115
    advantages and limitations, 83–84
    CPA (see Cerebellopontine angle (CPA))
    EEA, 81, 83
    endoscopic management, 81
    management of ventral posterior fossa, 81
    outcomes, petroclival meningiomas, 81
    pathological anatomy
        clival meningiomas, 83
        foramen magnum meningiomas, 83
        petroclival meningiomas, 82–83
    PC (see Petroclival (PC) meningiomas)
    preoperative radiological assessment, 82
    radiation therapy, 81
    tentorial meningiomas (see Tentorial meningiomas)
    ventral posterior fossa, 81
Meningitis, 49
Metastasis
    brain imaging, 177
    breast cancer patient, 179
    cerebellum, 177, 178
    clinical presentation, 179
    CT and MRI, 180
    necrotic and cystic lesions, 180
    perioperative care, 184
    preoperative care, 185
    recursive partitioning analysis, 185
    SBM, 178–180
    SRS, 181
    surgical techniques, 184
    treatment, 182, 183
    WBRT, 181
Metastatic lesions, 188, 189
Microneurosurgical skull base techniques, 89
Microsurgery
    AVMs, 214

cavernous malformations, 214
dissection, 75
posterior circulation aneurysms
    AICA, 214
    basilar and vertebral, 212
    BRAT, 211–214
    ISAT, 211–214
    PCA, 213, 214
    SCA, 214
Microsurgical treatment
    diagnostic imaging, 204
    DSA, 205
    ICG, 205
    neurological examination, 204
    neuromonitoring, 205
    patient history, 204
Middle cerebellar peduncle (MCP), 212
Middle cerebral artery (MCA), 208
Middle clivus, 76
Middle fossa, 49, 50
    bone flap, 41
    complications
        CSF leak, 49
        hemorrhage, 49
        meningitis, 49
        neurological, 50
        sigmoid sinus thrombosis, 49, 50
        VTE, 50
    dura, 41, 42
    facial nerve, 40, 48
    GSPN, 41
    IAC, 39, 42
    ipsilateral scalp, 40
    Layla retractor, 41
    postoperative pain, 47
    skin incision, 40
    symptomatic control, 47
    vestibular nerve, 37
Middle fossa approach (MFA)
    axial, 156
    axial T2-weighted and coronal T1-weighted MRI,
        151, 158
    bony exposure, 152–155
    cadaveric dissection, 152
    dural opening techniques, 155, 156
    fallopian canal, 150
    IAC, 151, 152
    indications, 150
    intracanalicular tumor with cisternal extension, 154
    limitations, 156, 157
    otolaryngologists, 150
    surgical anatomy, 150, 151
    surgical outcome, 157
    surgical risk and complications, 157
    tumor dissection techniques, 155, 156
Middle meningeal artery (MMA), 151, 155
Middle petrous face meningiomas (MPFM), 103, 104,
    106–108
Midline approach, 186
Midline suboccipital craniotomy, 167, 173

Motor evoked potentials (MEP), 56
MR angiography, 92
MRI technologies, 80
MR venogram, 104
MR venography, 92
Multimodality management, 89, 99
Muscle dissection, 66, 68

N
Nasal/nasopharyngeal mucosa postoperative morbidity, 138
Nasopharynx, 76, 77
Nerve sheath tumor, 145
Neural foramina, 4
Neurological complications, 50
Neuromonitoring and mapping, 205
Neuronavigation assistance, 97

O
Occipital artery, 66
Occipital bone, 3–5, 20
Occipital condyle lesion, 181
Occipital condyle syndrome, 180
Occipital transtentorial approach, 13
Occipito-transcondylar, 70, 73
Orbitozygomatic approach, 208
Otological structures, 12, 13
Otorhinolaryngologist, 97

P
Paracondylar, 65, 71–73
Paramedian approach, 187
Parasellar region, 89
Petroclival (PC) meningiomas, 82, 96, 103
    cerebral revascularization, 92
    classification, 89
    clinical presentation, 90
    clival, 89
    cranial nerves, 89
    decision-making process, 93
    deficit-free survival, 89
    description, 89
    intraoperative electrophysiological
        neuromonitoring, 93
    management, 89
    microneurosurgical skull base techniques, 89
    natural history, 90
    preoperative hearing status, 92
    radiological imaging, 90–92
    safe anesthetic techniques, 93
    SRS, 89
    surgical approaches, 94–96
    synchondrosis, 89
    transpetrosal approaches (*see* Transpetrosal
        approaches)
    treatment outcomes in multimodality management,
        99–101
    treatment strategies, 93–94

Petroclival region, 12
Petroclival synchondrosis, 80
Petro-occipital suture, 103
Petrosal approach
    and combined, 56
    craniotomy, 57, 58
    patient positioning, 56
    skin incision, 57, 58
Petrosal nerve, 42
Petrous, 103, 104
    apex, 81, 116
    bone, 151, 152
    face meningiomas, 112
Pharmacological cardiac arrest, 206
PICA, *see* Posterior inferior cerebellar artery (PICA)
Pneumatization of skull base, 90
Porus acusticus, 149, 152, 156, 159
Posterior cerebral artery (PCA), 198, 199
Posterior circulation, 200
    AICAs, 198
    aneurysms (*see* Aneurysms)
    PCAs, 198
    PCoA, 198
    PICA, 196
    SCAs, 198
    VA, 196
Posterior communicating arteries (PCoA), 198
Posterior fossa, 3, 4, 6, 14, 15, 75
    AICA, 11
    anterior, 22
    anterolateral, 22
    arteries, 9
    brainstem, 6
    cavernous sinus, 11
    cerebral peduncles, 6
    clivus, 12, 13
    complications, 189
    craniotomy, 185
    CSF, 189
    EEA (*see* Endoscopic endonasal approach (EEA))
    enclosure
        neural foramina, 4
        skull base, 3, 4
        surgery obstacles, 6
        tentorium, 4
        venous sinuses, 4, 6
    iMRI, 186
    internal auditory meatus, 12, 13
    jugular foramen, 13
    lateral, 22
    medulla oblongata, 7
    metastatic lesions, 191
    midline vermis, 185
    occipital transtentorial, 13
    patient positioning, 185, 187
    petroclival region, 12
    PICA, 11
    pons, 7
    posterolateral, 15
        presigmoid (*see* Presigmoid)

Posterior fossa (*cont.*)
    retrosigmoid, 14, 15
  postoperative care, 189
  radiosurgical treatment, 184
  SCA, 11
  SCIT, 13
  SRS, 191
  stereotactic radiosurgery, 190, 191
  suboccipital craniotomy, 14
  veins, 11
  WBRT, 190
Posterior fossa, 201
  AVM (*see* Arteriovenous malformations (AVM))
  EEA
    extradural, 77–81
    indications, 83
    intradural, 81–84
Posterior inferior cerebellar artery (PICA), 11, 68,
    196, 197
Posterior interhemispheric transtentorial approach,
    125–127
Posterior petrous face meningiomas (PPFM), 103, 104,
    106–109, 111
Posterior spinal artery, 68
Posterior tentorium
  aggressive resection, 131–134
  operative approach, 128
  suboccipital approach, 129–131
  surgical management, 128
  surgical planning, 128–129
Posterior transpetrosal approaches
  complications and avoidance, 98
  indications and limitations, 97
  surgical technique and nuances, 97–98
Posterolateral approach, 80, 137
Postoperative day (POD), 46
Prass electrode, 149
Preauricular curvilinear incision, 41
Pre-medullary region, 71
Presigmoid
  jugular foramen, 18, 20
  mastoidectomy, 15–18
  supra-/infratentorial petrosal, 18
  transcochlear, 18
  transcrusal, 18
  translabyrinthine, 18
  transotic, 18

R
Radiation therapy, 81
Radical tumor resection, 90
Radiological imaging, 90
Radiological surveillance, 90
Rankin Scale score, 214
Recurrence-free survival, 79
Recursive partitioning analysis (RPA), 182, 185
Resection
  BAER, 149

  MFA and retrosigmoid approaches, 145
  neurosurgeons, 150
  VS, 157, 159, 161
Retrolabyrinthine approach, 98
Retrosigmoid approaches, 14, 15, 116, 118, 120,
    125–129, 167, 188, 210–212
  indications, 145
  surgical outcome, 150
  surgical risks and complications, 150
  surgical technique, 146–149
Retrosigmoid craniectomy
  asterion, 32
  CN, 29
  sigmoid sinus, 33
Retrosigmoid craniotomy
  anatomy
    CN, 29
    cranial and extradural, 27
    flocculus, 29
    intradural, 28
    SCA, 28
  complications, 34
  indications, 27
  surgical technique
    closure, 33, 34
    CSF, 33
    dura, 32
    Kerrison rongeurs, 31
    positioning, 29–31
    reconstruction, 33, 34
    sigmoid-transverse junction, 31
Retrosigmoid suboccipital approach, 95, 96

S
Safe anesthetic techniques, 93
SCA, *see* Superior cerebellar artery (SCA)
Scalp-based fiducials, 104
Schwannomas, 75, 76
Sella, 89
Sigmoid sinus, 128, 129
Sigmoid sinus thrombosis, 49, 50
Simpson Grade I resection, 84
Simulating acoustic tumors, 103
Skin incision, 57
Skull base, 3–4
  approaches, 75, 207
  lesions, 55, 56
  reconstruction, 75, 84
Skull base metastasis (SBM), 178
Somatosensory evoked potentials
    (SSEP), 56
Sphenoethmoid complex, 77
Sphenoid bone, 3, 12
Sphenoid sinus, 76
Spheno-occipital bones, 79
Spheno-occiput, 77
Spinocranial meningiomas, 83
Squamous epithelium, 165

S-shaped incision, 66
Stereotactic radiosurgery (SRS), 89, 93, 94, 101, 173, 190, 191
Sternocleidomastoid muscle, 66
Subarachnoid aneurysm trial (ISAT), 212
Subarachnoid hemorrhage (SAH), 200
Suboccipital, 213
    approaches, 95, 96, 129–131
    craniotomy, 68, 135, 185, 188
Subperiosteal dissection, 66
Superficial muscles, 66
Superior cerebellar approach, 188
Superior cerebellar artery (SCA), 11, 198, 199
Superior petrosal sinus (SPS), 56, 96
Superior sagittal sinus, 131–134
Superior semicircular canal (SCC), 96, 97, 99, 151
Supra-/infratentorial petrosal approaches, 18
Supracerebellar-infratentorial (SCIT), 207
Supracondylar, 65, 70–73
Surgical approaches, PC meningiomas, 94, 95
Surgicel, 149

T
T2/FLAIR MRI, 90
Temporal bone, 4, 6, 12, 22
Temporo-occipital synchondrosis, 77
Tentorial incisura, 115–117
    anterior transpetrosal approach, 116, 117, 120
    combined transpetrosal approach, 117, 122
    interpeduncular, crural and ambient cisterns, 115
    retrosigmoid approach, 116, 118, 120
    surgical planning, 115–116
Tentorial meningiomas
    classification, 115, 116
    falcotentorial type, 117–125
    incisural type, 115–117
    intracranial, 115
    lateral tentorium, 125–128
    morphological features, 115
    posterior type, 128–134
Tentorium, 4
Three-quarter prone position, 66
Transbasal transplanum transclival approach, 94
Transclival approach, 76
Transcochlear approach, 18
Transcondylar, 65, 69, 70, 73
Transcranial approaches, 94
Transcrusal approach, 18, 98
Transfacial approaches, 94
Translabyrinthine approach, 18, 38, 49, 50, 98, 157
    Adson Cerebellar Retractors, 44
    bone removal, 45
    complications
        CSF leak, 49
        hemorrhage, 49

        meningitis, 49
        neurological, 50
        sigmoid sinus thrombosis, 49, 50
        VTE, 50
    cottonoids, 46
    facial nerve, 46, 48, 159
    hemostasis, 45, 46
    IAC, 45
    indications, 157
    labyrinthectomy, 44
    limitations of, 159
    mastoidectomy, 43
    morbidity and mortalities, 161
    patient counseling, 40
    perioperative considerations, 159–161
    surgical risks and complications, 159
    tumor removal techniques, 157–159
    vestibular schwannoma, 161
Transmastoid, 73
Trans-middle cerebellar peduncle approach, 212
Transpetrosal approaches, 92, 95, 116
    anterior (Kawase's), 96–97
    combined, 98–99
    posterior, 97–98
Trans-superior fovea approach, 213
Trans-tumor corridor, 65
Transverse sinus, 129–131
Trapezius muscle, 66
Tuberculum jugulare meningioma, 84
Tuberculum sella meningiomas, 138
Tumor dissection techniques, 155, 156
Tumor embolization, 92
Tumor growth index, 90
Tumor removal techniques, 157–159
Tumor resection, 60, 61

U
Ultrasonic aspirators, 140
Upper clivus, 76

V
Vascular anatomy (VA), 196
Vascular lesions, 65, 206–211
Vascular relationships, 82
Vascular tumors, 189
Veins, 11
Venous drainage system, 91
Venous sinuses, 4–6
Venous thromboembolism (VTE), 50
Ventral medulla, 209
Ventral midbrain/posterior fossa, 206–207
Ventral pons, 209
Ventral posterior fossa intradural epidermoid and dermoid cysts, 75
Vermial/medial hemispheric lesions, 186

Vertebral artery, 66, 138
Vertebrobasilar system, 136
Vestibular schwannomas (VSs), 145–161
    management, 145
    MFA (*see* Middle fossa approach (MFA))
    microsurgical approach, 145
    postoperative CT scan brain, 162
    resection of, 145
    retrosigmoid approach
        indications, 145
        resection, 147, 149
        surgical outcome, 150
    surgical risks and complications, 150
    surgical technique, 146–149
    translabyrinthine approach (*see* Translabyrinthine
        approach)

W
WHO grade I residual tumors, 93

Z
Zygoma, 96

Printed in the United States
By Bookmasters